Update on General Medicine

Section 1

2005–2006

(Last major revision 2002–2003)

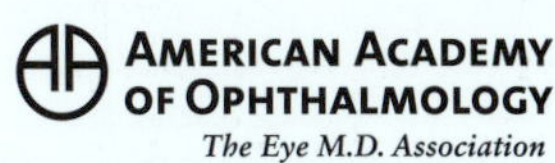

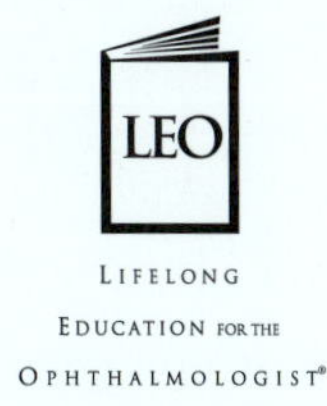

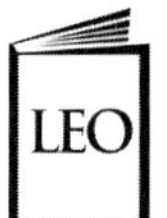

The Basic and Clinical Science Course is one component of the Lifelong Education for the Ophthalmologist (LEO) framework, which assists members in planning their continuing medical education. LEO includes an array of clinical education products that members may select to form individualized, self-directed learning plans for updating their clinical knowledge. Active members or fellows who use LEO components may accumulate sufficient CME credits to earn the LEO Award. Contact the Academy's Clinical Education Division for further information on LEO.

The Academy provides this material for educational purposes only. It is not intended to represent the only or best method or procedure in every case, nor to replace a physician's own judgment or give specific advice for case management. Including all indications, contraindications, side effects, and alternative agents for each drug or treatment is beyond the scope of this material. All information and recommendations should be verified, prior to use, with current information included in the manufacturers' package inserts or other independent sources, and considered in light of the patient's condition and history. Reference to certain drugs, instruments, and other products in this course is made for illustrative purposes only and is not intended to constitute an endorsement of such. Some material may include information on applications that are not considered community standard, that reflect indications not included in approved FDA labeling, or that are approved for use only in restricted research settings. The FDA has stated that it is the responsibility of the physician to determine the FDA status of each drug or device he or she wishes to use, and to use them with appropriate patient consent in compliance with applicable law. The Academy specifically disclaims any and all liability for injury or other damages of any kind, from negligence or otherwise, for any and all claims that may arise from the use of any recommendations or other information contained herein.

Basic and Clinical Science Course

Thomas J. Liesegang, MD, Jacksonville, Florida, *Senior Secretary for Clinical Education*
Gregory L. Skuta, MD, Oklahoma City, Oklahoma, *Secretary for Ophthalmic Knowledge*
Louis B. Cantor, MD, Indianapolis, Indiana, *BCSC Course Chair*

Section 1

Faculty Responsible for This Edition

William G. Tsiaras, MD, Chair, Providence, Rhode Island
Emily Y. Chew, MD, Bethesda, Maryland
Bernard F. Godley, MD, PhD, Consultant, Dallas, Texas
Eric P. Purdy, MD, Fort Wayne, Indiana
Michael J. Spedick, MD, Toms River, New Jersey
Glenn L. Stoller, MD, Rockville Center, New York
Daniel T. Weaver, MD, Billings, Montana
Patrick S. O'Connor, MD, San Antonio, Texas
    Practicing Ophthalmologists Advisory Committee for Education

Each author states that he or she has no significant financial interest or other relationship with the manufacturer of any commercial product discussed in the chapters that he or she contributed to this course or with the manufacturer of any competing commercial product.

Recent Past Faculty

John D. Bullock, MD

Andrew W. Danyluk, MD

Barry N. Hyman, MD

Edward K. Isbey, Jr, MD

Douglas A. Jabs, MD

Lee M. Jampol, MD

Marilyn C. Kay, MD

Jeffrey H. Levenson, MD

Travis A. Meredith, MD

James E. Puklin, MD

Mitchell B. Stein, MD

Brian Younge, MD

In addition, the Academy gratefully acknowledges the contributions of numerous past faculty and advisory committee members who have played an important role in the development of previous editions of the Basic and Clinical Science Course.

American Academy of Ophthalmology Staff

Richard A. Zorab, *Vice President, Ophthalmic Knowledge*

Hal Straus, *Director, Publications Department*

Carol L. Dondrea, *Publications Editor*

Christine Arturo, *Acquisitions Editor*

Ruth Modric, *Production Manager*

Stephanie Tanaka, *Medical Editor*

Katie Loftus, *Administrative Coordinator*

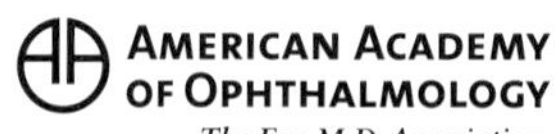

655 Beach Street

Box 7424

San Francisco, CA 94120-7424

Contents

2 Hypertension 63

3 Cerebrovascular Disease 81

4 Acquired Heart Disease 89

General Introduction

The Basic and Clinical Science Course (BCSC) is designed to meet the needs of residents and practitioners for a comprehensive yet concise curriculum of the field of ophthalmology. The BCSC has developed from its original brief outline format, which relied heavily on outside readings, to a more convenient and educationally useful self-contained text. The Academy updates and revises the course annually, with the goals of integrating the basic science and clinical practice of ophthalmology and of keeping ophthalmologists current with new developments in the various subspecialties.

The BCSC incorporates the effort and expertise of more than 80 ophthalmologists, organized into 13 section faculties, working with Academy editorial staff. In addition, the course continues to benefit from many lasting contributions made by the faculties of previous editions. Members of the Academy's Practicing Ophthalmologists Advisory Committee for Education serve on each faculty and, as a group, review every volume before and after major revisions.

Organization of the Course

The Basic and Clinical Science Course comprises 13 volumes, incorporating fundamental ophthalmic knowledge, subspecialty areas, and special topics:

1. Update on General Medicine
2. Fundamentals and Principles of Ophthalmology
3. Clinical Optics
4. Ophthalmic Pathology and Intraocular Tumors
5. Neuro-Ophthalmology
6. Pediatric Ophthalmology and Strabismus
7. Orbit, Eyelids, and Lacrimal System
8. External Disease and Cornea
9. Intraocular Inflammation and Uveitis
10. Glaucoma
11. Lens and Cataract
12. Retina and Vitreous
13. Refractive Surgery

In addition, a comprehensive Master Index allows the reader to easily locate subjects throughout the entire series.

References

Readers who wish to explore specific topics in greater detail may consult the journal references cited within each chapter and the Basic Texts listed at the back of the book.

These references are intended to be selective rather than exhaustive, chosen by the BCSC faculty as being important, current, and readily available to residents and practitioners.

Related Academy educational materials are also listed in the appropriate sections. They include books, audiovisual materials, self-assessment programs, clinical modules, and interactive programs.

Study Questions and CME Credit

Each volume of the BCSC is designed as an independent study activity for ophthalmology residents and practitioners. The learning objectives for this volume are given on page xv. The text, illustrations, and references provide the information necessary to achieve the objectives; the study questions allow readers to test their understanding of the material and their mastery of the objectives. Physicians who wish to claim CME credit for this educational activity may do so by mail, by fax, or online. The necessary forms and instructions are given at the end of the book.

Conclusion

The Basic and Clinical Science Course has expanded greatly over the years, with the addition of much new text and numerous illustrations. Recent editions have sought to place a greater emphasis on clinical applicability, while maintaining a solid foundation in basic science. As with any educational program, it reflects the experience of its authors. As its faculties change and as medicine progresses, new viewpoints are always emerging on controversial subjects and techniques. Not all alternate approaches can be included in this series; as with any educational endeavor, the learner should seek additional sources, including such carefully balanced opinions as the Academy's Preferred Practice Patterns.

The BCSC faculty and staff are continuously striving to improve the educational usefulness of the course; you, the reader, can contribute to this ongoing process. If you have any suggestions or questions about the series, please do not hesitate to contact the faculty or the editors.

The authors, editors, and reviewers hope that your study of the BCSC will be of lasting value and that each section will serve as a practical resource for quality patient care.

Objectives

Upon completion of BCSC Section 1, the reader should be able to:

- Describe the ophthalmic manifestations of the major systemic diseases covered in this volume

- Summarize the most common human pathogens and their manifestations

- Review the newer antiviral, antifungal, and antibacterial agents and their benefits

- Classify levels of hypertension by blood pressure measurements

- List the major classes of antihypertensive medications and some of their characteristics and side effects

- Describe the various diagnostic procedures used in the evaluation of patients with coronary artery disease

- Review the current treatment options for atrial fibrillation, atrial flutter, and ventricular tachycardia

- Discuss the indications for dietary and pharmacologic treatment of hypercholesterolemia

- Distinguish between obstructive and restrictive, reversible and irreversible, pulmonary diseases and give examples of each type

- Describe the classification, pathophysiology, presentation, and diagnostic criteria for diabetes mellitus

- Review the various therapeutic approaches for diabetes mellitus, including new insulins and oral agents

- List the most prevalent types of cancer for men and for women together with the appropriate screening methods for detecting them

- Review current concepts about the etiologies of most malignancies

- Describe both the traditional and more novel approaches to the treatment of cancers

- Summarize the major behavioral disorders and possible therapeutic modalities for these conditions (including the ocular side effects of psychoactive medications)

- List some of the factors associated with a patient's compliance or noncompliance with medical regimens

- Explain the rationale for and value of screening programs for various systemic diseases

- Summarize the major disease processes affecting most of the adult populations and how preventive measures may reduce the morbidity and mortality they cause

- Identify the different types of epidemiologic studies and the appropriateness of each for a particular research question

- Assess medical literature more critically in regard to appropriate study design and validity of conclusions

- Explain the importance of the randomized, controlled clinical study in evaluating the effects of new treatments

- Differentiate between statistically significant results from observational studies and cause and effect

Introduction

For many patients, the ophthalmologist may be their initial or most frequent contact with a physician. In addition, many systemic diseases—and the drugs used to treat them—have significant ocular manifestations. For these reasons, ophthalmologists must be aware of the general medical concerns of their patients.

Only by keeping current with the larger world of general medicine can ophthalmologists maintain their standing as physicians rather than as focused technicians. Ocular manifestations of systemic diseases, as well as the systemic interactions of ocular therapeutics, form the basis of the ophthalmologist's relationship with fellow physicians.

The authors hope that this book will provide both the resident and the ophthalmologist with current information on the medical conditions that may affect their practice and, most important, their patients.

CHAPTER 1

Infectious Disease

Recent Developments

- Vancomycin-resistant strains of enterococci and reduced-sensitivity staphylococci have emerged in recent years as a cause of life-threatening infection in hospitalized patients.
- DNA probes using polymerase chain reaction (PCR) provide new, more sensitive diagnostic tools for the detection of gonorrhea, syphilis, Lyme disease, and infections caused by *Chlamydia,* mycobacteria, and many viruses.
- Newer nucleoside analogues and protease inhibitors provide potent drug combinations that are improving survival in HIV-infected patients.
- Cidofovir and fomivirsen join ganciclovir and foscarnet in the pharmacologic treatment of cytomegalovirus (CMV) retinitis.
- New antibiotics, such as meropenem, cefepime, linezolid, quinupristin/dalfopristin, evernimicin, telithromycin, daptomycin, grepafloxacin, and teicoplanin, provide expanded antimicrobial coverage and offer treatment options for multidrug-resistant infections.

General Microbiology

Despite formidable immune and mechanical defense systems, we harbor an extensive, well-adapted population of microorganisms on the skin and in the gastrointestinal, vaginal, and upper respiratory tracts. The organisms maintain their foothold on these epithelial surfaces chiefly by adherence, and they indirectly benefit the host by excluding pathogenic bacterial colonization and by priming the immune system. If antimicrobial agents alter this host–microbe interplay by eliminating the normal flora, the host's susceptibility to normally excluded pathogenic microorganisms is increased. When the mechanical defenses of the epithelial layers are breached so as to expose normally sterile areas, or if a critical component of the immune system that normally prevents microbial invasion fails, severe infections can result from the normal microbial flora.

However, even when both the mechanical and immune defense systems are intact, pathogenic microbes can cause infections by means of specific virulent characteristics that allow the microbes to invade and multiply. These virulent traits vary among different species.

Following are several mechanisms of virulence:

- *Attachment. Neisseria gonorrhoeae* and *Neisseria meningitidis* breach epithelial barriers by adhering to host epithelial cell surface receptors by means of a ligand located on the bacteria's pili. The presence of the cell surface receptors is genetically determined.
- *Polysaccharide encapsulation. Streptococcus pneumoniae, N meningitidis, Haemophilus,* and *Bacteroides* evade phagocytosis in the absence of antibody and complement because of their polysaccharide coating.
- *Blocking lysosomal fusion.* Intracellular existence, as well as protection from humoral immune mechanisms, is a characteristic of *Chlamydia, Toxoplasma, Legionella,* and *Mycobacterium.*
- *Antigenic surface variation.* Antigenic shifts in the cell wall of *Borrelia recurrentis* incapacitate the humoral immune system, which has a lag time in antibody production. Similar antigenic shifts are found in *Chlamydia* and influenza viruses.
- *IgA protease. Haemophilus influenzae, N gonorrhoeae,* and *N meningitidis* eliminate the IgA antibody normally found on mucosal surfaces, which would otherwise prevent the microbes' adherence.
- *Endotoxin.* A normal constituent of the gram-negative bacterial cell wall, endotoxin produces dramatic systemic physiologic responses ranging from fever and leukocyte margination to disseminated intravascular coagulation and septic shock.
- *Exotoxin.* Exotoxins are a diverse set of proteins with specific actions on target tissues that can cause severe systemic effects in such diseases as cholera or tetanus.

The immune system, which makes possible the host's adaptive response to colonization and infection, is classically divided into the humoral and cellular immune systems. The *humoral immune system,* composed of cells derived from the B lymphocyte series, is responsible for antibody-mediated opsonization, complement-mediated bacterial killing, antitoxin, and mediation of intracellular infections. The *cellular immune system,* determined by the T lymphocytes, is responsible for interaction and stimulation of the humoral immune system, direct cytotoxicity, release of chemical messengers, and control of chronic infections. The successful interplay between the humoral and cellular immune systems mitigates and usually eradicates the infection, allowing for repair and healing. See BCSC Section 9, *Intraocular Inflammation and Uveitis,* for in-depth discussion.

Staphylococcus

Staphylococcus aureus colonizes the anterior nares and other skin sites in 15% of community isolates. Of the tertiary-care hospital isolates, 25% are resistant to all β-lactam antibiotics. Transmission of organisms is usually by direct contact. Resistance of organisms to antimicrobials is usually plasmid determined and varies by institution. The increasing prevalence of methicillin-resistant *S aureus* (MRSA) in tertiary referral hospitals appears to be related to the population of high-risk patients at such centers. The natural history of staphylococcal infections indicates that immunity is of short duration and incomplete. Delayed hypersensitivity reactions to staphylococcal products may be responsible for chronic staphylococcal disease.

Conditions caused by staphylococcal infections include stye, furuncle, acne, bullous impetigo, paronychia, osteomyelitis, septic arthritis, deep-tissue abscesses, bacteremia, endocarditis, enterocolitis, pneumonia, wound infections, scalded skin syndrome, toxic shock syndrome, and food poisoning.

Acute serious staphylococcal infections require immediate intravenous antibiotic therapy. A penicillinase-resistant penicillin or first-generation cephalosporin is normally used, pending the results of susceptibility tests. With the emergence of methicillin-resistant staphylococci, vancomycin has become the drug of choice in life-threatening infections, pending susceptibility studies. The increasing emergence of vancomycin-resistant enterococci has led to concern about cases of vancomycin-resistant *S aureus* infection, mediated through plasmid transfer. In fact, since 1997, infections due to strains of *S aureus* with reduced susceptibility to vancomycin (glycopeptide-intermediate *S aureus*) have been identified in the United States, Japan, and Europe. Many of the cases occurred after prolonged inpatient treatment with intravenous vancomycin. Some reported cases have been successfully treated with various forms of combination therapy, including rifampin and trimethoprim-sulfamethoxazole; vancomycin, gentamicin, and rifampin; and vancomycin and nafcillin. Other agents with activity against vancomycin-intermediate *S aureus* are ampicillin-sulbactam (Unasyn) and some newer antibiotics: trovafloxacin, daptomycin, evernimicin (Ziracin), linezolid (Zyvox), and quinupristin/dalfopristin (Synercid). In July 2002, the first case of true vancomycin-resistant *S aureus* (VRSA) was reported, and additional cases have been described since then.

Staphylococcus epidermidis is an almost universal inhabitant of the skin, present in up to 90% of skin cultures. It can cause infection when local defenses are compromised. Its characteristic adherence to prosthetic devices makes it the most common cause of prosthetic heart valve infections, and it is a common infectious organism of intravenous catheters and cerebrospinal fluid shunts.

Most isolates are resistant to methicillin and cephalosporin; therefore, the drug of choice is vancomycin, occasionally in combination with rifampin or gentamicin. Unfortunately, there have also been recent reports of vancomycin-resistant infections caused by coagulase-negative staphylococcus. In one recent report, the standard disk diffusion antibiotic sensitivity method was unable to detect these isolates with decreased susceptibility to vancomycin. In addition to antibiotic therapy, management often involves removal of the infected prosthetic device or vascular catheter.

Del' Alamo L, Cereda RF, Tosin I, et al. Antimicrobial susceptibility of coagulasenegative staphylococci and characterization of isolates with reduced susceptibility to glycopeptides. *Diagn Microbiol Infect Dis.* 1999;34:185–191.

Smith TL, Pearson ML, Wilcox KR, et al. Emergence of vancomycin resistance in Staphylococcus aureus. Glycopeptide-Intermediate Staphylococcus aureus Working Group. *N Engl J Med.* 1999;340:493–501.

Srinivasan A, Dick JD, Perl TM. Vancomycin resistance in staphylococci. *Clin Microbiol Rev.* 2002;15:430–438.

Vancomycin-resistant *Staphylococcus aureus*—Pennsylvania, 2002. *MMWR Morb Mortal Wkly Rep.* 2002;51:902.

Streptococcus

Group A β-hemolytic streptococci *(Streptococcus pyogenes)* cause a variety of acute suppurative infections through droplet transmission. The infection is modulated by an opsonizing antibody, which provides a type-specific immunity that lasts for years and is directed against the protein in the cell wall pili. Suppurative streptococcal infections in humans include pharyngitis, impetigo, pneumonia, erysipelas, wound and burn infections, puerperal infections, and scarlet fever. Genetically mediated humoral and cellular responses to certain strains of group A streptococci play a role in the development of the postinfectious syndromes of glomerulonephritis and rheumatic fever, both of which represent delayed, nonsuppurative, noninfectious complications of group A streptococcal infections.

S pyogenes remains highly susceptible to penicillin G; however, in the presence of allergy, erythromycin or (if no cross-allergy exists) cephalosporin is substituted. In recent years, macrolide-resistant strains of group A β-hemolytic streptococci have been reported. Antibiotic prophylaxis against recurrent rheumatic fever is administered for procedures that may result in transient bacteremia. However, such prophylaxis may not prevent acute glomerulonephritis.

Streptococcus pneumoniae organisms are lancet-shaped diplococci that cause α-hemolysis on blood agar. Although 10%–30% of the normal population carry one or more serologic types of pneumococci in the throat, the incidence and mortality of pneumococcal pneumonia increases sharply after age 50, with a fatality rate approaching 25%. Pneumococcal virulence is determined by its complex polysaccharide capsule, of which there are more than 80 distinct serotypes. The polysaccharide capsule inhibits macrophage engulfment of the organism. Infection is modulated by the development of anticapsular antibodies after 5–7 days; these antibodies allow phagocytosis of the organism by polymorphonuclear leukocytes.

Conditions caused by *S pneumoniae* include pneumonia, sinusitis, meningitis, otitis media, and peritonitis. Pneumococci are usually highly susceptible to penicillin, other β-lactams, erythromycin, or the newer fluoroquinolones. Routine susceptibility testing should be performed on patients with meningitis, bacteremia, or other life-threatening infections. Penicillin-resistant strains of *S pneumoniae* have been reported with increasing frequency in recent years. In several regions, over 25% of isolates are penicillin resistant; many of these are also resistant to cephalosporins and macrolides. Multidrug resistance was present in 19% of isolates in one recent study. Treatment of highly resistant strains may require vancomycin or meropenem. Prophylaxis is available through use of the 23-valent vaccine (see Chapter 13, Preventive Medicine).

α-Hemolytic streptococci and staphylococci cause the majority of cases of subacute bacterial endocarditis. Patients with prosthetic cardiac valves and most congenital or acquired cardiac structural or valvular defects should receive prophylaxis for subacute bacterial endocarditis (SBE) whenever they undergo invasive procedures involving the oral, nasopharyngeal, respiratory, gastrointestinal, or genitourinary regions. Prophylaxis for subacute bacterial endocarditis is usually not considered necessary for routine ocular surgery in an uninfected patient but should be provided for surgery involving the nasolacrimal drainage system or sinuses (Tables 1-1 through 1-4).

Table 1-1 Cardiac Conditions Associated With Endocarditis

=== **Endocarditis Prophylaxis Recommended** ===

High-risk category
Prosthetic cardiac valves, including bioprosthetic and homograft valves
Previous bacterial endocarditis
Complex cyanotic congenital heart disease (eg, single ventricle states, transposition of the great
  arteries, tetralogy of Fallot)
Surgically constructed systemic pulmonary shunts or conduits
Moderate-risk category
Most other congenital cardiac malformations (other than above and below)
Acquired valvar dysfunction (eg, rheumatic heart disease)
Hypertrophic cardiomyopathy
Mitral valve prolapse with valvar regurgitation and/or thickened leaflets

=== **Endocarditis Prophylaxis Not Recommended** ===

Negligible-risk category (no greater risk than the general population)
Isolated secundum atrial septal defect
Surgical repair of atrial septal defect, ventricular septal defect, or patent ductus arteriosus
  (without residua beyond 6 mo)
Previous coronary artery bypass graft surgery
Mitral valve prolapse without valvar regurgitation
Physiologic, functional, or innocent heart murmurs
Previous Kawasaki disease without valvar dysfunction
Previous rheumatic fever without valvar dysfunction
Cardiac pacemakers (intravascular and epicardial) and implanted defibrillators

(Reprinted from Dajani AS, Taubert KA, Wilson W, et al. Prevention of bacterial endocarditis. Recommendations by the American Heart Association. *JAMA*. 1997;277:1795. © American Medical Association.)

Dajani AS, Taubert KA, Wilson W, et al. Prevention of bacterial endocarditis. Recommendations by the American Heart Association. *JAMA*. 1997;277:1794–1801.

Mason EO Jr, Lamberth LB, Kershaw NL, et al. Streptococcus pneumoniae in the USA: in vitro susceptibility and pharmacodynamic analysis. *J Antimicrob Chemother*. 2000;45:623–631.

Tan TQ. Antibiotic resistant infections due to *Streptococcus pneumoniae:* impact on therapeutic options and clinical outcome. *Curr Opin Infect Dis*. 2003;16:271–277.

Clostridium difficile

Clostridium difficile is an endemic anaerobic gram-positive bacillus that is part of the normal gastrointestinal flora. It has acquired importance because of its role in the development of pseudomembranous enterocolitis following the use of antibiotics. Typically, within 1–14 days of starting antibiotic therapy, patients develop fever and diarrhea. The diarrhea occasionally becomes bloody and typically contains a cytopathic toxin that is elaborated by *C difficile*. At present, a tissue-culture assay for the toxin is the best diagnostic test. Newer enzyme immunoassay tests allow rapid detection, but these have lower sensitivity than toxigenic tissue culture. Also, PCR has been used to detect *C difficile* toxins A and B. The most frequently associated antibiotics include clindamycin, ampicillin, chloramphenicol, tetracycline, erythromycin, and the cephalosporins. Initial treat-

Table 1-2 Surgical Procedures and Endocarditis Prophylaxis

Endocarditis Prophylaxis Recommended

Respiratory tract
Tonsillectomy and/or adenoidectomy
Surgical operations that involve respiratory mucosa
Bronchoscopy with a rigid bronchoscope
Gastrointestinal tract*
Sclerotherapy for esophageal varices
Esophageal stricture dilation
Endoscopic retrograde cholangiography with biliary obstruction
Biliary tract surgery
Surgical operations that involve intestinal mucosa
Genitourinary tract
Prostatic surgery
Cystoscopy
Urethral dilation

Endocarditis Prophylaxis Not Recommended

Respiratory tract
Endotracheal intubation
Bronchoscopy with a flexible bronchoscope, with or without biopsy[†]
Tympanostomy tube insertion
Gastrointestinal tract
Transesophageal echocardiography[†]
Endoscopy with or without gastrointestinal biopsy[†]
Genitourinary tract
Vaginal hysterectomy[†]
Vaginal delivery[†]
Cesarean section
In uninfected tissue:
　Urethral catheterization
　Uterine dilatation and curettage
　Therapeutic abortion
　Sterilization procedures
　Insertion or removal of intrauterine devices
Other
Cardiac catheterization, including balloon angioplasty
Implanted cardiac pacemakers, implanted defibrillators, and coronary stents
Incision or biopsy of surgically scrubbed skin
Circumcision

* Prophylaxis is recommended for high-risk patients; optional for medium-risk patients.
† Prophylaxis is optional for high-risk patients.

(Reprinted from Dajani AS, Taubert KA, Wilson W, et al. Prevention of bacterial endocarditis. Recommendations by the American Heart Association. *JAMA.* 1997;277:1797. ©American Medical Association.)

ment includes discontinuing the causative antibiotic and administering oral metronidazole for 10 days. Vancomycin is also effective, but its use should be limited to decrease the development of vancomycin-resistant organisms such as enterococci and staphylococci. It is also much more expensive than metronidazole. Vancomycin should be limited to those who cannot tolerate or have not responded to metronidazole, or when metronidazole use is contraindicated, such as during the first trimester of pregnancy. A new

Table 1-3 Prophylactic Regimens for Dental, Oral, Respiratory Tract, or Esophageal Procedures

Situation	Agent	Regimen*
Standard general prophylaxis	Amoxicillin	Adults: 2.0 g; children: 50 mg/kg orally 1 h before procedure
Unable to take oral medications	Ampicillin	Adults: 2.0 g intramuscularly (IM) or intravenously (IV); children: 50 mg/kg IM or IV within 30 min before procedure
Allergic to penicillin	Clindamycin *or*	Adults: 600 mg; children: 20 mg/kg orally 1 h before procedure
	Cephalexin[†] or cefadroxil[†] *or*	Adults: 2.0 g; children: 50 mg/kg orally 1 h before procedure
	Azithromycin or clarithromycin	Adults: 500 mg; children: 15 mg/kg orally 1 h before procedure
Allergic to penicillin and unable to take oral medications	Clindamycin *or*	Adults: 600 mg; children: 20 mg/kg IV within 30 min before procedure
	Cefazolin[†]	Adults: 1.0 g; children: 25 mg/kg IM or IV within 30 min before procedure

* Total children's dose should not exceed adult dose.

[†] Cephalosporins should not be used in individuals with immediate-type hypersensitivity reaction (urticaria, angioedema, or anaphylaxis) to penicillins.

(Reprinted from Dajani AS, Taubert KA, Wilson W, et al. Prevention of bacterial endocarditis. Recommendations by the American Heart Association. *JAMA*. 1997;277:1798. ©American Medical Association.)

toxin-binding polymer is being investigated as an alternative therapy, and trials are in progress with a new toxoid vaccine.

Karasawa T, Nojiri T, Hayashi Y, et al. Laboratory diagnosis of toxigenic Clostridium difficile by polymerase chain reaction: presence of toxin genes and their stable expression in toxigenic isolates from Japanese individuals. *J Gastroenterol*. 1999;34:41–45.

Stoddart B, Wilcox MH. *Clostridium difficile. Curr Opin Infect Dis*. 2002;15:513–518.

Haemophilus influenzae

H influenzae is a common inhabitant of the upper respiratory tract in 20%–50% of healthy adults and 80% of children. *H influenzae* is divided into six serotypes, based on differing capsular polysaccharide antigens. Both encapsulated and unencapsulated species cause disease, but systemic spread is typical of the encapsulated strain, whose capsule protects it against phagocytosis. The exact mechanism of invasion is unknown, but an acute suppurative response results, with eventual humoral immunologic modulation of the infection. Long-term immunity follows with the development of bactericidal antibodies to the type B capsule in the presence of complement. Infants are usually protected for a few months by passively acquired maternal antibodies; thereafter, active antibody levels increase with age, being inversely related to the risk of infection. Of the patients with meningitis, roughly 14% develop significant neurologic damage. Other infections

Table 1-4 Prophylactic Regimens for Genitourinary and Gastrointestinal Procedures

Situation	Agents*	Regimen†
High-risk patients	Ampicillin plus gentamicin	Adults: ampicillin 2.0 g intramuscularly (IM) or intravenously (IV) plus gentamicin 1.5 mg/kg (not to exceed 120 mg) within 30 min of starting the procedure; 6 h later, ampicillin 1 g IM/IV or amoxicillin 1 g orally Children: ampicillin 50 mg/kg IM or IV (not to exceed 2.0 g) plus gentamicin 1.5 mg/kg within 30 min of starting the procedure; 6 h later, ampicillin 25 mg/kg IM/IV or amoxicillin 25 mg/kg orally
High-risk patients allergic to ampicillin/amoxicillin	Vancomycin plus gentamicin	Adults: vancomycin 1.0 g IV over 1–2 h plus gentamicin 1.5 mg/kg IV/IM (not to exceed 120 mg); complete injection/ infusion within 30 min of starting the procedure Children: vancomycin 20 mg/kg IV over 1–2 h plus gentamicin 1.5 mg/kg IV/IM; complete injection/infusion within 30 min of starting the procedure
Moderate-risk patients	Amoxicillin or ampicillin	Adults: amoxicillin 2.0 g orally 1 h before procedure, or ampicillin 2.0 g IM/IV within 30 min of starting the procedure Children: amoxicillin 50 mg/kg orally 1 h before procedure, or ampicillin 50 mg/kg IM/IV within 30 min of starting the procedure
Moderate-risk patients allergic to ampicillin/amoxicillin	Vancomycin	Adults: vancomycin 1.0 g IV over 1–2 h; complete infusion within 30 min of starting the procedure Children: vancomycin 20 mg/kg IV over 1–2 h; complete infusion within 30 min of starting the procedure

* Total children's dose should not exceed adult dose.
† No second dose of vancomycin or gentamicin is recommended.

(Reprinted from Dajani AS, Taubert KA, Wilson W, et al. Prevention of bacterial endocarditis. Recommendations by the American Heart Association. *JAMA.* 1997;277:1799. ©American Medical Association.)

include epiglottitis, orbital cellulitis, arthritis, otitis media, bronchitis, pericarditis, sinusitis, and pneumonia.

Treatment of acute infections has been complicated by the emergence of ampicillin-resistant strains, with an incidence approaching 50% in some geographic areas. Current recommendations are to start empirical therapy with amoxicillin trihydrate–clavulanate potassium (Augmentin), trimethoprim-sulfamethoxazole (Bactrim), a quinolone such as ciprofloxacin, or a third-generation cephalosporin, pending susceptibility testing of the organism. Nearly all isolates of *H influenzae* are now resistant to macrolides. Serious or life-threatening infections should be treated with an intravenous third-generation cephalosporin with known activity against *H influenzae,* such as ceftriaxone or cefotaxime, while results of sensitivity testing are pending. Recent reports note an increase of isolates with reduced sensitivity to cephalosporins, especially in patients with chronic pulmonary disease. A recent case of ofloxacin resistance illustrated the possible emergence of quinolone resistance during prolonged therapy.

The US Food and Drug Administration has approved two *H influenzae* type B conjugate vaccines for use in infants. Both have demonstrated their effectiveness in protecting infants and older children against meningitis and other invasive diseases caused by *H influenzae* type B. In studies of fully immunized populations, *H influenzae* infection has been nearly eradicated since the *H influenzae* type B vaccines were introduced. Also, the incidence of meningitis, orbital cellulitis, and other infections caused by *H influenzae* have been reduced significantly since *H influenzae* type B conjugate vaccines became available.

Ambati BK, Ambati J, Azar N, et al. Periorbital and orbital cellulitis before and after the advent of Haemophilus influenzae type B vaccination. *Ophthalmology.* 2000;107:1450–1453.

Jacobs MR, Bajaksouzian S, Zilles A, et al. Susceptibilities of Streptococcus pneumoniae and Haemophilus influenzae to 10 oral antimicrobial agents based on pharmacodynamic parameters: 1997 U.S. Surveillance study. *Antimicrob Agents Chemother.* 1999;43:1901–1908.

Neisseria

Most *Neisseria* organisms are normal inhabitants of the upper respiratory and alimentary tracts; however, the commonly recognized pathogenic species are the meningococci and the gonococci.

Meningococci can be cultured in up to 15% of healthy persons in nonepidemic periods. Virulence is determined by the polysaccharide capsule and the potent endotoxic activity of the cell wall, which can cause cardiovascular collapse, shock, and disseminated intravascular coagulation. Resolution of the infection is related to circulating group-specific opsonizing antibodies and complement. Complement-deficient or asplenic persons are at risk for clinical infection. Prolonged immunity is usually acquired through a subclinical or carrier state and becomes more prevalent with increasing age. Diagnostic testing may include Gram stain, blood and cerebrospinal fluid cultures, counterimmunoelectrophoresis, enzyme-linked immunosorbent assay (ELISA), and PCR.

The range of infections includes meningitis; mild to severe upper respiratory infections; and, less often, endocarditis, arthritis, pericarditis, and endophthalmitis. A less common infection is chronic meningococcemia, characterized by fever, headache, rash, and arthralgia over a period of days to weeks. This infection occurs sporadically, with the rare development of localized infections. Chronic meningococcemia represents an altered host–organism relationship that is poorly understood. Meningitis with a petechial or puerperal exanthem is the classic presentation, although each may occur in isolation.

The treatment of choice for meningococcal meningitis Historically has been high-dose penicillin or, in the case of allergy, chloramphenicol or a third-generation cephalosporin. However, in a recent European study, 39% of asymptomatic carriers and 55.3% of infected patients had isolates with decreased susceptibility to penicillin. Rifampin or minocycline is used as chemoprophylaxis for family members or intimate personal contacts of the infected individual. Polysaccharide vaccines for groups A, C, Y, and W-135 strains have been developed and are most effective in older children and adults. The routine administration of meningococcal vaccines is not recommended except in patients who have undergone splenectomy, complement-deficient persons, military personnel, travelers to endemic regions, and close contacts of infected patients.

Gonococci are not normal inhabitants of the respiratory or genital flora, and their major reservoir is the asymptomatic patient. Among infected women, 50% are asymptomatic, whereas 95% of infected men have symptoms. Asymptomatic patients are infectious for several months, with a transmissibility rate of 20%–50%. Nonsexual transmission is rare. Following a 13-year decline, the number of reported gonorrhea cases in the United States increased by 9% in 1998. The key to prevention is identification and treatment of asymptomatic carriers and their sexual contacts. Symptomatic infection is characterized by a purulent response, with systemic manifestations of endotoxemia only in the bacteremic phase of the disease. Immunity to gonococcal infection is poorly understood, and repeated infections are common. *C trachomatis* coexists with gonorrhea in 25%–50% of women with endocervical gonorrhea and 20%–33% of men with gonococcal urethritis. Diagnosis of gonococcal infections, as well as infections caused by many other bacteria, mycobacteria, viruses, and mycoplasma, has been enhanced with the development of highly sensitive DNA probes that use DNA amplification through PCR techniques.

The range of gonococcal infections includes cervicitis, urethritis, pelvic inflammatory disease, pharyngitis, conjunctivitis, ophthalmia neonatorum, and disseminated gonococcal disease with fever, polyarthralgias, and rash.

Because penicillin- and tetracycline-resistant gonococcal strains have become common in many areas of the United States, treatment should be tailored to their local prevalence. Most of the original resistant isolates have been traced abroad, where there is a very high incidence of penicillinase-producing strains. Tetracycline is effective for susceptible strains, penicillin-allergic persons, or concurrent chlamydial infections. Ceftriaxone (via intramuscular injection) is a drug of choice for penicillinase-resistant strains; thus far, reduced susceptibility to this antibiotic is extremely rare. Other alternatives include oral cefixime; cefuroxime; azithromycin (a newer macrolide); and the quinolones ciprofloxacin, ofloxacin, and sparfloxacin. These drugs are so effective against gonococci that single oral-dose therapy has become a recommended treatment protocol. The macrolides and quinolones have the added benefit of excellent activity against concomitant *C trachomatis* infection. Not surprisingly, the emergence of gonococcal isolates with reduced sensitivity to quinolones has been reported.

Arreaza L, de LaFuente L, Vazquez JA. Antibiotic susceptibility patterns of Neisseria meningitidis isolates from patients and asymptomatic carriers. *Antimicrob Agents Chemother.* 2000;44:1705–1707.

Centers for Disease Control and Prevention. Gonorrhea—United States, 1998. *MMWR.* 2000;49:538–542.

Ison CA, Martin IM. Susceptibility of gonococci isolated in London to therapeutic antibiotics: establishment of a London surveillance programme. London Gonococcal Working Group. *Sex Transm Infect.* 1999;75:107–111.

Pseudomonas aeruginosa

P aeruginosa is a gram-negative bacillus found free living in moist environments. Together with *Serratia marcescens*, *P aeruginosa* is one of the two most consistently antimicrobial-resistant pathogenic bacteria. Infection usually requires either a break in the first-line defenses or altered immunity resulting in a local pyogenic response. The virulence of this organism is related to extracellular toxins, endotoxin, and a polysaccharide protection from phagocytosis. Systemic spread can result in disseminated intravascular coagulation, shock, and death. Humoral immune production of antitoxin is correlated with improved survival in bacteremic patients; however, eradication of infection is probably a multifactorial immune process.

Usual sites of infection include the respiratory system, skin, eye, urinary tract, bone, and wounds. Systemic infections caused by a resistant organism carry a high mortality rate and are usually associated with depressed immunity, often in a hospital setting.

Up to half of *P aeruginosa* isolates are now resistant to aminoglycosides. Therefore, treatment of serious infections relies on combined antimicrobial coverage with either a semisynthetic penicillin or a third-generation cephalosporin with an aminoglycoside. Ceftazidime has been the most effective cephalosporin for pseudomonal infections. Imipenem and piperacillin/tazobactam also remain highly effective against most isolates, but resistance to imipenem has been rising gradually. The initial choice of antimicrobials depends on local susceptibility prevalence and should be guided by susceptibility testing. A recent study revealed that multidrug-resistant *P aeruginosa* arises in a stepwise manner following prolonged exposure to antipseudomonal antibiotics and results in adverse outcomes, with high mortality.

The use of vaccines incorporating multiple *P aeruginosa* serotypes is under investigation for use in patients with severe burns, cystic fibrosis, or immunosuppression. Oral ciprofloxacin has also been useful as a prophylactic agent in patients with cystic fibrosis.

Bonfiglio G, Marchetti F. In vitro activity of ceftazidime, cefepime and imipenem on 1,005 Pseudomonas aeruginosa clinical isolates either susceptible or resistant to beta-lactams. *Chemotherapy.* 2000;46:229–234.

Jang IJ, Kim IS, Park WJ, et al. Human immune response to a Pseudomonas aeruginosa outer membrane protein vaccine. *Vaccine.* 1999;17:158–168.

Treponema pallidum (Syphilis)

The spirochete *T pallidum* is exclusively a human pathogen. It dies rapidly on drying and is readily killed by a wide variety of disinfectant agents and soaps. After a low of 6000 cases in 1956, the number of cases reported annually has risen to about 25,000 per year in the United States. Infection usually follows direct sexual contact. Less commonly, infection occurs after nongenital contact with an infected lesion or accidental inoculation with infected material. Transplacental transmission from an untreated pregnant woman to her fetus before 16 weeks' gestation results in *congenital syphilis.*

Stages

Initial inoculation occurs through intact mucous membranes or abraded skin and, within 6 weeks, results in a broad, ulcerated, painless papule called a *chancre*. The chancre is infiltrated with lymphocytes, plasma cells, histiocytes, and spirochetes, which readily enter the lymphatic system and blood stream. The ulcer heals spontaneously, and signs of dissemination appear after a variable quiescent period of several weeks to months.

The secondary stage is heralded by fever, malaise, adenopathy, and patchy loss of hair. Meningitis, uveitis, optic neuritis, and hepatitis are less common. Maculopapular lesions may develop into wartlike condylomata in moist areas, and oral mucosal patches sometimes appear, all of which are highly infectious. The secondary lesions usually resolve in 2–6 weeks, although up to 25% of patients may experience relapse in the first 2–4 years. Without treatment, these persons enter the latent stage of disease.

Latent syphilis, characterized by positive serologic results without clinical signs, is divided into two stages. The *early latent stage* is within 1 year of infection. During this time, the disease is potentially transmissible because relapses associated with spirochetemia are possible. The *late latent stage* is associated with immunity to relapse and resistance to infectious lesions.

Tertiary manifestations can occur from 2 to 20 years after infection, and one third of untreated cases of latent disease progress to this stage. The remaining two thirds of cases are either subclinical or resolve spontaneously. *Tertiary disease* is characterized by destructive granulomatous lesions with a typical endarteritis that can affect the skin, bone, joints, oral and nasal cavities, parenchymal organs, cardiovascular system, eye, meninges, and central nervous system. Few spirochetes are found in lesions outside the central nervous system.

Immune mechanisms modulating syphilitic infection can contribute to the manifestations of the later stages of the disease. High titers of treponemal and nontreponemal antibodies are present throughout the secondary stage, conferring immunity to reinfection. The manifestations of the tertiary stage are those of a cellular response; however, the paucity of organisms suggests a delayed hypersensitivity to the spirochete products or an autoimmune-type reaction. Pathologically, obliterative endarteritis with a perivascular infiltrate of lymphocytes, monocytes, and plasma cells is a feature of all active stages of syphilis. Gummas of tertiary syphilis are evidenced by a central area of caseating necrosis with a surrounding granulomatous response.

Diagnosis

Most cases of syphilis are diagnosed serologically. *Nontreponemal tests,* such as the VDRL (*V*enereal *D*isease *R*esearch *L*aboratory) test or RPR (*r*apid *p*lasma *r*eagin) test, depend on the patient's nontreponemal serum antibodies causing immune flocculation of cardiolipin in the presence of lecithin and cholesterol. Nontreponemal test results are usually positive during the early stages of the primary lesion, uniformly positive during the secondary stage, and progressively nonreactive in the later stages. In neurosyphilis, the serum VDRL test result may be negative and the cerebrospinal fluid VDRL result may be positive. These patients require careful evaluation and aggressive treatment with close follow-up. Nontreponemal test results become predictably negative after successful therapy and can be used to assess the efficacy of treatment. Nontreponemal test results can be falsely positive in a variety of autoimmune diseases, especially systemic lupus erythematosus. False-positive results can also occur in diseases with a substantial amount of tissue destruction, liver disease, pregnancy, or infections caused by other treponemae.

The *fluorescent treponemal antibody absorption test* (FTA-ABS) involves specific detection of antibody to *T pallidum* after the patient's serum is treated with nonpathogenic treponemal antigens to avoid nonspecific reactions. Hemagglutination tests specific for treponemal antibodies also have high sensitivity and specificity for detecting syphilis. These tests include the hemagglutination treponemal test for syphilis (HATTS), the *T pallidum* hemagglutination assay (TPHA), and the microhemagglutination test for *T pallidum* (MHA-TP). Treponemal antibody detection tests are more specific than nontreponemal tests, but the titers do not decrease with successful treatment; thus, such tests should be considered as confirmatory tests, especially in later stages of disease (Table 1-5).

Results of treponemal tests can be falsely positive in 15% of patients with systemic lupus erythematosus, in patients with other treponemal infections or Lyme disease, and rarely in patients who have lymphosarcoma or are pregnant, although the fluorescent staining is typically weak.

Newer, more sensitive diagnostic tests for syphilis are under investigation, including direct antigen, ELISA, and DNA PCR techniques. These methods may also improve our ability to diagnose congenital syphilis and neurosyphilis. Laboratory diagnosis of treponemal infection may also involve dark-field microscopy of scrapings from primary and secondary lesions. Scrapings of oral lesions are prone to misinterpretation because spirochetes may be present in normal mouth flora.

Management

Treatment of syphilis is determined by stage and central nervous system involvement. *T pallidum* is exquisitely sensitive to penicillin, which remains the antimicrobial of choice (Table 1-6). Erythromycin, azithromycin, chloramphenicol, tetracycline, and the cepha-

Table 1-5 Percent Positive Tests in Untreated Syphilis

	VDRL	FTA-ABS
Primary	70%	80%
Secondary	100%	100%
Tertiary	70%	98%

Table 1-6 Treatment of Syphilis

Syphilis	Drug of Choice and Dosage
Early <1 yr	Penicillin G 2.4 million U IM × 1
Late >1 yr, no CNS	Penicillin G 2.4 million U IM weekly × 3 wks
Neurosyphilis	Penicillin G 2-4 million U IV q 4 hr × 10 days

losporins are acceptable alternatives to penicillin. Lumbar puncture should be performed to determine cerebrospinal fluid involvement in latent syphilis of more than 1 year's duration, suspected neurosyphilis, treatment failure, HIV coinfection, high RPR titers (>1:32), or evidence of other late manifestations (cardiac involvement, gumma). Penicillin G or a single oral dose of azithromycin have been recommended for treatment of patients recently exposed to a sexual partner with infectious syphilis.

Many reports have described an accelerated clinical course of syphilis in patients infected with HIV; furthermore, such patients may experience an incomplete response to standard therapy. An HIV-infected patient with syphilis often requires a longer and more intensive treatment regimen, ongoing follow-up to assess for recurrence, and complete neurologic work-up with an aggressive cerebrospinal fluid investigation for evidence of neurosyphilis. In a recent study, ceftriaxone compared favorably with intravenous penicillin for the treatment of neurosyphilis in HIV-infected patients. Patients with any stage of clinical syphilis should also be tested for HIV status.

Hook EW III, Stephens J, Ennis DM. Azithromycin compared with penicillin G benzathine for treatment of incubating syphilis. *Ann Intern Med.* 1999;131:434–437.

Larsen SA, Steiner BM, Rudolph AH. Laboratory diagnosis and interpretation of tests for syphilis. *Clin Microbiol Rev.* 1995;8:1–21.

Marra CM, Boutin P, McArthur JC, et al. A pilot study evaluating ceftriaxone and penicillin G as treatment agents for neurosyphilis in human immunodeficiency virus-infected individuals. *Clin Infect Dis.* 2000;30:540–544.

Borrelia burgdorferi (Lyme Disease)

Borrelia burgdorferi is a large, microaerophilic, plasmid-containing spirochete. When transmitted to humans and domestic animals through the bite of the *Ixodes* genus of ticks, this organism can cause both acute and chronic illness, now known as *Lyme disease.* First recognized in 1975, Lyme disease is the most common vector-borne infection in the United States. Although cases have been reported in 43 states, clusters are apparent in the northeast Atlantic, the upper Midwest, and the Pacific southwest, areas corresponding to the distribution of the *Ixodes* tick population. The range of the disease extends throughout Europe and Asia. In the United States, the number of reported cases has increased fivefold since 1982, partly because of the rapid growth in the deer population in rural and suburban areas and partly as a result of increased awareness of the disease. One recent innovative approach to reducing proliferation of the tick vector was the placement of insecticide applicators around the opening of deer feeding troughs in endemic areas.

The life cycle of the spirochete depends on its horizontal transmission through a mouse. Early in the summer, an infected *Ixodes* tick nymph bites a mouse, which becomes infected; then, in late summer, the infection is transmitted to an immature uninfected larva after it bites the infected mouse. This immature larva then molts to become a nymph, and the cycle is repeated. Once a nymph matures to an adult, its favorite host is the white-tailed deer, although it can survive with other hosts. Recently, it has been discovered that two other tick-borne zoonoses (babesiosis and human granulocytic ehrlichiosis) can be cotransmitted with Lyme disease.

Stages

Lyme disease usually occurs in three stages following a tick bite: *localized (stage 1), disseminated (stage 2),* and *persistent (stage 3).* Localized disease (stage 1), present in 86% of infected patients, is characterized by skin involvement, initially as a red macule or papule, which later expands in a circular manner, usually with a bright red border and a central clear indurated area, known as *erythema chronicum migrans.*

Hematogenous dissemination (stage 2) can then occur within days to weeks and is manifested as a flu-like illness with headaches, fatigue, and musculoskeletal aching.

More profound symptoms occur as the infection localizes to the nervous, cardiac, and musculoskeletal systems (stage 3). Neurologic complications such as meningitis, encephalitis, cranial neuritis (including Bell palsy), radiculopathy, and neuropathy occur in 15% of patients. Cardiac manifestations include myopericarditis and variable heart block in 5%. Unilateral asymmetrical arthritis occurs in up to 80% of untreated patients.

Late persistent manifestations are usually confined to the nervous system, skin, and joints. Late neurologic signs include encephalomyelitis as well as demyelinating and psychiatric syndromes. Joint involvement includes asymmetrical pauciarticular arthritis and skin involvement characterized by localized scleroderma-type lesions or acrodermatitis chronica atrophicans.

Other systemic manifestations during the initial dissemination or the late persistent state include lymphadenopathy, conjunctivitis, keratitis, neuritis, uveitis, hematuria, and orchitis. In some studies, serologic testing of patients with chronic fatigue syndrome has shown an increased incidence of positive *B burgdorferi* antibodies.

Diagnosis

During the early stages of infection, the immune response is minimal, with little cellular reactivity to *B burgdorferi* antigens and nonspecific elevation of IgM. The spirochete is most easily seen and cultured from the skin lesions during this early stage. During the disseminated phase, cellular antigenic response is markedly increased and specific IgM is followed by a polyclonal B cell activation, with development of specific IgG antibody within weeks of the initial infection. The infection is immunologically mediated by both serum-mediated complement lysis and cellular phagocytosis. Histopathology demonstrates lymphocytic tissue infiltration, often in a perivascular distribution. Late manifestations may be either HLA-mediated autoimmune damage or prolonged latency followed by persistent infection.

Laboratory diagnosis of *B burgdorferi* infection depends on serodiagnosis: there is a poor recovery rate from blood, cerebrospinal fluid, and synovial fluid during the early stages of infection. The expensive laboratory media needed and the several weeks required for incubation of the organism diminish the practical value of culture-proven infection. Skin-biopsy specimens with monoclonal antibody staining have demonstrated good sensitivity in identifying the organism. Although serodiagnosis remains the practical solution for establishing the diagnosis, laboratory methodology is not standardized. Variations in antigen preparation, adsorption of cross-reacting antibodies, types of assays employed, and intralaboratory quality control have resulted in significant inter- and intralaboratory discrepancies with the same serum sample.

The most commonly used serologic tests are the *immunofluorescence antibody* assay or the more sensitive *ELISA*. Other immunologic tests recently available are the *indirect hemagglutination antibody* test and the *immunodot* assay. The ELISA is 50% sensitive during the early stages of the disease, and almost all symptomatic patients are seropositive during the latter disseminated and persistent phases of the infection. These tests should be used only to support a clinical diagnosis of Lyme disease, not as the primary basis for making diagnostic or treatment decisions. Serologic testing is not useful early in the course of Lyme disease because of the low sensitivity of tests in early disease. Serologic testing is more helpful in later disease, when the sensitivity and specificity are greater. Early administration of antibiotics can cause antibody titers to remain below the threshold level; however, cellular reactivity to *Borrelia* antigens remains high. False-positive results can occur in patients with syphilis, Rocky Mountain spotted fever, yaws, pinta, *B recurrentis,* and various rheumatologic disorders. Western blot analysis has been advocated in identifying false-positive results; however, up to 10% of infected patients may be asymptomatic. PCR has been used to detect *B burgdorferi* DNA in serum and cerebrospinal fluid, but its sensitivity in neuroborreliosis is no better than that of the ELISA methods. Although the FTA-ABS test result for syphilis may be positive in patients with Lyme disease, the VDRL test should be nonreactive.

Management

Treatment of *B burgdorferi* infection depends on the stage and the severity of the infection. The organism is highly sensitive in vitro to tetracycline, ampicillin, erythromycin, ceftriaxone, and imipenem; it is less sensitive to penicillin. Early Lyme disease is typically treated with oral doxycycline, amoxicillin, cefuroxime, or erythromycin. Mild disseminated disease is treated with oral doxycycline or amoxicillin. Serious disease (with cardiac or neurologic manifestations) is typically treated with ceftriaxone or high-dose penicillin G intravenously for up to 6 weeks. Patients who do not respond to the initial regimen may require alternate or combination therapy. Up to 15% of patients may develop a *Jarisch-Herxheimer reaction,* in which symptoms worsen during the first day of treatment.

A new recombinant outer surface protein A vaccine for *B burgdorferi* has been developed and studied. It has an acceptable adverse effect profile and effectively prevents Lyme disease. This vaccine is only recommended for persons aged 15 to 70 who are living, working, or traveling outdoors extensively in endemic areas. Efforts to decrease the incidence of the disease by pesticide spraying have met with limited success. In endemic areas, adults may be able to reduce their risk by applying insect-repellent sprays containing diethyltoluamide (DEET).

Brown SL, Hansen SL, Langone JJ. Role of serology in the diagnosis of Lyme disease. *JAMA.* 1999;282:62–66.

Hayney MS, Grunske MM, Boh LE. Lyme disease prevention and vaccine prophylaxis. *Ann Pharmacother.* 1999;33:723–729.

Loewen PS, Marra CA, Marra F. Systematic review of the treatment of early Lyme disease. *Drugs.* 1999;57:157–173.

Ravishankar J, Lutwick LI. Current and future treatment of Lyme disease. *Expert Opin Pharmacother.* 2001;2:241–251.

Terkeltaub RA. Lyme disease 2000. Emerging zoonoses complicate patient work-up and treatment. *Geriatrics.* 2000;55:34–35, 39–40, 43–44.

Chlamydia trachomatis

Chlamydia is a small, obligate, intracellular parasite that contains DNA and RNA and has a unique biphasic life cycle. This prokaryote uses the host cell's energygenerating capacity for its own reproduction. *C trachomatis* can survive only briefly outside the body and is transmitted by close contact. *C trachomatis* is the most common sexually transmitted infection, with 4 million new cases per year. Over 15% of infected pregnant women and 10% of infected men are asymptomatic.

Infection is initiated by local inoculation and ingestion of the organism by phagocytes, followed by intracellular reproduction and eventual spread to other cells. The mechanism for immunologic eradication of *Chlamydia* is uncertain but appears to involve cell-mediated immunity. Infections in humans include trachoma, inclusion conjunctivitis, nongonococcal urethritis, epididymitis, mucopurulent cervicitis, proctitis, salpingitis, infant pneumonia syndrome, and lymphogranuloma venereum. Genital *C trachomatis* infection can result in pelvic inflammatory disease, tubal infertility, and ectopic pregnancy.

Diagnostic techniques include culture, direct immunofluorescent antibody testing of exudates, enzyme immunoassay, and newer DNA probes utilizing PCR, such as the Amplicor PCR test.

Chlamydial infections are readily treated with tetracycline, erythromycin, or one of the quinolones or newer macrolides. Although single-dose therapy of urethritis and cervicitis with azithromycin or sparfloxacin has been proven effective in some studies, treatment for at least 7 days is usually recommended to ensure complete eradication.

Stokes T, Schober P, Baker J, et al. Evidence-based guidelines for the management of genital chlamydial infection in general practice. (Leicestershire Chlamydia Guidelines Group.) *Fam Pract.* 1999;16:269–277.

Tanaka M, Nakayama H, Sagiyama K, et al. Evaluation of a new amplified enzyme immunoassay (EIA) for the detection of Chlamydia trachomatis in male urine, female endocervical swab, and patient obtained vaginal swab specimens. *J Clin Pathol.* 2000;53:350–354.

Fungal Infections

Candida albicans is a yeast that is normally present in the oral cavity, lower gastrointestinal tract, and female genital tract. Under conditions of disrupted local defenses or depressed immunity, overgrowth and parenchymal invasion occur, with the potential for systemic spread. Increased virulence of *Candida* is related to its mycelial phase, when it is more resistant to the host's cellular immune system, which acts as the primary modulator of infection. Recently, DNA PCR techniques have been used to diagnose candidemia. Infections include oral lesions (thrush) and vaginal, skin, esophageal, and urinary tract involvement. Chronic mucocutaneous lesions may occur in persons with specific T cell defects. Disseminated disease can involve any organ system, most commonly the kidneys, brain, heart, and eye.

Some other important invasive fungal infections are cryptococcosis, histoplasmosis, blastomycosis, aspergillosis, and coccidioidomycosis. Invasive fungal infections have become a major problem in immunocompromised patients. Treatment of serious systemic infections has traditionally involved the use of intravenous amphotericin B, sometimes in combined therapy with either flucytosine or an imidazole. Recently, lipid complex and liposome-encapsulated formulations of amphotericin B (AmBisome, Amphotec) have been developed to reduce the drug's nephrotoxicity and myelosuppression. A recent controlled study revealed that intravenous amphotericin B prophylaxis reduced the incidence of systemic fungal infections in immunocompromised patients with leukemia. Newer imidazoles, such as fluconazole, itraconazole, and voriconazole, are less toxic and better-tolerated alternatives. In fact, itraconazole has replaced ketoconazole as the treatment of choice for nonmeningeal, non–life-threatening cases of histoplasmosis, blastomycosis, and paracoccidioidomycosis. Itraconazole is also effective in patients with cryptococcosis and coccidioidomycosis, including those with meningitis.

Carrillo-Munoz AJ, Quindos G, Tur C, et al. Comparative in vitro antifungal activity of amphotericin B lipid complex, amphotericin B and fluconazole. *Chemotherapy.* 2000; 46:235–244.

Evertsson U, Monstein HJ, Johansson AG. Detection and identification of fungi in blood using broad-range 28S rDNA PCR amplification and species-specific hybridisation. *APMIS.* 2000;108:385–392.

Polak A. Antifungal therapy—state of the art at the beginning of the 21st century. *Prog Drug Res.* 2003;spec no:59–190.

Mycobacteria

Mycobacteria include a range of pathogenic and nonpathogenic species distributed widely in the environment. *Mycobacterium tuberculosis* is the most significant human pathogenic species. *M tuberculosis* infects an estimated 1.86 billion persons worldwide (32% global prevalence) and causes about 2 million deaths each year. There were 8 million new cases of tuberculosis in 1997 alone, most of these occurring in Africa and Southeast Asia. *Nontuberculous mycobacteria* may be responsible for up to 5% of all clinical mycobacterial infections. Atypical mycobacterial infections are more prevalent in immunosuppressed patients and those with AIDS. Infections caused by nontuberculous mycobacteria include lymphadenitis, pulmonary infections, skin granulomas, prosthetic valve infections, and bacteremia. Despite their low virulence, atypical mycobacterial infections are difficult to treat because of resistance to standard antituberculous regimens.

Tuberculosis

Infection usually occurs through inhalation of infective droplets and rarely by way of the skin or gastrointestinal tract. The organism is able to multiply within macrophages with a minor inflammatory response. Cell-mediated hypersensitivity to tuberculoprotein develops 3–9 weeks after infection, with a typical granulomatous response that slows or contains bacterial multiplication. Most organisms die during the fibrotic phase of the response. Reactivation is usually associated with depressed immunity and aging. Systemic spread occurs with reactivation and results in a granulomatous response to the infected foci. Acquired immunity is cell mediated but incomplete, and the role of delayed hypersensitivity is complex: high degrees of sensitivity to tuberculoprotein can cause caseous necrosis, which leads to spread of the disease. Infections include pulmonary involvement, which can lead to systemic spread with involvement of any organ system.

Laboratory diagnosis involves culture of infective material on Lowenstein-Jensen medium for 6–8 weeks and use of the acid-fast type of Ziehl-Neelsen stain or fluorescent antibody staining of infected material. In addition, ELISA as well as DNA probes using PCR techniques for *M tuberculosis* and other mycobacteria are now available.

The tuberculin skin test measures delayed hypersensitivity to tuberculoprotein. Purified protein derivative (PPD) produced from a culture filtrate of *M tuberculosis* is standardized and its activity expressed as tuberculin units (TU). Usually, intermediate strength (5 TU) is used; however, if a high degree of sensitivity to tuberculoprotein is suspected, low strength (1 TU) is used to avoid the risk of excessive reaction locally or at the site of an infected focus. A positive high-strength (250 TU) reaction with a doubtful intermediate-strength reaction suggests infection with atypical mycobacteria and resultant cross-sensitization.

A positive PPD reaction is defined as an area of induration 10 mm or greater in the area of intradermal injection of 0.1 mL of PPD read 48–72 hours later. Ninety percent of persons demonstrating 10 mm of induration to 5 TU are infected with *M tuberculosis*. A positive response indicates an infection, although the infection might not be currently active. Induration of 5 mm in persons with HIV infection is sufficient to warrant chemoprophylaxis. For children, the tine test is an easily administered alternative to the PPD.

Among patients in whom skin testing yields positive results, the overall risk of reactivation of the disease is 3%–5%. A positive PPD test result should be considered in light of the individual patient's radiologic and clinical data as well as age to determine the need for prophylactic treatment. Administration of isoniazid daily for 1 year reduces the risk of reactivation by 80%; however, the risk of isoniazid hepatotoxicity increases with age and alcohol use. Patients with a positive tuberculin skin test result who require long-term high-dose steroids or other immunosuppressive agents should be treated prophylactically with isoniazid for the duration of their immunosuppressive therapy to prevent reactivation of tuberculosis.

Treatment of active infection involves use of two or three drugs because of the emergence of resistance and of delay in culture susceptibility studies. Standard regimens employ multiple drugs for 18–24 months, but with the addition of newer agents, 6–9 months of treatment have been found equally effective. Drugs currently used include isoniazid, rifampin, rifabutin, ethambutol, streptomycin, pyrazinamide, aminosalicylic acid, ethionamide, and cycloserine. All of the agents currently used have toxic side effects, especially hepatic and neurologic, which should be carefully monitored during the course of therapy. Isoniazid and ethambutol can cause optic neuritis in a small percentage of patients, and rifampin may cause pink-tinged tears and blepharoconjunctivitis. The BCG (*bacille Calmette-Guérin*) vaccine causes false-positive reactions to the PPD skin test and thus interferes with the efficacy of the PPD skin test as a diagnostic and epidemiologic tool.

Outbreaks of nosocomial and community-acquired multidrug-resistant tuberculosis (MDRTB) have been reported recently, particularly in the presence of concurrent HIV infection. MDRTB in patients infected with HIV is associated with widely disseminated disease, poor treatment response, and substantial mortality. Infection has also been documented in health care workers exposed to these patients. MDRTB represents a serious public health threat that will require an aggressive governmental and medical response to limit its spread.

Dye C, Scheele S, Dolin P, et al. Consensus statement. Global burden of tuberculosis: estimated incidence, prevalence, and mortality by country. WHO Global Surveillance and Monitoring Project. *JAMA.* 1999;282:677–686.

Pottumarthy S, Wells VC, Morris AJ. A comparison of seven tests for serological diagnosis of tuberculosis. *J Clin Microbiol.* 2000;38:2227–2231.

Herpesvirus

As a class, viruses are strictly intracellular parasites, relying on the host cell for their replication. Herpesviruses, which are large-enveloped, double-stranded DNA viruses, are one of the most common human infectious agents, responsible for a wide spectrum of acute and chronic diseases. The major members of the group are herpes simplex viruses (HSV-1 and HSV-2), varicella-zoster virus, cytomegalovirus (CMV), and Epstein-Barr virus.

Herpes Simplex

HSV has two antigenic types, each with numerous antigenic strains. Each type has different epidemiologic patterns of infection. Seroepidemiologic studies demonstrate a high prevalence of HSV-1 antibodies with a lower prevalence of HSV-2 antibodies. Many people with HSV antibodies are asymptomatic. Infection is modulated by a predominantly cellular response. The presence of high titers of neutralizing antibodies to HSV does not seem to retard the cell-to-cell transmission of the virus. The virus can spread within nerves and cause a latent infection of sensory and autonomic ganglia. Latent infection does not result in death of the host cell, and the exact mechanism of viral genome interaction with the host genome is incompletely understood. Reactivation of HSV from the trigeminal ganglia may be associated with asymptomatic excretion or with the development of mucosal herpetic ulceration. Serologic testing, DNA PCR testing, and viral culture can assist in the diagnosis of difficult cases, particularly central nervous system infections.

Herpes simplex type 1 is associated with mucocutaneous superficial infections of the pharynx, skin, oral cavity, vagina, eye, and brain. Herpes encephalitis carries a 30% mortality rate. *Herpes simplex type 2* is an important sexually transmitted disease that is associated with genital infections, aseptic meningitis, and congenital infection. *Neonatal herpes infection* involves multiple systems and carries a 70% untreated mortality rate.

The drug of choice for treating acute systemic infections is acyclovir. Localized disease can be treated with oral acyclovir. Topical treatment of skin or mucocutaneous lesions with acyclovir ointment decreases the healing time. Oral acyclovir can also be used prophylactically for severe and recurrent genital herpes. Long-term suppressive oral acyclovir also reduces the recurrence of herpes simplex epithelial keratitis and stromal keratitis.

Two newer antiviral agents, famciclovir and valacyclovir, are approved for the treatment of herpes zoster and herpes simplex. These agents have better bioavailability and achieve higher blood levels than acyclovir. HSV is also sensitive to vidarabine. Cidofovir, a new antiviral drug used for CMV infections, is also very effective against acyclovir-resistant herpes simplex.

Varicella-Zoster

Varicella-zoster virus (VZV) produces infection in a manner similar to herpes simplex. After a primary infection, the virus remains latent in dorsal root ganglia, with host cellular immune interaction inhibiting reactivation. Primary infection usually occurs in childhood in the form of chickenpox (varicella), a generalized vesicular rash accompanied by mild constitutional symptoms. Reactivation may be heralded by pain in a sensory nerve distribution, followed by a unilateral vesicular eruption occurring over one to three dermatomic areas. New crops of lesions appear in the same area within 7 days. Resolution of the lesions may be followed by postherpetic neuralgia, the mechanism of which is incompletely understood. Other neurologic syndromes following herpes zoster involvement include segmental myelitis, Guillain-Barré syndrome, and Ramsay Hunt syndrome. The incidence of herpes zoster is two to three times higher in patients over age 60. Postherpetic neuralgia occurs after herpes zoster infection in approximately 50% of patients older than 50 years. The pain of postherpetic neuralgia can be severe and debilitating and may persist for months or even years. Immunosuppressed persons experience recurrent lesions; the incidence of disseminated disease in such patients may be 10 times that of immunocompetent persons.

Treatment of acute infection in immunocompromised patients or those with visceral involvement is with acyclovir, famciclovir, or valacyclovir. Newer drugs being evaluated for resistant VZV strains or concomitant HIV infection include sorivudine, brivudine, fialuridine, fiacitabine, netivudine, lobucavir, foscarnet, and cidofovir. A live attenuated varicella vaccine (Varivax) is available for prevention of primary disease, and it appears to also reduce the incidence of recurrent *H zoster* infection and neuralgia. This vaccine is recommended for children, patients with chronic diseases or leukemia, and patients receiving immunosuppressive therapy. In some patients, tricyclic antidepressants, carbamazepine, gabapentin, and topical capsaicin cream have reduced the pain of postherpetic neuralgia. For refractory cases, transcutaneous electronic nerve stimulation or nerve blocks are sometimes used.

Johnson RW, Dworkin RH. Treatment of herpes zoster and postherpetic neuralgia. *BMJ.* 2003;326:748–750.

Oral acyclovir for herpes simplex virus eye disease: effect on prevention of epithelial keratitis and stromal keratitis. Herpetic Eye Disease Study Group. *Arch Ophthalmol.* 2000;118:1030–1036.

Ormrod D, Scott LJ, Perry CM. Valacyclovir: a review of its long term utility in the management of genital herpes simplex virus and cytomegalovirus infections. *Drugs.* 2000;59:839–863.

Cytomegalovirus

CMV is a ubiquitous human virus: 50% of adults in developed countries harbor antibodies, which are usually acquired during the first 5 years of life. The virus can be isolated from all body fluids, even in the presence of circulating neutralizing antibody, for up to several years after infection. Cytopathic effects following infection are similar to those of HSV. Serologic and PCR testing are available to assist in the diagnosis of CMV infection.

Clinical syndromes with greatest morbidity include congenital CMV disease, with a 20% incidence of hearing loss or mental retardation and 0.1% incidence of various other congenital disorders, including jaundice, hepatosplenomegaly, anemia, microcephaly, and chorioretinitis. Infections in adults include heterophilenegative mononucleosis, pneumonia, hepatitis, and Guillain-Barré syndrome. In immunocompromised patients, CMV interstitial pneumonia carries a 90% mortality rate. Disseminated spread to the gastrointestinal tract, central nervous system, and eye is common in patients with AIDS. Latent infection within leukocytes accounts for transfusion-associated disease. CMV replication itself can further suppress cell-mediated immunity, with resultant depressed lymphocyte response and development of severe opportunistic infections.

CMV retinitis and colitis have been successfully treated with the nucleoside derivative ganciclovir. This drug is available for intravenous, oral, or intravitreal routes. A slow-release intraocular ganciclovir insert is also available for the treatment of CMV retinitis. It should be noted that the intravitreal and intraocular methods of administration are effective only for CMV retinitis and will not treat colitis or other systemic manifestations. Intravenous foscarnet and cidofovir have also been effective in the treatment of CMV retinitis. A recent study showed that intravitreal cidofovir given at 6 week intervals was highly effective for treating CMV retinitis. Valganciclovir is a new oral agent that is highly effective in the treatment of CMV infection, including retinitis.

Segarra-Newnham M, Salazar MI. Valganciclovir: a new oral alternative for cytomegalovirus retinitis in human immunodeficiency virus–seropositive individuals. *Pharmacotherapy.* 2002;22:1124–1128.

Tong CY, Cuevas LE, Williams H, et al. Prediction and diagnosis of cytomegalovirus disease in renal transplant recipients using qualitative and quantitative polymerase chain reaction. *Transplantation.* 2000;69:985–991.

Epstein-Barr Virus

Epstein-Barr virus (EBV) antibodies are found in 90%–95% of all adults. Childhood infections are usually asymptomatic, with symptomatic disease occurring in young adults. Infectious mononucleosis is the usual clinical disease in most symptomatic adults. Transplant recipients on cyclosporine or patients with AIDS may develop lymphoproliferative disorders. EBV is epidemiologically associated with Burkitt lymphoma and nasopharyngeal carcinoma. EBV's host range is restricted to B lymphocytes, nasopharyngeal epithelial, and uterine epithelial cells; however, latent infection appears to be limited to B cells. The virus does not generally produce cytopathic effects in cells, and the viral DNA remains in a circular nonintegrated form within the cell. Lymphoblastoid cell lines infected with EBV can be cultured indefinitely in vitro. The lymphocytosis of mononucleosis is thought to result from a T cell reaction to infected B cells.

Treatment of acute disease is largely supportive, although the EBV DNA polymerase is sensitive to acyclovir and ganciclovir, which decrease viral replication in tissue culture. No vaccine is presently available against EBV, but research is ongoing toward developing a cytotoxic T-cell–based vaccine.

Bharadwaj M, Moss DJ. Epstein-Barr virus vaccine: a cytotoxic T-cell–based approach. *Expert Rev Vaccines*. 2002;1:467–476.

Influenza

See Chapter 13 for a discussion of influenza.

Hepatitis

Hepatitis A

Hepatitis A is usually transmitted by the oral route and may be acquired from contaminated water supplies and unwashed or poorly cooked foods. Patients at high risk (travelers to endemic areas, military personnel, drug abusers, family contacts of infected patients, and laboratory workers exposed to the virus) should be given the hepatitis A vaccine (Havrix). Many adults in the United States are already immune, so antibody testing can be performed first, followed by vaccination if antibodies are not present.

Hepatitis B

See Chapter 13 for a discussion of hepatitis B.

Hepatitis C

Approximately 20%–40% of acute viral hepatitis reported in the United States is of the non-A, non-B type; of the group, the majority is caused by the hepatitis C virus (HCV). Worldwide prevalence is about 1%. Current estimates suggest that approximately 170,000 new cases of HCV occur annually in the United States; 50%–80% of these patients develop evidence of chronic hepatitis, and 20% of these patients develop cirrhosis. Only 6% of reported cases of hepatitis C are transfusion related. Other recognized risk factors for hepatitis C transmission include parenteral drug use, hemodialysis, and occupational exposure to blood. Although the role of sexual activity in the transmission of HCV remains to be fully elucidated, this mode is clearly not a predominant source of transmission. Of all the hepatitis viruses, HCV causes the most damage in immunocompetent hosts because of direct hepatocyte cytotoxicity and may result in cirrhosis, fulminant hepatitis, and hepatocellular carcinoma. At present, cirrhosis from HCV infection is the most common indication for liver transplantation in the United States. Treatment of chronic active hepatitis C includes α-interferon and ribavirin; management of chronic persistent hepatitis C is largely supportive. No vaccine is presently available against HCV, but researchers are hopeful that a vaccine will soon be developed.

Chronic delta hepatitis is a severe form of chronic liver disease caused by hepatitis delta virus (hepatitis D virus) infection superimposed on chronic hepatitis B. Lamivudine has been effective for treating hepatitis B as well as chronic delta hepatitis.

Hepatitis E virus is an RNA virus that is transmitted enterically and causes sporadic as well as epidemic acute viral hepatitis in many developing countries.

Hepatitis G virus may cause coinfection with hepatitis B virus or HCV but usually does not increase their pathogenicity. GBVC and the hepatitis G virus (GBVC/HGV) are variants of the same RNA flavivirus, which was recently found to be a lymphotropic virus that replicates primarily in the spleen and bone marrow.

Transfusion-transmitted virus (TTV) is a new virus identified in a small percentage of patients with non–A, G post-transfusion hepatitis. The virus causes coinfection in some patients with hepatitis C. TTV DNA is common in high-risk populations, such as patients with hemophilia, those on hemodialysis, and intravenous drug abusers.

Radkowski M, Kubicka J, Kisiel E, et al. Detection of active hepatitis C virus and hepatitis G virus/GB virus C replication in bone marrow in human subjects. *Blood.* 2000;95:3986–3989.

Thomas DL, Astemborski J, Rai RM, et al. The natural history of hepatitis C virus infection: host, viral, and environmental factors. *JAMA.* 2000;284:450–456.

Watanabe H, Saito T, Kawamata O, et al. Clinical implications of TT virus superinfection in patients with chronic hepatitis C. *Am J Gastroenterol.* 2000;95:1776–1780.

Acquired Immunodeficiency Syndrome

During the 1980s, AIDS emerged as a major public health problem. AIDS was originally described in 1981 when *Pneumocystis carinii* pneumonia (PCP) and Kaposi sarcoma were noted to occur in homosexual men and intravenous drug abusers. Since then, the number of cases has increased exponentially. In 1983, it was discovered that AIDS was caused by the retrovirus HIV. Subsequently, it became evident that HIV caused a spectrum of disease, including an asymptomatic carrier state, the AIDS-related complex (ARC), and AIDS itself.

As of December 2001, 816,149 AIDS cases in the United States had been reported to the Centers for Disease Control and Prevention (CDC). Adult and adolescent AIDS cases totaled 807,074, with 666,026 cases in males and 141,048 cases in females. Through the same time period, 9074 AIDS cases were reported in children under age 13. Total cumulative deaths of persons reported with AIDS were 467,910, including 5257 children under age 15. It is estimated that between 600,000 and 800,000 Americans are currently infected with HIV. More than 200,000 of these are unaware that they are infected. On the positive side, improved antiretroviral therapy in recent years has resulted in a significant decline in the number of AIDS cases in the United States and a 70% reduction in deaths due to AIDS since 1995. Also, AIDS is no longer the leading cause of death in young adults in the United States.

Worldwide, AIDS continues to take a devastating toll, particularly in countries of sub-Sahara Africa and in Asian nations with large, impoverished populations. According to the Joint United Nations Program on HIV/AIDS, as of the end of 2002, 42 million people are estimated to be living with HIV/AIDS. Of these, 19.2 million are women, and

3.2 million are children under age 15. An estimated 28 million people have died from AIDS since the epidemic began, including 12 million women and 5.5 million children under age 15. During 2002, AIDS caused the deaths of an estimated 3.1 million people, including 1.2 million women and 610,000 children under age 15. Women are increasingly more affected by HIV. Approximately 50%, or 19.2 million, of the 38.6 million adults now living with HIV or AIDS worldwide are women. The overwhelming majority of people with HIV, approximately 95% of the global total, are in developing countries. It is estimated that there are about 16,000 new infections occurring worldwide each day. Over 50% of the infections are in young adults between the ages of 15 and 25. Only 10% of the world's HIV-infected people know that they are infected. Over 13 million children have been orphaned by HIV infection of one or both of their parents.

Etiology and Pathogenesis

AIDS is caused by infection with HIV (HIV-1), previously known as the human T cell lymphotropic virus type III, lymphadenopathy-associated virus, and AIDS-related virus. Thus far, there are nine known serotypes of HIV-1 group M, and one of HIV-1 groups O and N. In the United States, HIV group M, serotype B is the most common form of HIV.

Another human T cell lymphotropic virus, HIV-2, has been isolated from West Africans and is associated with AIDS as well. HIV-2 is closely related to simian immunodeficiency virus. HIV belongs to a family of viruses known as retroviruses. A retrovirus encodes its genetic information in RNA and uses a unique viral enzyme called *reverse transcriptase* to copy its genome into DNA. Other members of this retrovirus family include the human T cell lymphotropic retrovirus type I, which can cause adult T cell leukemia and chronic progressive myelopathy with atrophy of the spinal cord. HTLV II is associated with hairy cell leukemia.

HIV preferentially infects T cells, especially T-helper (CD4+) lymphocytes. The virus infects mature T cells in vitro, although other cells can serve as targets. CD4 is the phenotypic marker for this subset and is identified by monoclonal antibodies OKT4 and Leu-3.

The hallmark of the immunodeficiency in AIDS is a depletion of the CD4+ helper/inducer T lymphocytes. HIV selectively infects these lymphocytes as well as macrophages; with HIV replication, the helper T cell is killed. Because of the central role of the helper T lymphocyte in the immune response, loss of this subset results in a profound immune deficiency, leading to the life-threatening opportunistic infections indicative of AIDS. This selective depletion of CD4+ helper T cells leads to the characteristic inverted CD4+/CD8+ ratio (also known as T4/T8 ratio). Years may pass between the initial HIV infection and the development of these immune abnormalities.

In addition to the cellular immune deficiency, patients with AIDS have abnormalities of B cell function. These patients fail to mount an antibody response to novel T cell–dependent B cell challenges, although they have B cell hyperfunction with polyclonal B cell activation, hypergammaglobulinemia, and circulating immune complexes. This B cell hyperfunction may be a direct consequence of HIV infection: studies have demonstrated that polyclonal activation can be induced in vitro by adding HIV to B cells.

HIV has also been documented to infect the brains of patients with AIDS. It is thought that HIV infection of the brain is responsible for the HIV encephalopathy syndrome. HIV-infected cells in the brain have generally been identified as macrophages.

Clinical Syndromes

The clinical syndrome of AIDS consists of recurrent severe opportunistic infections or unusual neoplasms. In 1982, the CDC published an original case definition of AIDS as the presence of a reliably diagnosed disease at least moderately indicative of an underlying cellular immune deficiency (Kaposi sarcoma in a patient less than 60 years old, PCP, or other opportunistic infection) and the absence of known causes of an underlying immune deficiency or of any other stage of resistance reported to be associated with the disease (immunosuppressive therapy, lymphoreticular malignancy). This original surveillance case definition has been modified by the CDC as new data have become available.

AIDS is now diagnosed when a person presents with one or more of the indicator diseases outlined in the following list. These diseases are indicative of an underlying cellular immunodeficiency, and the most common presentations are with PCP or with Kaposi sarcoma.

These conditions are included in the current AIDS surveillance case definition:

- Candidiasis of bronchi, trachea, or lungs
- Candidiasis, esophageal
- Cervical cancer, invasive
- Coccidioidomycosis, disseminated or extrapulmonary
- Cryptococcosis, extrapulmonary
- Cryptosporidiosis, chronic intestinal (>1 month's duration)
- CMV disease (other than liver, spleen, or nodes)
- Herpes simplex: chronic ulcer(s) (>1 month's duration); or bronchitis, pneumonitis, or esophagitis
- Histoplasmosis, disseminated or extrapulmonary
- HIV encephalopathy
- Isosporiasis, chronic intestinal (>1 month's duration)
- Kaposi sarcoma
- Lymphoma, Burkitt (or equivalent term)
- Lymphoma, immunoblastic (or equivalent term)
- Lymphoma, primary in brain
- *Mycobacterium avium* complex or *Mycobacterium kansasii,* disseminated or extrapulmonary
- *M tuberculosis,* any site (pulmonary or extrapulmonary)
- PCP
- Pneumonia, recurrent
- Progressive multifocal leukoencephalopathy
- *Salmonella* septicemia, recurrent
- Toxoplasmosis of brain
- Wasting syndrome due to HIV

AIDS represents the most severe end of the spectrum of HIV infection. Acute infection with HIV often manifests as a transient mononucleosis-like syndrome. This syndrome has been called *primary HIV infection*, or *retroviral syndrome*, and the typical symptoms are fever, fatigue, weight loss, myalgias, headache, pharyngitis, and nausea. Primary HIV infection is diagnosed by a positive result with the plasma HIV RNA test obtained on the same day as a negative Western blot assay. A repeat HIV antibody test should be obtained 2–3 weeks after resolution of symptoms to confirm seroconversion.

Patients may then enter a prolonged asymptomatic carrier state (the majority of HIV-infected patients in the United States are in this condition). There is also a syndrome of persistent generalized lymphadenopathy, which is associated with depleted T-helper lymphocytes and HIV infection. Lymphadenopathy with other signs and symptoms has commonly been called the *lymphadenopathy syndrome* or *ARC*. Constitutional symptoms in patients with ARC include fever, weight loss, chronic diarrhea, oral thrush, and lymphadenopathy. Although these patients have immunologic defects similar to those found in patients with AIDS, those with ARC have not developed one of the AIDS-defining opportunistic infections or unusual neoplasms. The CDC has classified HIV infection into the three groups outlined in Table 1-7. The shaded boxes illustrate clinical conditions now defined as AIDS.

Seroepidemiology

Antibodies to HIV can be detected in HIV-infected persons. Such screening is now performed with commercially available kits, all of which are based on an ELISA using whole disrupted HIV antigens. The ELISA test for HIV antibodies is sensitive (99%) and specific (99%). However, false-negative results can occur, especially in the first weeks after HIV infection. Because of the possibility of false-positive ELISA results, the ELISA must yield positive results twice and be confirmed by Western blot analysis or immunofluorescence assay before a patient is said to have antibodies to HIV. Persons with antibodies to HIV should be considered infectious for HIV. Currently, HIV p24 antigen testing or HIV-1

Table 1-7 1992 Revised Classification System for HIV Infection and Expanded AIDS Surveillance Case Definition for Adolescents and Adults*

| | Clinical Categories | | |
| | A | B | C |
CD4+ CELL CATEGORIES	Asymptomatic, or PGL**	Symptomatic, not A or C conditions	AIDS-indicator conditions
1. $\geq$500/mm^3	A1	B1	C1
2. 200–499/mm^3	A2	B2	C2
3. <200/mm^3	A3	B3	C3

* The shaded cells illustrate the expansion of the AIDS surveillance case definition. Persons with AIDS-indicator conditions (category C) are currently reportable to the health department in every state and US territory. In addition to persons with clinical category C conditions (categories C1, C2, and C3), persons with CD4+ lymphocyte counts of less than 200/mm^3 (categories A3 or B3) are also reportable as AIDS cases in the United States, effective April 1, 1992.

** PGL = persistent generalized lymphadenopathy. Clinical category A includes acute (primary) HIV infection.

RNA analysis can be performed. These tests yield positive results earlier than anti-HIV antibody tests do.

Seroepidemiologic studies conducted in high-risk populations revealed an increasing prevalence of HIV infection from almost nil prior to 1979 to as high as 70% by 1988. The rate of increase of HIV infection slowed during the 1990s in the United States but accelerated in Africa and other developing regions. In the past, 100% of patients with HIV infection ultimately developed AIDS, but this percentage is gradually falling as many patients respond to highly active antiretroviral therapy (HAART), resulting in a corresponding decrease in the incidence of opportunistic infections. The median incubation period between acquisition of HIV infection and the development of AIDS is now estimated to be over 10 years.

Modes of Transmission

Modes of transmission of HIV infection are:

- Sexual contact
- Intravenous drug use
- Transfusion
- Perinatal transmission from an infected mother to her child

There have been no documented cases of transmission by casual contact. Furthermore, although HIV infection may be transmitted by blood or blood products, the risk of transmission by accidental needle stick appears quite low (<0.5%). Studies of nonsexual household contacts of patients with AIDS have revealed that these people are at minimal or possibly no risk of infection with HIV.

At the beginning of the AIDS epidemic, almost all the cases were confined to gay men in the United States, but that proportion has been steadily decreasing, along with corresponding increases in intravenous drug users and in patients infected through heterosexual contact. Furthermore, in Africa the male/female ratio is 1:1, and epidemiologic data have suggested that the disease is transmitted predominantly by heterosexual activity, parenteral exposure to blood transfusion and unsterilized needles, and perinatally from infected mothers to their newborns.

Prognosis and Treatment

Currently, AIDS is an incurable and fatal disease. Nevertheless, infected patients are living longer and have had better quality of life in recent years because of significant improvements in antiviral therapy. The risk factors most closely associated with decreased survival in patients with AIDS are reduced CD4 levels, length of time since diagnosis, low serum albumin levels (<0.30 g/L), previous opportunistic infections, high viral load, and new "clinical progression" events. CD4 counts are good predictors of risk of opportunistic infection. Plasma HIV RNA levels are even better predictors of progression than CD4 counts and are the best single predictors of response to therapy.

Recommended laboratory studies with a newly diagnosed case of HIV infection often include complete blood count with manual differential, CD4 count, HIV viral load testing (RNA level), electrolytes, renal and liver function tests, urinalysis, PPD (tuberculosis test), anergy panel, and serologic tests for syphilis, hepatitis B virus and HCV, *Toxoplasma*, CMV, and VZV. Female patients should undergo a Pap smear because of the high risk of invasive cervical cancer in HIV-infected persons. The recommended vaccinations in HIV-positive patients are diphtheria/tetanus (every 5 years), inactivated polio, measles, *Pneumococcus* (every 5 years), hepatitis B virus, hepatitis A virus (especially if the patient is HCV-positive), and influenza virus (yearly). *H influenzae* B vaccine is optional.

In 1986, the drug *zidovudine* (also known as azidothymidine, AZT, or Retrovir), a synthetic analogue of thymidine, became available for the treatment of AIDS. Zidovudine is incorporated into DNA by the DNA polymerase (reverse transcriptase) of HIV and prevents further viral DNA synthesis. A controlled trial conducted in 1986 demonstrated significantly decreased mortality during the study period among patients with AIDS and ARC treated with zidovudine compared with those taking a placebo. Episodes of opportunistic infections also decreased. The major limiting side effect of this therapy was bone marrow suppression, often requiring repeated transfusions.

In recent years, the treatment of AIDS has advanced significantly. Multicenter clinical trials demonstrated that half-dose zidovudine (100 mg orally every 4 hours) was as effective as full-dose zidovudine (200 mg every 4 hours). This lower dose was associated with a lower incidence of side effects. More recent data revealed that 200 mg every 8 hours is as effective as more frequent dosing schedules. Currently, zidovudine is used primarily in combination therapy.

Data released from early zidovudine trials also showed that when symptomatic HIV-infected persons with ARC and asymptomatic HIV-infected persons with CD4 counts less than 500/mm^3 were treated with zidovudine, progression of the disease to later stages (ie, AIDS) was delayed. Furthermore, the data showed improved short-term survival and improved CD4 counts. Zidovudine was approved for use in HIV-positive adults and children in 1990 and for HIV-positive pregnant women and newborns in 1994. A new timed-release form of the drug, called AZTEC, was released to provide longer dosing intervals.

Some of the other nucleoside analogue reverse transcriptase inhibitors approved for the treatment of HIV infection are *didanosine* (dideoxyinosine, ddI, Videx), *zalcitabine* (dideoxycytidine, ddC, Hivid), *lamivudine* (3TC, Epivir), and *stavudine* (d4T, Zerit). These drugs have in vitro activity against HIV similar to that of zidovudine. The primary benefit of these drugs over zidovudine is reduced bone marrow toxicity, which makes them more useful in the setting of concurrent leukopenia or use of other marrow-toxic drugs (eg, ganciclovir). Lamivudine is available as a combination drug with zidovudine (Combivir). A new drug, abacavir (Ziagen), was the first clinically available guanosine analogue reverse transcriptase inhibitor. Trizivir is a combination drug containing abacavir, lamivudine, and zidovudine. Other new nucleoside analogues include adefovir (Preveon) and emtricitabine (FTC, Emtriva). They are active against isolates resistant to older nucleoside analogues. Tenofovir DF (PMPA, Viread) is a new *nucleotide* reverse transcriptase inhibitor.

The major treatment-limiting toxicity of didanosine is acute pancreatitis, and its use is therefore contraindicated in the setting of alcoholism or prior pancreatitis. In addition, didanosine should not be used concurrently with pentamidine. Zalcitabine may cause rapidly progressive, severe peripheral neuropathy, which may not be reversible upon discontinuing therapy. Lamivudine has been associated with neutropenia and peripheral neuropathy in a small percentage of patients. Stavudine causes peripheral neuropathy in 15%–20% of patients.

Several non-nucleoside reverse transcriptase inhibitors (NNRTIs)— *nevirapine* (Viramune), *delavirdine* (Rescriptor), and *atevirdine*—are available, but they share the disadvantage of rapid emergence of viral resistance. Therefore, they are currently used only in combination therapy. A promising new NNRTI, efavirenz (Sustiva), is taken once daily, has excellent activity against HIV, and has fewer side effects than other NNRTIs. Efavirenz is approved for combined therapy in adult and pediatric patients but should not be used by pregnant women. Efavirenz is well tolerated in most patients, and the reported side effects are dizziness, insomnia, abnormal dreams, and skin rash. Emivirine (Coactinon), capravirine, and calanolide are new investigational NNRTIs.

The protease inhibitors are a class of antiretroviral drugs that prevent the cleavage of precursor proteins into viral elements needed for viral assembly. This results in the production of nonfunctional, noninfectious virions. The protease inhibitors currently approved for the treatment of HIV infection include *saquinavir* (Invirase, Fortovase), *indinavir* (Crixivan), *ritonavir* (Norvir), *nelfinavir* (Viracept), *amprenavir* (Agenerase), *atazanavir* (Reyataz), and a *lopinavir/ritonavir combination* (Kaletra). Tiprinavir is a new protease inhibitor involved in clinical trials. The protease inhibitors are used primarily in multidrug therapy along with one or more nucleoside analogues. Potential side effects include hyperlipidemia, pancreatitis, renal failure, lipodystrophy, rhabdomyolysis, and hepatitis.

Fusion inhibitors are a completely new class of investigational antiviral agents that block fusion of HIV with the human cell by blocking the function of the gp120 envelope glycoprotein. *Enfuvirtide* (T-20, Fuzeon) was approved by the FDA for treatment of HIV infection in March 2003. *T-1249* and *AMD-3100* are investigational peptide fusion inhibitors that appear to be very effective in reducing HIV viral load in early studies.

In response to the extremely high prices of many AIDS drugs, several states have established AIDS Drug Assistance Programs. Also, many AIDS drug manufacturers now offer patient assistance programs to help patients locate sources for reimbursement or provide drugs free to patients who have no means of obtaining them.

Multidrug therapy, currently known as HAART, is now the standard of care and usually involves drug regimens with three or more agents. To prevent early drug resistance, it is important that the drugs all be initiated simultaneously rather than sequentially. Most of the recent clinical trials recommend a drug regimen that includes a potent protease inhibitor in combination with two nucleoside analogue reverse transcriptase inhibitors or two protease inhibitors combined with one or two nucleoside analogue reverse transcriptase inhibitors. Recently, some alternative treatment regimens have omitted protease inhibitors *(protease-sparing regimen)*. This is a departure from the standard treatment that has included protease inhibitors since their introduction in the 1990s. Protease inhibitors remain among the most effective and important treatments developed, but some persons experience significant problems, including cross-resistance and patient intolerance. Protease-sparing regimens such as abacavir/AZT/3TC and drug combinations that include efavirenz appear to be as effective as regimens that contain protease inhibitors.

HAART has been shown to result in dramatic reduction of HIV viral load, increased CD4 cell counts, delay of disease progression, reduction of opportunistic infections, decreased hospitalizations, and prolonged survival. Some statistics show up to an 82% decline in opportunistic infections in patients on HAART. These advantages are translating into improved survival and enhanced quality of life for HIV-infected patients. It is interesting to note that the number of AIDS cases in the United States peaked in 1993 and has been gradually decreasing since then. The HIV mortality rate has declined over 70% since 1995, mostly because of HAART. From 1995 to 1997, the AIDS mortality rate decreased from 29.4 to 8.8 per 100 person-years. Unfortunately, the benefits of HAART have not reached the 42 million HIV-infected patients in the developing world. The number of AIDS cases and the AIDS-related mortality rate continue to rise relentlessly in these regions, partially because of the socioeconomic barriers to expensive therapy.

At present, the most common treatment endpoint or goal of HAART is reduction of HIV RNA levels, preferably to undetectable levels (<500 copies/mL). In some studies, HAART reduced HIV RNA to undetectable levels in up to 78% of patients. Baseline levels should be checked before the initiation or change of antiretroviral therapy, again at 1 month after treatment begins to show efficacy, and then every 3 or 4 months. Available HIV RNA assays include branched DNA (Multiplex) and PCR (Amplicor HIV-1 Monitor). Although both tests provide similar information, concentrations of HIV RNA obtained with the PCR test are about two times higher than those obtained by the branched DNA method. Thus, for consistency, all HIV RNA testing in a single patient should be obtained via the same assay.

Discontinuation of HAART after 1 year of successful treatment is usually followed by a rapid rebound of viral load. Viral antigen quickly returns to undetectable levels following reintroduction of HAART. For patients in whom HAART fails because of drug resistance, some recent studies have offered alternative aggressive salvage therapy regimens with five or more agents. HIV drug sensitivity testing is now available for most of the approved antiretroviral agents and should be performed in patients with suspected drug-resistant infections. In some patients, HAART is interrupted because of drug toxicity.

The immunomodulators are a diverse group of drugs and immunologic adjuvants being evaluated for their efficacy in enhancing the host immune response to HIV and related opportunistic infections. This list includes agents that enhance or stimulate T cell and macrophage response: ditiocarb, ampligen, CD4-IgG, human granulocyte colony stimulating factor, sargramostim, lentinan, levamisol, thymosin-α_1, and thymic humoral factor.

Some agents induce humoral as well as cellular immune responses: interleukin-2 and zinc replacement therapy. Other drugs inhibit viral replication, such as β-interferon, interleukin-10, hydroxyurea, and thalidomide.

These immunomodulators have been primarily used as a supplement to antiretroviral agents in combined therapy study protocols and have been discussed much less in the literature since the availability of HAART. *Hematopoietic agents,* such as erythropoietin and interleukin-3, enhance the proliferation of blood cells and are useful in the treatment of cytopenias. Thalidomide is also beneficial for the treatment of HIV wasting syndrome.

A small percentage of the population appears to be naturally immune to HIV infection. These persons have defective genes for CCR-5, a surface receptor that HIV requires to attach to T cells. Also, about 50% of long-term survivors of HIV are heterozygous for the CCR5 defect. This has led to some speculation concerning the possibilities for genetic therapy in which anti-HIV genes could be "injected" into a patient's chromosomes with a harmless viral vector. Also, one drug company is now testing a CCR5 receptor antagonist in clinical trials.

Although no highly successful HIV vaccines have been developed, clinical trials of several vaccines are in progress. Viral components, such as gp120 and gp160 envelope glycoproteins, and p17 and p24 viral antigens have been incorporated into vaccines that generate limited immune protection. One recent study demonstrated improved CD4 levels in patients with AIDS given recombinant envelope glycoprotein gp160 vaccine. Two DNA vaccines are currently being investigated. HIV-1 delta 4 is a vaccine in development that uses a mutated form of the virus. However, there is reluctance to use vaccines made up of whole inactivated virions or live attenuated HIV because of the perceived possible risk of transmitting the infection through the vaccine. Another obstacle for vaccine development is the need to provide protection for the 10 or so known subtypes of HIV now in existence around the world as well as the new mutations that continue to arise.

Many health care providers who have been exposed occupationally to HIV have used zidovudine prophylactically immediately after such exposure. The typical dose has been 200 mg orally every 4 hours for 6 weeks. Treatment with zidovudine may reduce the risk of HIV infection following percutaneous exposure by as much as 80%. Recommendations by the CDC incorporate combination therapy that includes some of the newer antiviral drugs into the prophylactic regimen (Table 1-8). The combination of ritonavir + lamivudine + zidovudine has been recommended as one of the most effective prophylactic drug regimens.

Opportunistic Infections

Treatment of Pneumocystis carinii *pneumonia*

PCP ultimately affects approximately 75% of patients with AIDS and is a major cause of mortality in these patients. However, therapy and prophylaxis of PCP have been improving in recent years. PCP is generally treated with IV trimethoprim-sulfamethoxazole (TMP-SMX—Bactrim, Septra) or IV pentamidine. Inhaled pentamidine prevents the recurrence of PCP (secondary prophylaxis) and appears to be efficacious for primary prophylaxis when used in patients with HIV infection and CD4 counts less than $200/mm^3$. The regimen for inhaled pentamidine is generally 300 mg every 4 weeks using a nebulizer. This form of therapy avoids the toxicity of systemically administered pentamidine.

Recent data indicate that oral TMP-SMX prophylaxis is more effective than aerosolized pentamidine for PCP prophylaxis in those patients who can tolerate it. This regimen may also provide systemic prophylaxis against toxoplasmosis infection. Adverse reactions, however, are frequent in HIV-infected patients. Dapsone, effective for primary and secondary prophylaxis against PCP, is tolerated by most patients who develop rashes with TMP-SMX. A new combination drug with dapsone and trimethoprim is currently

Table 1-8 Provisional Public Health Service Recommendations for Chemoprophylaxis After Occupational Exposure to HIV

Type of Exposure	Source Material	Antiretroviral Prophylaxis	Antiviral Regimen*
Percutaneous	**Blood**		
	Highest risk[1]	Recommend	AZT plus 3TC plus IDV
	Increased risk[2]	Recommend	AZT plus 3TC ± IDV
	No increased risk[3]	Offer	AZT plus 3TC
	Fluid containing visible blood, other potentially infectious fluid,[4] or tissue	Offer	AZT plus 3TC
	Other body fluid (urine)	Not offer	
Mucous Membrane	**Blood**	Offer	AZT plus 3TC ± IDV
	Fluid containing visible blood, other potentially infectious fluid,[4] or tissue	Offer	AZT ± 3TC
	Other body fluid (urine)	Not offer	
Skin, Increased Risk	**Blood**	Offer	AZT plus 3TC ± IDV
	Fluid containing visible blood, other potentially infectious fluid,[4] or tissue	Offer	AZT ± 3TC
	Other body fluid (urine)	Not offer	

Dosages for Antiviral Regimens

Drug	Dosage
AZT	200 mg PO TID × 4 weeks
3TC	150 mg PO BID × 4 weeks
IDV	800 mg PO TID × 4 weeks
or	
Saquinavir (substituted for IDV)	600 mg PO TID × 4 weeks

* Abbreviations: AZT = zidovudine (Retrovir); 3TC = lamivudine (Epivir); IDV = indinavir (Crixivan) or saquinavir (Invirase) substituted for IDV.
1. Highest risk = **Both** larger volume of blood (eg, deep injury with a large diameter hollow needle previously in a patient's vein or artery, especially involving an injection of source-patient's blood) **and** blood containing a high titer of HIV (eg, source with acute retroviral illness or end-stage AIDS; viral load measurement may be considered, but its use in relation to postexposure prophylaxis has not been evaluated).
2. Increased risk = **Either** exposure to larger volume of blood **or** blood with a high titer of HIV.
3. No increased risk = **Neither** exposure to larger volume of blood **nor** blood with a high titer of HIV (eg, solid suture needle injury from source patient with asymptomatic HIV infection).
4. Includes semen; vaginal secretions; cerebrospinal, synovial, pleural, peritoneal, pericardial, and amniotic fluids.

(Reprinted from Gerberding JL. Prophylaxis for occupational exposure to HIV. *Ann Intern Med.* 1996;125: 497–501.)

in clinical trials for PCP prophylaxis. Primaquine, clindamycin, and atovaquone (Mepron) have been used successfully in treating PCP, but these drugs are reserved for use in patients intolerant of TMP-SMX or pentamidine. Judicious use of steroids may help reduce morbidity in patients with severe pulmonary inflammation caused by PCP.

Treatment of CMV infections

Ganciclovir is still used in the treatment of CMV retinitis and colitis in immunocompromised patients. Studies of ganciclovir suggest a response in 80%–100% of patients treated with ganciclovir for CMV retinitis and remissions in 60%–80% of these patients. Oral ganciclovir is effective and has fewer side effects than the intravenous form. Oral ganciclovir is usually recommended for maintenance therapy after intravenous induction.

In patients with AIDS, cessation of ganciclovir therapy is universally associated with relapse of the CMV retinitis. Ganciclovir's major toxicity is a reversible bone marrow suppression. One third of patients develop significant granulocytopenia, requiring them to discontinue the drug. Because ganciclovir and zidovudine have similar toxicities, most patients are not able to tolerate systemic therapeutic doses of these drugs simultaneously. Therapy with intravitreal ganciclovir injections has met with increasing popularity in recent years. Unfortunately, most cases require intravitreal injection of ganciclovir three to four times a week indefinitely to prevent progression of CMV retinitis. A slow-release ganciclovir implant (Vitrasert) is also approved for the treatment of CMV retinitis. These implants are surgically inserted within the vitreal cavity and attached at the pars plana. Combination therapy with oral ganciclovir and the ganciclovir implant is more effective than the implant alone.

Foscarnet (Foscavir) was approved by the FDA in 1992 for the treatment of CMV infections. Foscarnet inhibits the DNA polymerase of herpesvirus and HIV and demonstrates in vitro activity against CMV, herpes simplex, varicella-zoster, and HIV at concentrations readily achieved with intravenous therapy. Oral bioavailability is poor, and thus chronic intravenous therapy is required for suppression of CMV retinitis in HIV disease. Foscarnet's primary value is that it is not generally myelosuppressive and therefore may be used without discontinuing zidovudine therapy. Foscarnet's primary dose-limiting side effect is nephrotoxicity; aggressive pretreatment hydration may reduce this effect significantly.

Cidofovir (HPMPC, Vistide) is a potent antiviral agent with activity against herpes simplex, herpes zoster, CMV, adenovirus, EBV, and HIV. Cidofovir blocks DNA synthesis by viral DNA polymerase. Cidofovir provides a prolonged antiviral activity lasting up to several weeks, which allows infrequent dosing. Intravenous (3–5 mg/kg, every other week) and intravitreal cidofovir (20 µg per eye, every 5–6 weeks) have been used successfully in the treatment of CMV retinitis. In one recent study, intravitreal cidofovir led to healing of CMV retinitis in all 53 patients. During the follow-up period, none of the patients with no previous anti-CMV therapy experienced disease progression, and only 14% of the patients with previous anti-CMV therapy experienced disease progression.

Recently, *fomivirsen* (Vitravene), a new antisense drug that targets CMV mRNA, has been shown to be effective in controlling early or advanced CMV retinitis. Valganciclovir is a new oral agent that is as effective as IV ganciclovir for the treatment of CMV retinitis.

A recent study revealed that the incidence and frequency of recurrence of CMV retinitis decreased from 1995 to 1997, largely because of enhanced immune system function resulting from HAART.

Treatment of spore-forming intestinal protozoa

Spore-forming intestinal protozoa are a frequent cause of gastrointestinal infections in patients with AIDS. This group of infections includes cryptosporidiosis (caused by *Cryptosporidium parvum*), microsporidiosis *(Microsporida)*, isosporiasis *(Isospora belli)*, and cyclosporiasis *(Cyclospora cayetanensis)*. Cryptosporidiosis can be treated with clarithromycin, azithromycin, rifabutin, albendazole, or metronidazole. In many patients, symptoms can be successfully controlled, but eradication of the organism can be extremely difficult. Isosporiasis and cyclosporiasis have been treated successfully with TMP-SMZ. There are no curative drugs for invasive microsporidiosis, but recent studies have revealed that albendazole or fumagillin may control disease symptoms.

It is important to realize that chronic diarrhea in HIV-infected patients also may be caused by many other nonprotozoan pathogens, particularly *Salmonella, Shigella, Campylobacter, C difficile, Vibrio parahaemolyticus, Escherichia coli, M avium,* and CMV.

Treatment of tuberculosis and atypical mycobacteria

Multidrug resistance has become an increasing problem in patients with AIDS who have tuberculosis or atypical mycobacterial *(M avium, M kansasii)* infections. Delay in diagnosis and multidrug resistance are strong risk factors for mortality. These factors, along with poor compliance with patient isolation methods, were thought to be responsible for an outbreak of tuberculosis in 1994. This infection was caused by strain W, was resistant to seven antituberculous drugs, and was documented in 367 patients.

Standard drugs used in treating mycobacterial infections include isoniazid, rifampin, ethambutol, streptomycin, para-aminosalicylic acid, ethionamide, pyra-zinamide, cycloserine, kanamycin, and amikacin. Some of the newer drugs found to be effective in treating these refractory infections are clofazimine (also used in treating leprosy), capreomycin, rifabutin, azithromycin, clarithromycin, and the quinolones (ciprofloxacin, ofloxacin, and sparfloxacin). The quinolones are promising because they possess a high level of antimycobacterial activity with few adverse effects. In recent studies, combined therapy with rifampin or rifabutin, ethambutol, clofazimine, and clarithromycin or ciprofloxacin has been successful in treating atypical mycobacterial infections in patients with AIDS. Isoniazid prophylaxis has been recommended in HIV-positive patients at high risk for tuberculosis. Prophylactic therapy with azithromycin, clarithromycin, rifabutin, or combined therapy may help prevent disseminated *M avium* complex in patients with AIDS.

Treatment of other opportunistic infections

Other opportunistic infections encountered in patients with AIDS include central nervous system toxoplasmosis, disseminated fungal infections, and herpes simplex or herpes zoster infections. Although toxoplasmosis has traditionally been treated with sulfadiazine, pyrimethamine, or clindamycin, more recent data suggest that TMP-SMZ may be equally effective, with far fewer side effects. Also, TMP-SMZ has been used as prophylactic therapy to try to prevent PCP as well as toxoplasmosis. Treatment of disseminated fungal infections is evolving with the availability of the newer imidazoles, fluconazole and itraconazole. Amphotericin B continues to be important in treating advanced invasive fungal disease. New formulations of amphotericin B in lipid complexes or liposomes reduce systemic toxicity. The new antiviral agents valacyclovir and famciclovir, as well as other antiviral agents such as cidofovir, offer alternatives to acyclovir in the treatment of AIDS in patients with refractory or disseminated herpes simplex or herpes zoster infections.

Treatment of AIDS-related malignancies

Kaposi sarcoma is usually a localized disease that can be treated with radiotherapy, but metastatic or disseminated disease may require combined chemotherapy such as doxo-rubicin, bleomycin, and vincristine. In addition, immunotherapy with β-interferon has been used in some patients with Kaposi sarcoma. B cell lymphomas in patients with AIDS often involve the lymph nodes, central nervous system, and lungs and may require treatment with multidrug chemotherapy, sometimes with regional radiotherapy.

Ophthalmologic Considerations

The ocular manifestations of AIDS are discussed in BCSC Section 9, *Intraocular Inflammation and Uveitis.*

HIV has been demonstrated in tears, conjunctival epithelial cells, corneal epithelial cells, aqueous, retinal vascular endothelium, and retina. Although transmission of AIDS or HIV infection by ophthalmic examinations or ophthalmic equipment has not been documented, the following precautions are recommended.

Health care professionals performing eye examinations or other procedures involving contact with tears should wash their hands immediately after the procedure and between patients. Hand washing alone should be sufficient, but when practical and convenient, disposable gloves may be worn. The use of gloves is advisable when the hands have cuts, scratches, or dermatologic lesions.

Instruments that come into direct contact with external surfaces of the eyes should be wiped clean and disinfected by a 5- to 10-minute exposure to (1) a fresh solution of 3% hydrogen peroxide, (2) a fresh solution containing 5000 ppm free available chlorine— a one tenth dilution of common household bleach (sodium hypochlorite), (3) 70% ethanol, or (4) 70% isopropanol. The device should be thoroughly rinsed in tap water and dried before use.

Contact lenses used in trial fitting should be disinfected between fittings with a commercially available hydrogen peroxide contact lens disinfecting system or with the standard heat disinfection regimen (78°–80°C for 10 minutes).

The demonstration of HIV in corneal epithelium has led to the recommendation that all corneal donors be screened for antibodies to HIV and that all potential donor corneas from HIV antibody–positive persons be discarded.

For more specific recommendations, see the AAO Information Statement entitled "Updated Recommendations for Ophthalmic Practice in Relation to the Human Immunodeficiency Virus and Other Infectious Agents."

AIDS Epidemic Update 2003. Joint United Nations Programme on HIV/AIDS. Available at: http://www.unaids.org/en/resources/epidemiology.asp. Accessed December 17, 2003.

Centers for Disease Control and Prevention. *HIV/AIDS Surveillance Report.* 2001;13:1–44.

Daniel V, Susal C, Melk A, et al. Reduction of viral load and immune complex load on CD4+ lymphocytes as a consequence of highly active antiretroviral treatment (HAART) in HIV-infected hemophilia patients. *Immunol Lett.* 1999;69:283–289.

Davis MA. Primary HIV infection; primary care of HIV-infected adults; diarrhea in HIV-infected patients; antiretroviral therapy. *J AIDS/HIV*. 2001;8966:4225–4681.

De Clercq E. New anti-HIV agents and targets. *Med Res Rev*. 2002;22:531–565.

Deeks SG, Smith M, Holodniy M, et al. HIV-1 protease inhibitors. A review for clinicians. *JAMA*. 1997;277:145–153.

de Roda Husman AM, Koot M, Cornelissen M, et al. Association between CCR5 genotype and the clinical course of HIV-1 infection. *Ann Intern Med*. 1997;127:882–890.

Doan S, Cochereau I, Guvenisik N, et al. Cytomegalovirus retinitis in HIV-infected patients with and without highly active antiretroviral therapy. *Am J Ophthalmol*. 1999;128:250–251.

Gallant JE. Strategies for long-term success in the treatment of HIV infection. *JAMA*. 2000; 283:1329–1334.

Gerberding JL. Prophylaxis for occupational exposure to HIV. *Ann Intern Med*. 1996;125:497–501.

Goedert JJ, Cote TR, Virgo P, et al. Spectrum of AIDS-associated malignant disorders. *Lancet*. 1998;351:1833–1839.

Guidelines for using antiretroviral agents among HIV-infected adults and adolescents. Recommendations of the Panel on Clinical Practices for Treatment of HIV. *MMWR*. 2002;vol 52, no. RR7. Available at: http://www.cdc.gov/mmwr/PDF/RR/RR5107.pdf. Accessed December 17, 2003.

HIV/AIDS Surveillance Report. Centers for Disease Control and Prevention. National Center for HIV, STD, and TB Prevention. Atlanta: US Department of Health and Human Services; 2001.

Hu DJ, Vitek CR, Bartholow B, et al. Key issues for a potential human immunodeficiency virus vaccine. *Clin Infect Dis*. 2003;36:638–644.

Kahn J, Lagakos S, Wulfsohn M, et al. Efficacy and safety of adefovir dipivoxil with antiretroviral therapy: a randomized controlled trial. *JAMA*. 1999;282:2305–2312.

Katlama C, Clotet B, Plettenberg A, et al. The role of abacavir (ABC, 1592) in antiretroviral therapy-experienced patients: results from a randomized, double-blind, trial. CNA3002 European Study Team. *AIDS*. 2000;14:781–789.

McElrath MJ, Corey L, Montefiori D, et al. A phase II study of two HIV type 1 envelope vaccines, comparing their immunogenicity in populations at risk for acquiring HIV type 1 infection. AIDS Vaccine Evaluation Group. *AIDS Res Hum Retroviruses*. 2000;16:907–919.

Mellors JW, Munoz A, Giorgi JV, et al. Plasma viral load and CD4+ lymphocytes as prognostic markers of HIV-1 infection. *Ann Intern Med*. 1997;126:946–954.

Yeni PG, Hammer SM, Carpenter CC, et al. Antiretroviral treatment for adult HIV infection in 2002: updated recommendations of the International AIDS Society—USA Panel. *JAMA*. 2002;288:222–235.

Update on Antibiotics

For half a century, the main trend in infectious disease management has been the evolution and refinement of antibiotic therapy. Factors that have stimulated the development of new antibiotics include a spate of resistant bacteria, economics, and the desire to eliminate undesirable side effects. During the last couple of decades, emphasis gradually shifted from *aminoglycosides* to *β-lactams* and the development of new classes of antibiotics such as *carbapenems* and *monobactams*. In addition, *vancomycin, TMP-SMZ, erythromycin,* and *rifampin* have enjoyed a popular resurgence and new applications. Quinolones offer the possibility of treating serious infections on an outpatient basis. Antiviral drugs such as *acyclovir, ganciclovir, zidovudine,* and *ribavirin* are all *nucleoside analogues,* which inhibit viral DNA polymerase (reverse transcriptase) and interrupt the growing viral DNA chain. In addition, several new imidazole compounds have been introduced for treatment of systemic fungal infections. (For the characteristics of selected antibiotics, see Table 1-9. Antiretroviral agents are discussed in detail under the earlier heading, Acquired Immunodeficiency Syndrome.)

Antibacterial Agents

The various antibacterial agents act on bacteria in different ways. For example, unlike humans and other higher animals, most bacteria cannot utilize exogenous folic acid and must, therefore, synthesize their own in order to grow. For instance, sulfonamides and trimethoprim each block a different enzyme in this synthetic pathway. For this reason, bacteria susceptible to both agents are inhibited by lower concentrations of the two drugs acting together than are needed with either one alone. Therefore, these two agents often are administered as a fixed-combination drug.

The *quinolones* have a different mechanism of action. In order to function properly, the double-stranded DNA of the bacterial chromosome must be supercoiled by the enzyme DNA gyrase, and quinolones block this enzyme. A number of new *fluoroquinolones,* which have very broad spectra of activity against a wide range of gram-negative and gram-positive bacterial species, have become available.

To make proteins, bacteria begin by copying the code for each protein from its gene on the bacterial chromosome onto a newly synthesized strand of the specialized RNA known as *messenger RNA (mRNA).* The antituberculosis drug rifampin selectively blocks the enzyme that synthesizes this mRNA strand. Once synthesized, the strand of mRNA then threads its way through the bacterial ribosomes to direct each ribosome in the sequence of assembling amino acids into a protein. This process is blocked in different ways by the tetracyclines and by chloramphenicol, erythromycin, and clindamycin; however, the process resumes again if the drug is discontinued. Because their effect is reversible, these classes of agents are considered to be *bacteriostatic.* In contrast, the aminoglycosides belong to a class of antibiotics that irreversibly derange ribosomal protein synthesis; the process cannot resume even after the drugs are stopped. These drugs, therefore, are *bactericidal.*

The bacterial proteins themselves or their enzymatic products make up the rest of the bacterial cell, including the membrane that encloses the cell. Polymyxin and colistin damage the cell membrane, making it unable to perform essential barrier functions. Surrounding the bacterium and outside of the cell membrane is the bacterial cell wall. The components of the cell wall are synthesized within the bacterial cell, then transported to the outside through the cell membrane before being assembled on its surface. The drugs that block this transport include bacitracin, a topical polypeptide agent derived from a strain of *Bacillus subtilis,* and vancomycin, a glycopeptide.

The final, crucial step in bacterial growth is formation of the bacterial cell wall. The necessary cross-linking of its components is mediated by special enzymes that are unlike

Table 1-9 Characteristics of Selected Antibiotics

Antibiotic	Spectrum*	Route	Side Effects/Special Uses
		Antibacterial Agents	
Sulfonamides (bacteriostatic)			
Sulfisoxazole (Gantrisin)	Urinary tract infections, +, −, *Nocardia*, lymphogranuloma venereum, trachoma	PO	Crystalluria, allergic reactions (rashes, photosensitivity, and drug fever), kernicterus in newborns, renal damage, Stevens-Johnson syndrome (more likely with long-acting sulfonamides), blood dyscrasia (agranulocytosis), disseminated vasculitis.
Trimethoprim-sulfamethoxazole, TMP-SMX (Bactrim, Septra)	Urinary tract infections, +, −, shigellosis, *Nocardia*, *Pneumocystis* pneumonia	PO, IV	Same as above, plus nausea and vomiting, diarrhea, skin rashes, CNS irritability, bone-marrow toxicity. Liver damage and Stevens-Johnson syndrome may be fatal.
Penicillin G (bactericidal)			
Aqueous (many brands)	+, *Neisseria*, spirochetes, actinomycosis	IV only	Penicillin allergy,** CNS toxicity with high blood levels, Coombs-positive hemolytic anemia, rare nephritis.
Procaine (many brands)	Same as above	IM only	Same as above, plus -*caine* reactions.
Benzathine (Bicillin)	Spirochetes, *Streptococcus* prophylaxis	IM only	Prolonged penicillin allergy.**
Semisynthetic penicillins (bactericidal)			
Penicillin V (Pen-Vee K)	+, *Neisseria*, spirochetes, actinomycosis	PO	Much better absorption than penicillin G when given orally in the fasting state.
Nafcillin (Unipen)	Penicillinase-producing *Staph*	IV	Penicillin allergy,** phlebitis, interstitial nephritis, diarrhea; rare bone-marrow toxicity.
Cloxacillin (Tegopen)	+, especially *Staph*	PO	Penicillin allergy,** GI symptoms. Better absorbed and better tolerated than nafcillin and oxacillin given orally in the fasting state.
Dicloxacillin (Dynapen)	+, especially *Staph*	PO	Same as above.

* Symbols: + = gram-positive; − = gram-negative; *Staph* = penicillinase-producers.
** Penicillin allergy includes spectrum from anaphylaxis to serum sickness.

Table 1-9 Characteristics of Selected Antibiotics (Continued)

Antibiotic	Spectrum*	Route	Side Effects/Special Uses
Ampicillin (Polycillin)	+, especially *Enterococcus* (except *Staph*) and some −, especially *Haemophilus influenzae, Proteus mirabilis, Salmonella* sp, *Escherichia coli*	IV, PO	Penicillin allergy,** GI symptoms (from PO administration). Rash common in viral illnesses (maculopapular eruption that is not necessarily allergy).
Ampicillin-sulbactam (Unasyn)	Same as ampicillin plus beta-lactamase producers and some anaerobes	IV	Penicillin allergy,** diarrhea, elevated liver enzymes.
Amoxicillin (Amoxil)	Same as above, except *Shigella*	PO	Same as above. Better absorbed than oral ampicillin. Should replace *oral* ampicillin for everything except bacillary dysentery.
Amoxicillin–potassium clavulanate (Augmentin)	Same as amoxicillin plus beta-lactamase producers (*Haemophilus influenzae,Branhamella* sp, and *Staph* sp)	PO	Same as amoxicillin plus more diarrhea.
Ticarcillin (Ticar)	−, especially *Pseudomonas aeruginosa* and *Proteus sp,* abdominal anaerobes, and some +, except *Staph*	IV	Penicillin allergy,** rare bleeding diathesis, hypokalemia (4.0 mEq Na$^+$/gm), abnormal liver function tests, *Candida* overgrowth.
Ticarcillin-potassium clavulanate (Timentin)	Same as ticarcillin plus beta-lactamase producers (*Klebsiella* sp, *Bacteroides fragilis,* and *Serratia* sp)	IV	Same as ticarcillin plus more diarrhea and nausea. *Candida* overgrowth frequent.
Mezlocillin (Mezlin)	Same as ticarcillin	IV	Same as ticarcillin.
Piperacillin (Pipracil)	−, most active of all semi-synthetic penicillins against *Pseudomonas* and many other aerobic gram-negative rods including *Klebsiella;* abdominal anaerobes	IV	One half as much Na$^+$ as ticarcillin. Similar to ticarcillin, but approximately 25% of patients develop a hypersensitivity reaction and/or diarrhea. Must be used with an aminoglycoside. Rare bleeding diathesis.

* Symbols: + = gram-positive; − = gram-negative; *Staph* = penicillinase-producers.
** Penicillin allergy includes spectrum from anaphylaxis to serum sickness.

Table 1-9 Characteristics of Selected Antibiotics (Continued)

Antibiotic	Spectrum*	Route	Side Effects/Special Uses
Piperacillin-tazobactam (Zosyn)	Same as piperacillin with increased coverage of beta-lactamase producers and anaerobes	IV	Same as piperacillin.
Cephalosporins (bactericidal)			
First-generation cephalosporins			
Cefazolin (Kefzol, Ancef)	+ and some −; not a good *Staph* treatment	IM, IV	Thrombophlebitis or pain at injection site, skin rash, urticaria, eosinophilia, neutropenia.
Cephalexin (Keflex)	+, *Staph,* and some −	PO	Same as above plus GI symptoms.
Cephradine (Anspor, Velosef)	+, *Staph,* and some −	PO	Same as above.
Cefadroxil monohydrate (Duracef)	+, *Staph,* and some −	PO	Rash, urticaria, GI symptoms.
Second-generation (extended-spectrum) cephalosporins			
Cefamandole (Mandol)	+, especially *Staph,* and some −	IV	Less thrombophlebitis than above, skin rash, drug fever, eosinophilia, hypoprothrombinemia ± bleeding. Extremely effective prophylaxis for *Staph* including MRSE.
Cefoxitin (Mefoxin)	+, −, abdominal anaerobes (the best of all cephalosporins)	IV	Thrombophlebitis, fever, skin rash, eosinophilia, nausea, vomiting, diarrhea, bone-marrow and liver toxicity.
Cefonicid (Monocid)	− and some anaerobes	IV	Often used for prophylaxis with colorectal or gynecologic surgeries; may cause pain at injection site, eosinophilia, GI symptoms, rash.
Cefaclor (Ceclor, Distaclor)	+ and some −, *Haemophilus* sp	PO	Toxicity similar to other cephalosporins. Major uses are treating ENT infections in children and respiratory infections in adults with COPD.

* Symbols: + = gram-positive; − = gram-negative; *Staph* = penicillinase-producers.

Table 1-9 Characteristics of Selected Antibiotics (Continued)

Antibiotic	Spectrum*	Route	Side Effects/Special Uses
Cefuroxime sodium (IV: Zinacef, Kefurox); Cefuroxime axetil (PO: Ceftin)	+ and some −, *Haemophilus* sp	IV, PO	Rash, GI symptoms.
Cefotetan (Cefotan)	−, anaerobes	IM or IV	A long half-life cefoxitin. Hypoprothrombinemia, hemolytic anemia, and disulfiram-like reaction.
Third-generation (ultrabroad-spectrum) cephalosporins			
Cefotaxime (Claforan)	−, including many multidrug-resistant organisms	IV	Cephalosporin hypersensitivity reaction, thrombophlebitis. Good penetration into CSF in meningitis.
Cefoperazone (Cefobid)	−, including *Pseudomonas* sp and many multidrug-resistant organisms, some anaerobes	IM or IV	Cephalosporin hypersensitivity, hypoprothrombinemia, diarrhea. Can be given q 8–12h.
Ceftriaxone (Rocephin)	Like cefotaxime; gonorrhea, *Borrelia burgdorferi*	IM or IV	Very long half-life makes it attractive for outpatient therapy. Treatment of choice for gonorrhea. Effective for all forms of Lyme disease. Good CNS penetration for meningitis.
Ceftazidime (Fortaz, Tazidime, Tazicef)	−, especially *Pseudomonas* sp	IM, IV	Good anti-pseudomonal cephalosporin, long half-life: q 8–12h administration. The best all-purpose third-generation cephalosporin.
Ceftizoxime (Cefizox)	Many − and anaerobes	IV	Rash, GI symptoms, elevated liver enzymes.
Cefixime (Suprax)	+, some − (*Haemophilus influenzae, Branhamella catarrhalis*)	PO	Diarrhea, nausea, abdominal pain, flatulence. First oral third-generation cephalosporin.
Cefpodoxime proxetil (Vantin)	+, −, *Enterobacter, Pseudomonas, Serratia, Morganella, Enterococcus,* generally resistant infections	PO	Twice daily for ENT, respiratory, urinary, and soft tissue infections. Single dose for uncomplicated gonorrhea.
Cefprozil (Cefzil)	+, −, including *Haemophilus*	PO	Rash, GI symptoms.

* Symbols: + = gram-positive; − = gram-negative; *Staph* = penicillinase-producers.

Table 1-9 Characteristics of Selected Antibiotics (Continued)

Antibiotic	Spectrum*	Route	Side Effects/Special Uses
Ceftibuten (Cedax)	+, −, including *Haemophilus, Moraxella*	PO	No real advantages.
Cefdinir (Omnicef)	+, −, including *Haemophilus*	PO	Rash, GI symptoms.
Cefditoren (Spectracef)	+, −, including *Haemophilus*	PO	Very broad spectrum but not active against *Pseudomonas*.
Fourth-generation (super-duper broad spectrum) cephalosporins			
Cefepime (Maxipime)	+, −, some anaerobes	IV, IM	Expensive; slightly better gram-negative coverage than ceftazidime.
Cefpirome	+, −, some anaerobes	IV, IM	Effective for sepsis.
Carbacephems (bactericidal)			
Loracarbef (Lorabid)	+, − , including *Haemophilus*	PO	Rash, GI symptoms.
Cephamycins (bactericidal)			
Cefmetazole (Zefazone)	Similar to that of second-generation cephalosporins	IV	GI symptoms, rash, seizures in patients with renal insufficiency, more side effects than second-generation cephalosporins.
Monobactams (bactericidal)			
Aztreonam (Azactam)	Most −; no activity for + or anaerobes	IM, IV	First of this class of monocyclic beta-lactams. The spectrum of an aminoglycoside without oto- or nephrotoxicity. No cross-reaction in penicillin-allergic patients.
Carbapenems (bactericidal)			
Imipenem-cilastatin (Primaxin)	+, −, including *Pseudomonas* sp and multidrug-resistant strains, anaerobes	IV	Nausea, diarrhea, phlebitis, elevated serum glutamic-oxaloacetic transaminase (SGOT), elevated serum glutamic-pyruvic transaminase (SGPT), seizures. Prototype of carbapenems. *Candida* superinfection frequent. Extremely broad spectrum.

* Symbols: + = gram-positive; − = gram-negative; *Staph* = penicillinase-producers.

Table 1-9 Characteristics of Selected Antibiotics (Continued)

Antibiotic	Spectrum*	Route	Side Effects/Special Uses
Meropenem (Merrem)	Similar to imipenem, but less active against +, more active against −	IV	Does not require cilastatin component because more resistant to enzyme degradation; less problem with seizures.
Ertapenem	Similar to meropenem	IM, IV	Similar to meropenem; once-daily dosing.
Faropenem	Similar to meropenem	PO	Similar to meropenem
Macrolides (bacteriostatic)			
Erythromycin	+, spirochetes, *Mycoplasma, Legionella, Campylobacter*	PO, IV	GI upset, altered liver function test, hepatic damage, stomatitis, thrombophlebitis (with IV administration). Take with meals or a snack when given orally.
Clindamycin (Cleocin)	+, anaerobes, actinomycosis	PO, IV	GI toxicity can be severe and even lethal.
Azalides			
Clarithromycin (Biaxin) Azithromycin (Zithromax) Dirithromycin (Dynabec) Roxithromycin Spiramycin Josamycin	+, *Mycoplasma, Chlamydia, Legionella*	PO	Reversible dose-related hearing loss in high doses. Less GI than erythromycin.
Ketolides			
Telithromycin	+, *Mycoplasma, Chlamydia, Legionella.* Good for multidrug-resistant +	PO	Similar to above.
Glycopeptides (bactericidal)			
Vancomycin (Vancocin)	+, especially *Staph* and *Enterococcus, Clostridia,* and other beta-lactam-resistant +	IV, PO	Thrombophlebitis, leukopenia. Resistant enterococci and reduced-sensitivity *Staph* strains are increasing.

* Symbols: + = gram-positive; − = gram-negative; *Staph* = penicillinase-producers.

Table 1-9 Characteristics of Selected Antibiotics (Continued)

Antibiotic	Spectrum*	Route	Side Effects/Special Uses
Teicoplanin (Targocid)	Similar to vancomycin with better activity against *Streptococcus* and *Enterococcus*. Effective for some vancomycin-resistant strains of *Enterococcus*.	IV, IM	Longer half-life (allows daily dosing), lower toxicity, less nephrotoxicity, better tissue penetration than vancomycin.
Tetracyclines[†] (bacteriostatic) *In order of bacterial activity:*			
Minocycline (Minocin)	+ and − , spirochetes, *Mycoplasma*, lymphogranuloma venereum, psittacosis, *Rickettsia*	PO, IV	Most active. Useful as an alternative to vancomycin for treatment of methicillin-resistant staphylococci, particularly MRSE, and for meningococcal prophylaxis. Vertigo.
Doxycycline (Vibramycin)	Same as above	PO, IV	Hepatic excretion, so may be best in renal failure. Do not use in urinary tract infections. Phototoxic reactions.
Tetracycline	Same as above	PO, IV	Probably best choice for routine use. *Candida* overgrowth.
Aminoglycosides (bactericidal)			
Streptomycin	Tuberculosis, − , *Pasteurella* sp, *Franciscella* sp	IM only	Vestibular damage, drug fever, peripheral neuropathy.
Gentamicin (Garamycin)	Community-acquired −; not effective for + or anaerobes	IM or IV slowly	Vestibular damage, renal damage, curare-like effect.
Tobramycin (Nebcin)	− , especially *Pseudomonas* and *Aeromonas*	IM or IV slowly	Less nephrotoxic than gentamicin. Most active against *Pseudomonas*.
Netilmicin (Netromycin)	−, including some gentamicin/tobramycin-resistant organisms	IM or IV slowly	May be less toxic than gentamicin or tobramycin.

* Symbols: + = gram-positive; − = gram-negative; *Staph* = penicillinase-producers.

[†] *Side effects of tetracyclines:* GI disturbance; bone lesions; staining and deformity of teeth in children up to 8 years old and in newborns when given to pregnant women after the fourth month; malabsorption; enterocolitis; photosensitivity reaction (most frequent with demethylchlortetracycline). Parenteral doses may cause serious liver damage, especially in pregnant women and patients with renal disease; allergic reactions, blood dyscrasia, interference with protein metabolism, increased intracranial pressure in infants, Fanconi-like syndrome from deteriorated tetracyclines. Take with meals or a snack, but avoid milk and milk products.

Table 1-9 **Characteristics of Selected Antibiotics (Continued)**

Antibiotic	Spectrum*	Route	Side Effects/Special Uses
Amikacin (Amikin)	−, active against many gentamicin/tobramycin-resistant gram-negatives. Ideal for nosocomial gram-negative infection.	IM or IV slowly	Nephrotoxic and ototoxic (more deafness than vestibular effects). Curare-like effect.
Quinolones (bactericidal)	+, most −, including multidrug-resistant isolates, and MRSA and MRSE. Not good for *Enterococcus*.		Expensive, *Candida* overgrowth, photosensitivity reactions.
Norfloxacin (Noroxin)	Same as above	PO	Very broad treatment for complicated urinary-tract infections.
Ciprofloxacin (Cipro)	Same as above	PO	Very broad spectrum makes this a useful oral agent for mixed infections, infectious diarrhea, and multidrug-resistant organisms at any body site except CNS.
New quinolones			
Ofloxacin (Floxin) Sparfloxacin (Zagam) Enoxacin (Penetrex) Temafloxacin (Omniflox) Lomefloxacin (Maxaquin) Levofloxacin (Levaquin) Trovafloxacin (Trovan) Moxifloxacin (Avelox) Gatifloxacin (Tequin) Gemifloxacin (Factive) Clinafloxacin	Increased activity for + and −	PO	Same as above.
Miscellaneous agents			
Chloramphenicol (Chloromycetin)	+, −, anaerobes, *Rickettsia*; bacteriostatic	PO, IV	"Gray baby" syndrome in newborns, bone-marrow toxicity, optic atrophy, and peripheral neuropathy.
Metronidazole (Flagyl, Flagyl IV)	Anaerobes, *Campylobacter*, amoebae, *Trichomonas*, *C difficile*; bacteriostatic	PO, IV	GI upset, vertigo, ataxia, peripheral neuropathy, phlebitis, carcinogenic (?), Antabuse-like reaction.

* Symbols: + = gram-positive; − = gram-negative; *Staph* = penicillinase-producers.

Table 1-9 Characteristics of Selected Antibiotics (Continued)

Antibiotic	Spectrum*	Route	Side Effects/Special Uses
Rifampin (Rifadin)	TB, *Staph* (synergy), meningococcal prophylaxis; bactericidal	PO	Hepatotoxicity, flulike syndrome, discoloration of body secretions, drug interactions.
Pentamidine (Pentam300)	*Pneumocystis* pneumonia	IV, aerosol	Hypotension, hypoglycemia, abnormal liver function tests, azotemia, bone-marrow toxicity.
New Antibiotic Classes			
Streptogramins (bactericidal)			
Quinupristin/dalfopristin (Synercid)	Active against multidrug-resistant + organisms, even those with reduced sensitivity to vancomycin	IV	Bactericidal as a combined drug. No cross-resistance with other antibiotics. GI side effects, rash, myalgias.
Oxazolidinones (bactericidal)			
Linezolid (Zyvox) Eperezolid (investigational)	Similar to quinupristin/dalfopristin	IV, PO	Has monoamine oxidase (MAO) inhibitor effects, so drug interactions are possible.
Everninomicins (bactericidal)			
Evernimicin (Ziracin)	Similar to quinupristin/dalfopristin	IV	Effective for methicillin-resistant and vancomycin-intermediate-sensitivity organisms.
Avilamycin	Similar to quinupristin/dalfopristin	IV	Similar to above.
Lipopeptides (bactericidal)			
Daptomycin (investigational)	Similar to quinupristin/dalfopristin	IV, PO	Most bactericidal of all in a recent study of new antibiotics for drug-resistant + strain.

* Symbols: + = gram-positive; − = gram-negative; *Staph* = penicillinase-producers.

Table 1-9 Characteristics of Selected Antibiotics (Continued)

Antibiotic	Spectrum*	Route	Side Effects/Special Uses
Antifungal Agents (Fungistatic)			
Nystatin (Mycostatin)	*Candida*	PO tabs or suspension; topical cream, ointment, powder; GU irrigant, vaginal suppository	Useful for prevention of *Candida* overgrowth or for topical treatment of GI, mucosal, or skin candidiasis.
5-fluorocytosine (Ancobon, Ancotil)	*Candida, Cryptococcus*	PO	GI distress, leukopenia, hepatotoxicity. Particularly toxic in patients with compromised renal function.
Amphotericin B (Fungizone, Amphotec)	Most invasive fungi, oral candidiasis	IV for systemic use; PO only for oral candidiasis	Chills, fever, nausea, vomiting, thrombophlebitis, nephrotoxicity, hypokalemia, bone-marrow suppression, shock, cardiotoxicity.
Miconazole (Micatin, Monistat)	*Candida,* dermatophytes	Topical or vaginal cream; IV	Topical treatment of *Candida* and dermatophytes. When used IV thrombophlebitis, thrombocytosis, anemia.
Clotrimazole (Lotrimin, Gyne-Lotrimin, Mycelex)	*Candida,* dermatophytes	Topical solution, vaginal suppository; PO	Same as above.
Ketoconazole (Nizoral)	Many fungi	PO	Skin rash, pruritus, nausea, gynecomastia, liver toxicity, impaired fertility.
Newer imidazoles			
Fluconazole (Diflucan) Itraconazole (Sporanox) Croconazole	*Candida, Cryptococcus*	PO, IV	Less toxicity than amphotericin and flucytosine. Better tolerated than ketoconazole.
Allylamines			
Terbinafine (Lamisil)	Dermatophytes causing onychomycosis	PO	Headache, GI symptoms, rash.

* Symbols: + = gram-positive; − = gram-negative; *Staph* = penicillinase-producers.

Table 1-9 Characteristics of Selected Antibiotics (Continued)

Antibiotic	Spectrum*	Route	Side Effects/Special Uses
Benzylamines			
Butenafine (Mentax)	Dermatophyte skin and nail infections	Topical	Rash.
Antiviral Agents[†]			
Acyclovir (Zovirax)	HSV, varicella-zoster	IV, PO, topical	Nephrotoxicity, CNS toxicity, nausea, vomiting.
Famciclovir (Famvir)	HSV, varicella-zoster	PO	Less frequent dosing (q 8 hrs) than acyclovir.
Valacyclovir (Valtrex)	HSV, varicella-zoster	PO	Pro-drug for acyclovir. Less frequent dosing (q 8 hrs).
Ganciclovir (Cytovene)	CMV, EBV, HSV	IV, PO, intraocular	Bone-marrow toxicity, phlebitis, headache, disorientation, nausea, anorexia, myalgia, rash.
Foscarnet (Foscavir)	CMV, EBV, HSV	IV	Nephrotoxicity.
Cidofovir (Vistide)	CMV, EBV, HSV	IV, intraocular	Effective for CMV and acyclovir-resistant HSV; prolonged duration of action allows infrequent dosing (every other week for IV).
Fomivirsen (Vitravene)	CMV	Intraocular	Active against CMV strains that are resistant to other agents.
Amantadine (Symmetrel, Symadine)	Influenza A	PO	CNS toxicity, anticholinergic reactions.
Rimantadine (Flumadine)	Influenza A	PO	Fewer side effects than amantadine.
Zanamivir (Relenza)	Influenza A and B	Inhaled	An inhaled neuraminidase inhibitor. Approved for treatment and prophylaxis of contacts.
Oseltamavir (Tamiflu)	Influenza A and B	PO	Oral neuraminidase inhibitor. Fewer side effects and less resistance than with others. Approval for treatment and prophylaxis of contacts.
Ribavirin (Virazole)	Respiratory syncytial virus (RSV), hepatitis C; being studied for use with hantavirus	Inhaled, IV, PO	Synergistic with interferon A for hepatitis C.

* Symbols: + = gram-positive; − = gram-negative; *Staph* = penicillinase-producers.
† Antiretroviral agents for HIV infection are covered in the AIDS discussion in this chapter.

anything in the human cell. The antibiotics that selectively inhibit one or more of these enzymes include penicillin and its growing family of related agents. This family includes the semisynthetic penicillins, all of the cephalosporin-like drugs, and newly introduced β-lactams of novel structure such as imipenem. They are all grouped together under the label of *β-lactam* antibiotics because their structural formulas are marked by a distinctive four-atom structure known chemically as a *β-lactam ring*. When even a small number of one of these β-lactam molecules tag an infecting bacterium, gaps develop in its cell wall through which the organism ruptures and is destroyed.

Antibacterial agents can thus be separated into groups according to their specific targets on or within bacteria:

- β-Lactams and glycopeptides inhibit cell wall synthesis
- Polymyxins distort cytoplasmic membrane function
- Quinolones and rifampicins inhibit nucleic acid synthesis
- Macrolides, aminoglycosides, and tetracyclines inhibit ribosome function
- Trimethoprim and sulfonamides inhibit folate metabolism

All antibiotics facilitate the growth of resistant bacteria consequent to the destruction of susceptible bacteria. Although the wide use of antimicrobial agents for veterinary and agricultural purposes has contributed to the emergence of multiresistant microorganisms, the excessive use of antibiotics, especially in hospitals, has been the most significant catalyst for resistance. Bacteria resist antibiotics by inactivation of the antibiotic, decreased accumulation of the antibiotic within the microorganism, or alteration of the target site on the microbe. For example, resistance to penicillins and cephalosporins is initiated by β-lactamase enzymes that hydrolyze the β-lactam ring, thus destroying the antibiotic's effectiveness. Resistance can be mediated by chromosomal mutations or the presence of extrachromosomal DNA, also known as *plasmid resistance*. Plasmid resistance is more important from an epidemiologic point of view because it is transmissible, is usually highly stable, confers resistance to many different classes of antibiotics simultaneously, and is often associated with other characteristics that enable a microorganism to colonize and to invade a susceptible host.

Resistance-conferring plasmids have been identified in virtually all bacteria. Moreover, many bacteria contain transposons that can enter plasmids or chromosomes. Plasmids can therefore pick up chromosomal genes for resistance and transfer them to species not currently resistant.

Bacteria that have acquired chromosomal and plasmid-mediated resistance can neutralize or destroy antibiotics in three different ways (they can use one or more of these mechanisms simultaneously):

- By preventing the antibacterial agent from reaching its receptor site
- By modifying or duplicating the target enzyme so that it is insensitive to the antibacterial agent
- By synthesizing enzymes that destroy the antibacterial agent or modify the agent to alter its entry or receptor binding

Antimicrobial susceptibility testing permits a rational choice of antibiotics, although correlation of in vivo and in vitro susceptibility is not always precise. Disk-diffusion susceptibility testing has provided qualitative data about the inhibitory activity of commonly used antimicrobials against an isolated pathogen, and these data are usually sufficient. In serious infections, such as infective endocarditis, it is useful to quantify the drug concentrations that inhibit and kill the pathogen. The lowest drug concentration that prevents the growth of a defined inoculum of the isolated pathogen is the *minimal inhibitory concentration* (MIC); the lowest concentration that kills 99.9% of an inoculum is the *minimal lethal concentration* (MLC). For bactericidal drugs, the MIC and MLC are usually similar.

The antimicrobial activity of a treated patient's serum can be estimated via measurement of serum bactericidal titers. Clinical experience suggests that intravascular infections usually are controlled when the peak serum bactericidal titer is 1.8 or greater. Bactericidal therapy is preferred for patients with immunologic compromise or life-threatening infection. Other patients may be treated effectively with either bactericidal or bacteriostatic drugs. Although synergistic combinations are useful in certain clinical situations (eg, enterococcal endocarditis, gram-negative septicemia in granulocytopenic patients), combined antimicrobial therapy should be used judiciously to avoid potential antagonism and toxicity.

β-lactam antibiotics

The β-lactam group includes the penicillins, cephalosporins, and monobactams, all of which possess a β-lactam ring that binds to specific microbial binding sites and interferes with cell wall synthesis. The carbapenems and carbacephems are often grouped with β-lactams but have a slightly different ring structure. As new β-lactam agents emerge, it has become customary to refer to them by generation. The generation is not only a chronological classification but also connotes their antimicrobial spectrum. The majority of new agents have been created by side-chain manipulation of the β-lactam ring, which has improved resistance to enzymatic degradation. However, some of the newer antibiotics (such as third-generation cephalosporins) show diminished potency against gram-positive cocci, especially staphylococci.

Penicillins The first *natural penicillins*, types G and V, were degraded by the enzyme penicillinase. The *penicillinase-resistant penicillins*, such as methicillin, nafcillin, oxacillin, and cloxacillin, were developed for treatment of resistant *Staphylococcus* species, and except for a strain of methicillin-resistant *S epidermidis*, they were effective. The next generation of penicillins included the *aminopenicillins*, ampicillin and amoxicillin, created by placement of an amino group on the acyl side chain of the penicillin nucleus. This change broadened their effectiveness to include *H influenzae, E coli,* and *Proteus mirabilis.* The next advance was the *carboxypenicillins*, carbenicillin and ticarcillin, active against aerobic gram-negative rods such as *P aeruginosa, Enterobacter* species, and indole-positive strains of *Proteus.* Therefore, carboxypenicillins are particularly effective for intra-abdominal conditions such as cholangitis, diverticular rupture, and gynecologic infections. The fourth-generation penicillins, known as *acylureidopenicillins*, included azlocillin, mezlocillin, and piperacillin. Currently, their usefulness is for the treatment of Enterobacteriaceae, *P aeruginosa,* and febrile neutropenic patients as well as for infections secondary to a combination of flora found in skin, soft tissue, intra-abdominal, and pelvic infections. However, because of the possibility of emergence of resistance, the newer penicillins are usually administered with an aminoglycoside. Current data, however, do not indicate that they are superior to the older penicillins in such circumstances.

Allergic reactions are the chief side effects encountered with the use of the penicillins. In fact, among antimicrobial agents, the penicillins are the leading cause of allergy. Allergy to the penicillins may be present in 3%–5% of the general population and in as many as 10% of those who have previously received a penicillin. Furthermore, the reported mortality rate with penicillin-induced anaphylaxis is approximately 10%. Large doses or prolonged administration seems to be associated with a high frequency of untoward reaction. Allergic reactions to penicillin are less frequent when the drug is administered orally. Reactions are somewhat higher in frequency when aqueous crystalline penicillin G is given by injection and distinctly higher when procaine penicillin G is given intramuscularly. Cross-allergenicity among the semisynthetic and natural penicillins apparently reflects their common 6-aminopenicillanic acid nucleus and sensitizing derivatives. Cross-allergenicity to cephalosporins may occur in 3%–5% of patients and should be of particular concern when the allergic reaction to either group of antimicrobial agents has been of the immediate type, such as anaphylaxis, angioneurotic edema, or hives.

Cephalosporins The *first-generation cephalosporins* are active against β-lactamase–producing gram-positive cocci and gram-negative bacilli, which are responsible for most community-acquired infections. *Bacillus fragilis, P aeruginosa,* and *Enterobacter* species are typically resistant, as are methicillin-resistant staphylococci. None of the first-generation cephalosporins cross the meninges in concentrations sufficient for the treatment of meningitis.

The *second-generation extended-spectrum cephalosporins* have expanded coverage against gram-negative bacilli.

Third-generation cephalosporins have greater activity against gram-negative bacilli than the earlier cephalosporins, specifically inhibiting the majority of Enterobacteriaceae. Unfortunately, none of the third-generation cephalosporins is effective against enterococci. In general, third-generation cephalosporins are less active than their predecessors against gram-positive organisms, especially *S aureus*. Activity against *B fragilis* varies. Third-generation cephalosporins penetrate the cerebrospinal fluid and have been used successfully to treat meningitis caused by susceptible microorganisms. It is advisable to limit these expensive antibiotics to situations in which they offer a clear advantage, such as in gram-negative bacillary infections or in place of more toxic agents. With the possible exception of ceftazidime, none of these agents is effective enough to be used by itself against *P aeruginosa* or in a febrile neutropenic patient. Likewise, these agents are not to be used for surgical prophylaxis because of their limited activity against gram-positive organisms. Although several oral third-generation cephalosporins are now available, their antimicrobial spectrum is not as broad as that of the parenteral third-generation cephalosporins.

The fourth-generation cephalosporins, cefepime and cefpirome, have a very broad spectrum of activity and are active against most gram-positive bacteria, as well as *Pseudomonas* and other gram-negative organisms that are resistant to other β-lactam antibiotics. The fourth-generation cephalosporins also provide good coverage for most anaerobic infections. A new investigational cephalosporin, cefozopran, has similar activity and antibacterial spectrum.

In recent years, the benefits of continuous intravenous infusion of β-lactam antibiotics, such as nafcillin and ceftazidime, have been demonstrated. This method of dosing provides continuous and stable therapeutic blood and tissue levels of an antibiotic.

Parenteral cephalosporins have a direct effect on prothrombin production and on suppression of vitamin K–producing intestinal flora. The risk of hemorrhagic complications is increased in patients who are taking parenteral cephalosporins in conjunction with heparin, possibly the result of an additive or synergistic pharmacologic effect. The hypoprothrombinemic effects of oral anticoagulants may be increased by such cephalosporins as cefoxitin, leading to a coagulopathy. Acute intolerance to alcohol may occur in persons receiving cephalosporins that possess an N-methylthiotetrazole side chain, such as cefamandole or cefoperazone. Patients should avoid alcohol during therapy and for 2–3 days after completion.

Carbapenems Carbapenems are a new class of antibiotics with a basic ring structure similar to that of penicillins, except that a carbon atom replaces sulfur at the number 1 position. The antibacterial spectrum of the carbapenems is broader than that of any other existing antibiotic and includes *S aureus*, *Enterobacter* species, and *P aeruginosa*. However, an increase in carbapenem-resistant strains of *Staphylococcus* and *Pseudomonas* has been reported recently. Carbapenems also have excellent activity against anaerobic bacteria, including *Bacteroides fragilis.* Cross-resistance between the carbapenems and between carbapenems and piperacillin/tazobactam has been reported recently in *Pseudomonas* isolates. Carbapenems produce a postantibiotic killing effect against some organisms, with a delay in regrowth of damaged organisms similar to that seen with aminoglycosides but not with cephalosporins or acylureidopenicillins. This quality can be particularly important for settings in which host defenses are compromised, such as granulocytopenia or sequestered foci of infection.

Imipenem-cilastatin (Primaxin) combines imipenem, a carbapenem, with cilastatin, an inhibitor of renal dehydropeptidase. Cilastatin has no antimicrobial activity and is present solely to prevent degradation of imipenem by dehydropeptidase. Imipenem-cilastatin is an appropriate compound for monotherapy of mixed infections. Up to 50% of penicillin-allergic patients are also allergic to imipenem.

Meropenem (Merrem), *biapenem, panipenem, ertapenem, faropenem,* and *ritipenem* are newer penems that have increased stability against degradation by dehydropeptidases.

Loracarbef (Lorabid) is an oral *carbacephem,* a new class of antibiotic that is structurally similar to cephalosporins but that possesses a broader spectrum due to higher stability to both plasmid and chromosomally mediated β-lactamases. Loracarbef provides good coverage for most gram-positive and gram-negative aerobic bacteria. Newer parenteral carbacephems are currently being evaluated.

Clavulanic acid, sulbactam, and *tazobactam* are β-lactam molecules that possess little intrinsic antibacterial activity, but they are potent inhibitors of many plasmid-mediated β-lactamases. Currently, four combinations of β-lactam antibiotics plus β-lactamase inhibitors are available in the United States: *Augmentin* (oral amoxicillin and clavulanic acid), *Timentin* (intravenous ticarcillin and clavulanic acid), *Unasyn* (intravenous ampicillin and sulbactam), and *Zosyn* (intravenous piperacillin and tazobactam). These drugs have excellent activity against β-lactamase–producing gram-positive and gram-negative bacteria as well as many anaerobes.

Monobactams are a new monocyclic class of antibiotics utilizing only the β-lactam ring as their core structure. This group possesses excellent activity against aerobic gram-negative bacilli but is ineffective against both gram-positive cocci and anaerobes. The monobactams are similar in antimicrobial spectrum to the aminoglycosides and are generally better tolerated. However, the use of monobactams is limited by their narrow spectrum: many nosocomial infections are polymicrobial, involving gram-positive bacteria or anaerobes in addition to gram-negative aerobic bacilli. Despite the presence of a β-lactam ring, cross-allergenicity with penicillins and cephalosporins appears to be minimal. *Aztreonam*, the first approved monobactam antibiotic, has an excellent safety profile and good success rate in the therapy of infections caused by aerobic gram-negative bacilli. Aztreonam is generally combined with a semisynthetic antistaphylococcal penicillin or clindamycin in presumptive therapy of known mixed infections. Other new monobactams are currently under evaluation in microbiologic and clinical trials.

Aminoglycosides

The aminoglycoside antibiotics inhibit protein synthesis by binding to bacterial ribosomes. Gentamicin, tobramycin, amikacin, kanamycin, streptomycin, and netilmicin can be considered as a group because of their similar activity, pharmacology, and toxicity. Because of poor gastrointestinal absorption, parenteral administration is necessary to produce therapeutic levels.

Aminoglycosides are used for serious infections caused by gram-negative bacilli, including bacteremia in immunocompromised hosts, hospital-acquired pneumonia, and peritonitis. They may be combined with penicillin for the treatment of enterococcal endocarditis. Aminoglycosides are not effective against meningitis because they do not cross the blood–brain barrier. Aminoglycosides are not used for most gram-positive infections because the β-lactams are less toxic.

The major side effects of the aminoglycosides are nephrotoxicity and ototoxicity. Baseline blood urea nitrogen and creatinine levels should be measured, and serial studies should be performed twice a week. Aminoglycoside peak and trough serum levels should be obtained in patients with known renal disease. Combined administration of a loop diuretic such as furosemide with aminoglycosides has a synergistic ototoxic effect, potentially leading to permanent loss of cochlear function.

Penicillins may decrease the antimicrobial effectiveness of parenteral aminoglycosides, particularly in patients with impaired renal function. Aminoglycosides may exacerbate the neuromuscular blocking effects of nondepolarizing muscle relaxants such as tubocurarine. Their combined use during surgery can cause a prolonged respiratory depression accompanied by extended apnea. Oral aminoglycosides are used for bowel sterilization prior to gastrointestinal surgery; however, they may cause malabsorption of vitamin K, amplifying the effects of oral anticoagulants.

Once-daily aminoglycoside dosing regimens have been employed in recent years to decrease systemic toxicity, reduce variability in the timing of drug administration, and lower the costs associated with nursing care for intravenous antibiotic administration and drug level monitoring.

Macrolides

The macrolide *erythromycin* is often employed for the initial treatment of community-acquired pneumonia. This agent is effective against infections caused by pneumococci, group A streptococci, *Mycoplasma pneumoniae*, and *Chlamydia*. It is also effective against *Legionella* species, which have been recognized as a significant cause of community-acquired pneumonia. Erythromycin is used to treat upper-respiratory infections and sexually transmitted diseases in penicillin-allergic patients.

Clarithromycin (Biaxin), *azithromycin* (Zithromax), and *dirithromycin* (Dynabac) are newer macrolide antibiotics chemically related to erythromycin. All are well-tolerated alternatives to erythromycin and may offer particular advantages in the treatment of gonococcal and *Chlamydia* infections and in the treatment of *M avium* and other recalcitrant infections associated with AIDS. Azithromycin is subclassified as an *azalide*, and it possesses far fewer drug interactions than erythromycin. Increasing cross-resistance among the macrolides has been demonstrated. Additional new macrolide antibiotics, such as roxithromycin, spiramycin, and josamycin, are being evaluated and have similar antimicrobial spectra. Telithromycin, a new ketolide antibiotic that belongs to a new class of semisynthetic 14-membered-ring macrolides, is discussed later under New Antibiotic Classes.

Clindamycin has a gram-positive spectrum similar to that of erythromycin and is also active against most anaerobes, including *Bacteroides fragilis*. Except for anaerobic infection, it is rarely the drug of choice. Clindamycin is well absorbed orally, and parenteral formulations are available. Its major side effect is diarrhea, which may progress to pseudomembranous enterocolitis in some patients.

Glycopeptides

Vancomycin regained popularity because of the emergence of methicillin-resistant staphylococci and the recognition that *C difficile* is a cause of pseudomembranous colitis. Vancomycin has excellent activity against *Clostridium* and against most gram-positive bacteria, including methicillin-resistant staphylococci, diphtheroids, and other *Corynebacterium* species. Vancomycin has been used alone to treat serious infections caused by methicillin-resistant staphylococci. In cases of prosthetic-valve endocarditis caused by methicillin-resistant *S epidermidis*, a combination of vancomycin, rifampin, and gentamicin has been shown to be effective.

In recent years, several cases of vancomycin-resistant enterococcal infection have been reported. In one study of hospitalized patients, approximately 1% carried vancomycin-resistant enterococci in their gastrointestinal tract. These infections are very difficult or impossible to treat because of multidrug resistance. In vitro studies have shown that plasmid-mediated vancomycin resistance can be easily transferred to staphylococci; indeed, since July 2002, there have been reports of *S aureus* and *S epidermidis* infections resistant to vancomycin.

The CDC issued recommendations regarding appropriate use of vancomycin to help counteract the emergence of bacterial drug resistance. These guidelines include discouraging the use of vancomycin for routine surgical prophylaxis, avoiding its empirical use in febrile neutropenic patients unless there is strong evidence for a β-lactam–resistant gram-positive infection, and avoiding prophylactic therapy for patients with intravascular catheters or vascular grafts. The rationale for these recommendations is that inappropriate use of this drug will only hasten the emergence of new resistant bacterial strains. Similarly, many authors think that prophylactic use of vancomycin in routine ophthalmic surgery is not advisable from an infectious disease and public health standpoint.

Teicoplanin (Targocid) is a newer glycopeptide and has several advantages over vancomycin, including longer half-life, lower nephrotoxicity, and no requirement for monitoring drug levels. Teicoplanin is effective for staphylococcal infections including endocarditis, bacteremia, osteomyelitis, and septic arthritis. The once-daily or alternate-day dosage allows home administration of treatment of serious infections caused by MRSA and enterococci, with significant savings in hospital costs and enhanced quality of life. Teicoplanin may be preferable to vancomycin for surgical prophylaxis because of its excellent tissue penetration, lower toxicity, and long half-life, allowing single-dose administration in several surgical procedures. The antibacterial activity of teicoplanin is similar to that of vancomycin but with increased potency, particularly against *Streptococcus* and *Enterococcus*. Teicoplanin is active against vancomycin resistance caused by VanB and VanC resistant strains. Teicoplanin is an investigational drug and is available from the manufacturer for compassionate use. Another new investigational glycopeptide, ramoplanin, is highly active against vancomycin-resistant enterococcal infections.

Tetracyclines

The tetracyclines are bacteriostatic agents that reversibly inhibit ribosomal protein synthesis. Although they have a broad spectrum of activity (including *Rickettsia, Chlamydia, Nocardia,* and *Actinomyces*), resistance is widespread, especially among *S aureus* and gram-negative bacilli. The principal clinical uses of tetracyclines are in treatment of nongonococcal urethritis, Rocky Mountain spotted fever, chronic bronchitis, and sebaceous disorders such as acne rosacea. In addition, tetracyclines are an alternative for the penicillin-allergic patient with syphilis. Tetracyclines are well absorbed when taken on an empty stomach; however, their absorption is decreased when taken with milk, antacids, calcium, or iron. Tetracyclines are distributed throughout the extracellular fluid, but cerebrospinal fluid penetration is unreliable. Adverse effects include oral or vaginal candidiasis with prolonged use, gastrointestinal upset, photosensitivity, and elevation of the blood urea nitrogen. Tetracyclines should not be administered to pregnant women or to children under age 10 because of effects on developing bone and teeth.

Quinolones

In the early 1960s, *nalidixic acid* was discovered as an accidental byproduct of research on quinolones as antimalarial agents. Nalidixic acid has relatively good activity against aerobic gram-negative bacteria but only limited activity against gram-positive species. Nalidixic acid was adequate therapy for urinary tract infections, but it does not produce sufficient tissue concentrations after oral ingestion to treat systemic infections. When administered intravenously, it produces central nervous system and cardiac toxicity. Consequently, the quinolones were not considered an important class of drugs, particularly in the United States.

Recently, however, the introduction of a fluorine into the basic quinolone nucleus has produced compounds known as *fluoroquinolones,* which have excellent gram-positive activity. The subsequent addition of piperazine produced compounds such as *norfloxacin* (Noroxin) and *ciprofloxacin* (Cipro) that have a broad spectrum of activity, encompassing staphylococci and most of the significant gram-negative bacilli, including *Pseudomonas*. Ciprofloxacin is available in both oral and parenteral forms. It can be used to treat urinary tract infections, gonorrhea, and diarrheal diseases as well as respiratory, skin, and, particularly, bone infections. Fluoroquinolones introduced more recently into the United States market include *ofloxacin* (Floxin), *temafloxacin* (Omniflox), *lomefloxacin* (Maxaquin), *enoxacin* (Penetrex), *sparfloxacin* (Zagam), levofloxacin (Levaquin), moxifloxacin (Avelox), gatifloxacin (Tequin), trovafloxacin (Trovan), and gemifloxacin (Factive). Newer drugs awaiting FDA approval include clinafloxacin, sitafloxacin, and pazufloxacin. The new fluoroquinolones possess even greater activity against gram-positive and gram-negative bacteria. Moxifloxacin appears to be a good treatment choice for pneumococcal infections that are resistant to penicillin and the macrolides. Oral quinolones are an alternative form of therapy to β-lactams and aminoglycosides and have permitted physicians to treat more patients outside the hospital setting.

Miscellaneous Antibacterial Agents

Rifampin was originally developed as an antituberculosis agent but is also used to treat a host of intractable bacterial infections. Rifampin is usually employed adjunctively because bacteria develop resistance to the drug when it is used as a single agent. Rifampin often demonstrates higher effectiveness in vivo than in vitro, perhaps because it penetrates directly into leukocytes and kills phagocytosed bacteria. It also penetrates well into bone and abscess cavities. Rifampin in combination with other agents is used successfully in the treatment of *S aureus* and prosthetic-valve endocarditis caused by *S epidermidis*. Rifampin is effective in eradicating the carrier state of nasal *S aureus*. This drug is also effective prophylactically against *N meningitidis* and may be useful for treating oropharyngeal carriers of *H influenzae* type B.

Another oral antibiotic with potential for the treatment of deep-seated infections is TMP-SMX. After a single oral dose, the mean serum levels of trimethoprim and sulfamethoxazole are about 75% of the concentration that would be achieved through the intravenous route. In addition to its excellent pharmacokinetics, TMP-SMX has an extremely broad spectrum of activity (against Enterobacteriaceae, it is usually comparable to that of a third-generation cephalosporin or even an aminoglycoside). In addition, a number of unusual microorganisms that are resistant to cephalosporins are susceptible to TMP-SMX. One misconception is that TMP-SMX has limited activity against gram-positive bacteria; however, most streptococci, staphylococci, and *Listeria monocytogenes* are susceptible to this drug. Beyond the broad-spectrum effect of TMP-SMX, the concomitant use of *metronidazole* creates an antibiotic combination with activity against microorganisms surpassing that of a third-generation cephalosporin. TMP-SMX has seen increasing use in the treatment and prophylaxis of *Pneumocystis* infection and toxoplasmosis in recent years.

Chloramphenicol is a bacteriostatic agent that reversibly inhibits ribosomal protein synthesis. This drug is active against a wide variety of gram-negative and gram-positive organisms, including anaerobes. The major concern is hematopoietic toxicity, including reversible bone marrow suppression and irreversible aplasia. Aplastic anemia is an idiosyncratic late reaction to the drug and is usually fatal. Reversible leukopenia, thrombocytopenia, and suppression of erythropoiesis are dose related and can usually be avoided when peak serum levels are maintained at less than 25 µg/mL. Other side effects include hemolysis, allergy, and peripheral neuritis.

New Antibiotic Classes

Pharmacologic research is providing entirely new classes of antibiotics that offer additional treatment options for emerging resistant bacterial strains. Most of the new drugs that have been recently developed are targeted against resistant strains of gram-positive bacteria.

The first approved *streptogramin* antibiotic is *quinupristin/dalfopristin* (Synercid). Streptogramins, also called *synergistins*, represent a unique class of antibiotics notable for their outstanding antibacterial activity and their unique mechanism of action. These antibiotics are produced naturally by *Streptomyces* species and bind bacterial ribosomes and inhibit protein synthesis. Oral streptogramins have been available in Europe for years, but quinupristin/dalfopristin (Q/D) is the first parenteral drug in this class.

Synercid is composed of two semisynthetic pristinamycin derivatives, quinupristin and dalfopristin. Individually, each component drug has bacteriostatic activity; together, they exhibit synergy, resulting in bactericidal activity and up to 16 times more potency than either drug alone. Streptogramins have excellent activity against multidrug-resistant gram-positive organisms in vitro and in vivo. This class is noted for rapid bacterial killing and lacks cross-resistance with other antimicrobials. In one recent study, Q/D displayed excellent activity against all staphylococcal species tested regardless of the resistance pattern to other drug classes, including methicillin and macrolide-resistant strains. Q/D was two to four times more active than vancomycin. Q/D also has activity against mycoplasma, *N gonorrhoeae, H influenzae, Legionella*, and *Moraxella catarrhalis*. Despite a short half-life, an extended postantibiotic effect allows the drug to be administered every 8–12 hours. Side effects include skin rash, itching, diarrhea, vomiting, arthralgia, myalgias, and reversible elevation of serum alkaline phosphatase. Also, Q/D appears to be safe and effective in critically ill immunocompromised children with renal or hepatic impairment.

Linezolid (Zyvox) is the first approved *oxazolidinone* antibiotic and is highly active against multidrug-resistant strains of gram-positive bacteria. Linezolid is as effective as vancomycin for methicillin-resistant staphylococcal infections and active against vancomycin-resistant enterococci, penicillin- and multidrug-resistant pneumococci, and macrolide-resistant streptococci. In one study, linezolid was the most potent new antibiotic tested against gram-positive cocci, including multiresistant strains. It has monoamine oxidase inhibitor effects, so drug interaction precautions are necessary. *Furazolidone* (Furoxone) and newer experimental agents eperezolid and ranbezolid are other similar oxazolidinones.

Evernimicin (Ziracin) is a new *oligosaccharide* antibiotic of the everninomicin class. This drug offers outstanding activity against drug-resistant gram-positive strains. In a recent multicenter, multinational, in vitro study, evernimicin outperformed vancomycin and Q/D against methicillin-resistant *Staphylococcus* and all other gram-positive organisms tested. *Avilamycin* is another, newer member of this antibiotic family.

Telithromycin (HMR 3647) is a new *ketolide* that belongs to a new class of semisynthetic 14-membered-ring macrolides, which also have expanded activity against multidrug-resistant gram-positive bacteria. In some studies, these drugs are 8 to 10 times more potent than other macrolides. Telithromycin was specifically designed for the treatment of community-acquired respiratory infections and offers a wide spectrum of activity against common respiratory pathogens, such as *S pneumoniae, H influenzae, S pyogenes, M catarrhalis, Chlamydia pneumoniae, Legionella pneumophila,* and *M pneumoniae.* Telithromycin is active against β-lactam–resistant and macrolide-resistant bacteria and does not appear to induce cross-resistance to other antimicrobials. In one study, it was more effective than oral cephalosporins, macrolides, and quinolones. Orally administered telithromycin achieves good plasma levels and is highly concentrated in pulmonary tissues and leukocytes. In clinical trials, telithromycin given once daily for 5–10 days was effective for the treatment of community-acquired pneumonia, acute exacerbations of chronic bronchitis, acute sinusitis, and streptococcal pharyngitis.

Daptomycin, a new cyclic *lipopeptide* antibiotic, is also highly active against multidrug-resistant gram-positive bacteria. In one recent comparative study, daptomycin demonstrated greater bactericidal activity against MRSA and *S epidermidis,* vancomycin-resistant enterococci, and vancomycin-intermediate *S aureus* than vancomycin, linezolid, and Q/D. An added benefit of this drug is that it has been shown to reduce the nephrotoxicity of aminoglycosides, but the mechanism of this protection is unknown.

Other new antibiotics being evaluated for the treatment of multidrug-resistant infections include the glycycline antibiotic, tigecycline; the bacteriocins, nicin and sakacin; and the temporins, temporin A and temporin L.

Antifungal Agents

Fluconazole (Diflucan) and *itraconazole* (Sporanox) are newer antifungal *imidazoles* for treatment of cryptococcal meningitis, candidiasis, and other invasive fungal infections. These drugs are more effective and better tolerated than ketoconazole in the treatment of candidiasis and invasive fungal disease. Imidazoles function by inhibiting fungal cytochrome P-450–dependent enzymes, thereby blocking synthesis of the fungal cell membrane. The newer imidazoles offer a less toxic alternative to amphotericin B in the treatment of cryptococcal meningitis and may play a role in chronic suppression of *Cryptococcus* after remission of acute infection in severely immunocompromised patients. Additional new investigational imidazoles include *flutrimazole, croconazole, voriconazole* (Vfend), and *ravuconazole.*

Treatment of serious deep-seated systemic fungal infections may require the use of intravenous amphotericin B, sometimes in combined therapy with either flucytosine or an imidazole. Lipid complex and liposome-encapsulated formulations of amphotericin B (AmBisome, Amphotec) are available to reduce the drug's toxicity. Nystatin is classified as a topical antifungal agent and is structurally similar to amphotericin B. However, a new intravenous liposomal formulation of nystatin is currently in clinical trials for treatment of systemic fungal infections.

Terbinafine (Lamisil) is an *allylamine* oral antifungal agent that is effective in controlling onychomycosis due to chronic dermatophyte infections. Treatment must be continued for 6–12 weeks to eradicate the nail infection. Butenafine (Mentax) is a benzylamine that effectively treats skin and nail infections caused by dermatophytes.

Several novel antifungal agents in clinical trials include echinocandins (capsofungin), pneumocandins, and improved imidazoles. Promising new drugs in preclinical development include inhibitors of fungal protein, lipid, and cell wall synthesis.

Antiviral Agents

Acyclovir (Zovirax) is a nucleoside analogue that is effective against herpes simplex and varicella-zoster infections. It inhibits viral DNA replication. One phosphorylation step of acyclovir is catalyzed by the enzyme thymidine kinase. The viral-induced thymidine kinase is far more active than the host cell thymidine kinase. Therefore, acyclovir is very active against viruses within infected host cells and yet is generally well tolerated.

Acyclovir has proven effective in a variety of herpetic infections. A topical 5% ointment may be used in localized primary episodes of genital herpes. Oral acyclovir at a dose of 200 mg five times daily is effective in acute severe genital herpes. Chronic suppressive oral acyclovir has also demonstrated efficacy in immunocompetent patients with frequently recurring genital herpes. Intravenous acyclovir at a dose of 30 mg/kg every 8 hours is the treatment of choice for herpes simplex encephalitis. Acyclovir at a dose of 500 mg/M² every 8 hours has been used successfully for the treatment of herpes zoster infections in immunocompromised patients. This dose is also used in patients with acute retinal necrosis syndrome.

Oral acyclovir may be used to treat herpes zoster ophthalmicus: 800 mg five times daily is usually effective in reducing the incidence of ocular complications of herpes zoster ophthalmicus. However, postherpetic neuralgia is not affected by this therapy. A randomized, controlled study of acyclovir and oral corticosteroids demonstrated that the steroids did not help to reduce the incidence of postherpetic neuralgia when added to oral acyclovir.

Famciclovir (Famvir) and *valacyclovir* (Valtrex) are currently approved for the treatment of herpes zoster infections and have also been shown to be effective against herpes simplex in numerous studies. Both of these newer drugs allow less frequent dosing intervals (every 8–12 hours, depending on the indication). Valganciclovir is a new investigational antiviral agent currently in clinical trials.

Adefovir (Preveon) is a new nucleoside analogue and is a potent inhibitor of many viruses, such as HIV, HSV, human papillomavirus virus, and EBV.

Ganciclovir (Cytovene), foscarnet (Foscavir), cidofovir (Vistide), and fomivirsen (Vitravene) are antiviral agents used for the treatment of CMV infections, including retinitis. These drugs and the antiretroviral agents are discussed in more detail under the earlier heading, Acquired Immunodeficiency Syndrome.

Amantadine and rimantadine are M2 protein inhibitors effective for the treatment of influenza A and for the prophylactic treatment of contacts of infected patients. Rapid onset of drug resistance, ineffectiveness against influenza B, and central nervous system side effects have limited wide acceptance of these agents. Oseltamivir is a new oral neuraminidase inhibitor with excellent efficacy against influenza in humans. Oseltamivir provides about 90% protection for household contacts of patients with influenza. Recent studies have shown a very low incidence of viral resistance to this agent. It is approved for the treatment and prophylaxis of influenza. Another neuraminidase inhibitor, zanamivir, appears to be effective for influenza, but resistance has recently been reported.

Treatment of Hospital-Acquired Infections

Decisions concerning antibiotic administration in the treatment of serious hospital-acquired infections present important considerations for the prescribing physician. Three distinct stages of therapy tend to occur in such infections. (*Note:* Especially in the latter two stages, cost containment is enhanced by close monitoring of mode, level, and frequency of antibiotic dosing.)

The *first stage* of therapy typically lasts about 3 days, during which time uncertainty exists about the causative organism. Therapy is given empirically, often with the combination of an aminoglycoside and a β-lactam antibiotic.

The *second stage* begins about the fourth day, at which time definitive microbiological and clinical data are available that should allow for streamlining of antibiotic therapy, usually from combination therapy to less expensive monotherapy. It is at this stage in the patient's hospital stay that routine assessment of antibiotic management offers the first chance to reduce hospital antibiotic costs without compromising the clinical outcome.

The *third stage* of therapy typically begins around the seventh day, when the patient is usually clinically stable and afebrile. At this point, often the only reason the patient is kept hospitalized is to continue treatment with parenteral antibiotics. In many patients, however, therapy can be switched to daily intravenous dosing or oral antibiotics, facilitating outpatient therapy. Streamlining antibiotic therapy by changing modes and frequency of administration is a major step toward effective, responsible cost containment.

Asbel LE, Levison ME. Cephalosporins, carbapenems, and monobactams. *Infect Dis Clin North Am.* 2000;14:435–447.

Bronson JJ, Barrett JF. Quinolone, everninomycin, glycylcycline, carbapenem, lipopeptide and cephem antibacterials in clinical development. *Curr Med Chem.* 2001;8:1775–1793.

Brumfitt W, Salton MR, Hamilton-Miller JM. Nisin, alone and combined with peptidoglycan-modulating antibiotics: activity against methicillin-resistant *Staphylococcus aureus* and vancomycin-resistant enterococci. *J Antimicrob Chemother.* 2002;50:731–734.

Cassell GH, Mekalanos J. Development of antimicrobial agents in the era of new and re-emerging infectious diseases and increasing antibiotic resistance. *JAMA.* 2001;285:601–605.

Cercenado E, Garcia-Garrote F, Bouza E. In vitro activity of linezolid against multiply resistant gram-positive clinical isolates. *J Antimicrob Chemother.* 2001;47:77–81.

Cui L, Ma X, Sato K, et al. Cell wall thickening is a common feature of vancomycin resistance in *Staphylococcus aureus*. *J Clin Microbiol.* 2003;41:5–14.

Cunha BA. Ertapenem. A review of its microbiologic, pharmacokinetic and clinical aspects. *Drugs Today (Barc).* 2002;38:195–213.

Dalhoff A, Thomson CJ. The art of fusion: from penams and cephems to penems. *Chemotherapy.* 2003;49:105–120.

Decousser JW, Pina P, Picot F, et al. Comparative in vitro activity of faropenem and 11 other antimicrobial agents against 250 invasive *Streptococcus pneumoniae* isolates from France. *Eur J Clin Microbiol Infect Dis.* 2003;22:561–565.

Delgado G Jr, Neuhauser MM, Bearden DT, et al. Quinupristin-dalfopristin: an overview. *Pharmacotherapy.* 2000;20:1469–1485.

Hoellman DB, Lin G, Ednie LM, et al. Antipneumococcal and antistaphylococcal activities of ranbezolid (RBX 7644), a new oxazolidinone, compared to those of other agents. *Antimicrob Agents Chemother.* 2003;47:1148–1150.

Johnson MD, Perfect JR. Caspofungin: first approved agent in a new class of antifungals. *Expert Opin Pharmacother.* 2003;4:807–823.

Jones RN, Hare RS, Sabatelli FJ, et al. In vitro gram-positive antimicrobial activity of ever-nimicin (SCH 27899), a novel oligosaccharide, compared with other antimicrobials: a multicentre international trial. *J Antimicrob Chemother.* 2001;47:15–25.

Lee NL, Yuen KY, Kumana CR. Beta-lactam antibiotic and beta-lactamase inhibitor combinations. *JAMA.* 2001;285:386–388.

Lorenz J. Telithromycin: the first ketolide antibacterial for the treatment of community-acquired respiratory tract infections. *Int J Clin Pract.* 2003;57:519–529.

Mercier RC, Kennedy C, Meadows C. Antimicrobial activity of tigecycline (GAR-936) against *Enterococcus faecium* and *Staphylococcus aureus* used alone and in combination. *Pharmacotherapy.* 2002;22:1517–1523.

Montecalvo MA. Ramoplanin: a novel antimicrobial agent with the potential to prevent vancomycin-resistant enterococcal infection in high-risk patients. *J Antimicrob Chemother.* 2003;51;Suppl 3:31–35.

Namour F, Wessels DH, Pascual MH, et al. Pharmacokinetics of the new ketolide telithromycin (HMR 3647) administered in ascending single and multiple doses. *Antimicrob Agents Chemother.* 2001;45:170–175.

Polak A. Antifungal therapy—state of the art at the beginning of the 21st century. *Prog Drug Res.* 2003; spec no: 59–190.

Rybak MJ, Hershberger E, Moldovan T, et al. In vitro activities of daptomycin, vancomycin, linezolid, and quinupristin-dalfopristin against Staphylococci and Enterococci, including vancomycin-intermediate and -resistant strains. *Antimicrob Agents Chemother.* 2000;44:1062–1066.

Schaison G, Graninger W, Bouza E. Teicoplanin in the treatment of serious infection. *J Chemother.* 2000;12(Suppl 5):26–33.

Welliver R, Monto AS, Carewicz O, et al. Effectiveness of oseltamivir in preventing influenza in household contacts. A randomized controlled trial. *JAMA.* 2001;285:748–754.

Wright AJ. The penicillins. *Mayo Clin Proc.* 1999;74:290–307.

CHAPTER 2

Hypertension

Recent Developments

- Initial antihypertensive therapy should include diuretics or beta blockers.
- Low-dose fixed combinations may be appropriate for initial treatment.
- Blood pressure should be reduced even lower than 140/90 mm Hg in diabetic patients, and diastolic pressure can be safely reduced to levels below 85 mm Hg in patients with ischemic heart disease.
- Angiotensin-converting enzyme (ACE) inhibitors are probably better choices for therapy than calcium channel blockers in diabetic subjects.

Introduction

Hypertension is common in the United States, occurring in approximately 50 million persons over age 18. Most persons with hypertension have only mildly elevated pressures, but all are at greater risk for stroke, coronary artery disease, heart failure, peripheral vascular disease, and renal insufficiency. Ocular complications of hypertension include retinovascular disease and increased risk of glaucoma.

Definition

The Joint National Committee on Detection, Evaluation, and Treatment of Hypertension has defined hypertension as a systolic blood pressure greater than 140 and a diastolic blood pressure greater than 90 mm Hg. The readings should reflect resting values after the patient has been seated at least 5 minutes, with two readings taken at least 2 minutes apart. The appropriate cuff size must be used to ensure accurate measurement. The patient should not have used caffeine or nicotine within the half hour preceding the examination. Initial elevated readings should be confirmed on at least two subsequent visits during the following weeks. The risk of cardiovascular disease in hypertensive patients is determined by blood pressure level, presence or absence of target organ damage, and other risk factors as shown in Table 2-1.

Table 2-1 Components of Cardiovascular Risk Stratification in Patients With Hypertension

Major risk factors

Smoking
Dyslipidemia
Diabetes mellitus
Age >60 yr
Sex (men and postmenopausal women)
Family history of cardiovascular disease: women <65 yr or men <55 yr

Target organ damage/clinical cardiovascular disease

Heart diseases
   Left-ventricular hypertrophy
   Angina or prior myocardial infarction
   Prior coronary revascularization
   Heart failure
Stroke or transient ischemic attack
Nephropathy
Peripheral arterial disease
Retinopathy

(Reprinted from: Sixth report of the Joint National Committee on Prevention, Detection, Evaluation, and Treatment of High Blood Pressure. *Arch Intern Med.* 1997;157:2417. ©1997 American Medical Association.)

Classification

Hypertension in adults can be classified on the basis of blood pressure level (Table 2-2). All stages of hypertension warrant effective therapy. Over 70% of persons have mild (stage 1) hypertension. Patients in the high-normal category constitute an at-risk population. Frequent monitoring and modification of lifestyle factors in this group can reduce the risk of target organ disease. (See Table 2-3 for recommendations about follow-up based on initial blood pressure measurements.)

White Coat Hypertension

Twenty percent of patients with hypertension have *"white coat" hypertension*—that is, blood pressure that is increased only in a physician's office. These persons manifest an abnormal physiologic response that warrants further study because they are at greater risk for cardiovascular disease. Ambulatory blood pressure readings are used in identifying white coat hypertension.

Secondary Hypertension

Although 90% of hypertensive patients have *primary,* or *essential, hypertension,* in which the cause remains unknown, the remaining 10% have *secondary hypertension.* Secondary causes of hypertension include renovascular disease, pheochromocytoma, hyperaldosteronism, polycystic kidney disease, aortic coarctation, and Cushing syndrome. In addition to evaluating target organ disease, the initial physical assessment should not only evaluate

Table 2-2 Classification of Blood Pressure for Adults Aged 18 Years and Older*

Category	Blood Pressure, mm Hg		
	Systolic		Diastolic
Optimal[†]	<120	and	<80
Normal	<130	and	<85
High-normal	130–139	or	85–89
Hypertension[‡]			
Stage 1 (mild)	140–159	or	90–99
Stage 2 (moderate)	160–179	or	100–109
Stage 3 (severe)	≥180	or	≥110

* Not taking antihypertensive drugs and not acutely ill. When systolic and diastolic blood pressures fall into different categories, the higher category should be selected to classify the individual's blood pressure status. For example, 160/92 mm Hg should be classified as stage 2 hypertension, and 174/120 mm Hg should be classified as stage 3 hypertension. Isolated systolic hypertension is defined as systolic blood pressure 140 mm Hg or greater and diastolic blood pressure less than 90 mm Hg and staged appropriately (eg, 170/82 mm Hg is defined as stage 2 isolated systolic hypertension). In addition to classifying stages of hypertension on the basis of average blood pressure levels, clinicians should specify presence or absence of target organ disease and additional risk factors. This specificity is important for risk classification and treatment (see Table 2-4).

[†] Optimal blood pressure with respect to cardiovascular risk is less than 120/80 mm Hg. However, unusually low readings should be evaluated for clinical significance.

[‡] Based on the average of two or more readings taken at each of two or more visits after an initial screening.

(Reprinted from: Sixth report of the Joint National Committee on Prevention, Detection, Evaluation, and Treatment of High Blood Pressure. *Arch Intern Med.* 1997;157:2417. ©1997 American Medical Association.)

Table 2-3 Recommendations for Follow-up Based on Initial Blood Pressure Measurements for Adults

Initial Blood Pressure, mm Hg*		
Systolic	Diastolic	Follow-up Recommended[†]
<130	<85	Recheck in 2 yr
130–139	85–89	Recheck in 1 yr[‡]
140–159	90–99	Confirm within 2 mo[‡]
160–179	100–109	Evaluate or refer to source of care within 1 mo
≥180	≥110	Evaluate or refer to source of care immediately or within 1 wk depending on clinical situation

* If systolic and diastolic categories are different, follow recommendations for shorter follow-up (eg, 160/86 mm Hg should be evaluated or referred to source of care within 1 mo).

[†] Modify the scheduling of follow-up according to reliable information about past blood pressure measurements, other cardiovascular risk factors, or target organ disease.

[‡] Provide advice about lifestyle modifications.

(Reprinted from: Sixth report of the Joint National Committee on Prevention, Detection, Evaluation, and Treatment of High Blood Pressure. *Arch Intern Med.* 1997;157:2418. ©1997 American Medical Association.)

target-organ disease but also look for secondary causes of hypertension. Signs associated with secondary hypertension include:

- *Renovascular:* unilateral abdominal bruits in young females with marked hypertension; new-onset hypertension with severe end-organ disease

- *Hyperaldosteronism:* persistent hypokalemia
- *Pheochromocytoma:* markedly labile blood pressure with tachycardia and headaches
- *Polycystic kidney disease:* flank mass
- *Aortic coarctation:* delayed or absent femoral pulses
- *Cushing syndrome:* truncal obesity and abdominal striae

Secondary causes of hypertension should be suspected in persons who have accelerating hypertension, hypertension unresponsive to medication, or a sudden change in previously well-controlled blood pressure.

Epidemiology

More than 22% of adults in the United States have hypertension. The prevalence increases with age and tends to be familial. The rate of hypertension is higher in African Americans than in whites. The incidence of devastating complications is higher in lower socioeconomic groups, because of both greater prevalence and delayed detection.

Therapeutic Approaches

Treatment Goals

Morbidity and mortality from cardiovascular disease, renal disease, and stroke increase progressively with higher levels of blood pressure; accordingly, treatment of hypertension decreases the risk of these conditions. Lowering diastolic blood pressure by 5–6 mm Hg has been shown to reduce stroke incidence by 4%. Treatment of mild and moderate hypertension can decrease the myocardial infarction rate by 20%. The goals of successful hypertension management are normalizing the blood pressure, making beneficial lifestyle modifications, and controlling cardiovascular risk factors.

Lifestyle Factors

Although lifestyle modification is not as effective as pharmacologic approaches, certain modifiable factors can serve as either definitive or adjunctive therapy in the management of hypertension. Lifestyle modification is helpful both for hypertensive patients and for persons at risk for hypertension: such modification can reduce the risk of hypertensive complications in the first group and prevent hypertension in the second.

Controlling the risk factors for atherosclerotic disease is a crucial part of hypertension management. For example, smoking one pack of cigarettes a day increases the risk of coronary artery disease by five times; the risk increases more than 25 times in patients with mild hypertension. Hypercholesterolemia plays a direct role in the development of atherosclerosis; successful blood lipid normalization is key to reducing morbidity and mortality.

Obesity

Obesity or excess caloric intake is associated with increased blood pressure. Persons whose weight is in the top third of the population consistently have higher blood pressure than those in the bottom third. Weight loss, independent of sodium intake, consistently results in a drop in the blood pressure among persons who are more than 10% above their ideal body weight.

Exercise

Regular aerobic exercise involving moderately intense physical activity can effectively lower blood pressure as well as contribute to weight loss and reduced mortality. In sedentary normotensive persons, the risk of developing hypertension is 20%–50% greater than in their exercising counterparts.

Sodium

The average American consumes more than 150 mmol of sodium (approximately 6 g of salt) per day. A reduction of 50 mmol per day can lower systemic blood pressure by 7 mm Hg. Individuals vary in their responsiveness to dietary sodium; blacks, older people, and patients with hypertension are more sensitive. Processed food accounts for 75% of sodium intake.

Alcohol

Consumption of alcohol should be limited to less than 1 oz of ethanol (2 oz of 100 proof whiskey, 10 oz of wine, or 24 oz of beer) per day. Higher daily consumption is associated with both elevated blood pressure and resistance to antihypertensive therapy.

Smoking

Cigarette smoking appears to be related to hypertension only as a major risk factor for atherosclerotic vascular disease. However, this relationship is significant in that smoking multiplies the risk of coronary disease in hypertensive patients. The lower amounts of nicotine used in smoking cessation programs usually do not raise blood pressure.

Minerals

Maintaining an adequate intake of potassium, calcium, and magnesium also contributes to blood pressure normalization.

Pharmacologic Therapy

In considering the appropriate therapy for an individual patient, the physician should weigh multiple factors: hypertension class, target-organ disease, atherosclerotic risk factors, cost, compliance, side effects, and coexisting conditions. In general, the higher the stage, the greater the damage to target organs; and the greater the risk factors for cardiovascular disease, the sooner treatment should be initiated. For example, patients with severe hypertension and encephalopathy require emergent treatment, whereas those with mild hypertension may attempt lifestyle modification before drug therapy is initiated.

Approximately half of patients respond to monotherapy; the individual's treatment response dictates whether substitution of a drug of similar class or addition of a drug of a different class is indicated. Compliance and drug cost are directly related to treatment success. Successful compliance depends on minimal dose frequency and side effects. The sixth report of the Joint National Committee on Prevention, Detection, Evaluation, and Treatment of High Blood Pressure suggested the following:

- Diuretics or beta blockers should be the initial choice of therapy unless other medications are specifically indicated.
- Therapy should be started with low doses of a once-a-day medication and titrated.
- Low-dose fixed combinations may be appropriate for initial treatment.

More recent studies confirm that blood pressure should be reduced even lower than 140/90 in diabetic patients and that diastolic blood pressure can be safely reduced below 85 mm Hg in patients with ischemic heart disease. Overall, lowering blood pressure is probably more important in reducing morbidity and mortality than the specific medication used.

The major classes of antihypertensive drugs include diuretics, adrenergic inhibitors, direct vasodilators, calcium antagonists, ACE inhibitors, and angiotensin II receptor blockers (Table 2-4). Newly developed formulations, including combination agents, provide additional therapeutic choices (Table 2-5). Certain clinical situations require special consideration in individualizing antihypertension drug therapy, as outlined in Table 2-6.

Diuretics

Diuretics are divided into the thiazide, loop-acting, and potassium-sparing types.

Thiazide diuretics increase the sodium load on the kidney's distal tubules and, in the short term, decrease the plasma volume and cardiac output through natriuresis. As the renin-angiotensin-aldosterone system compensates for plasma volume, cardiac output returns to normal and peripheral vascular resistance is lowered.

Loop diuretics act on the ascending loop of Henle and inhibit electrolyte resorption, causing an initial decrease in plasma volume. As with the thiazide diuretics, blood pressure is eventually reduced because of decreased peripheral vascular resistance. Loop diuretics are used primarily in treating patients with renal insufficiency. Loop diuretics are not as useful on a chronic basis in patients with good kidney function.

Potassium-sparing diuretics are competitive antagonists of the mineralocorticoids, thereby preventing potassium loss in the distal tubule. Their mechanism of action is similar to that of thiazide diuretics, although less potent. Potassium-sparing diuretics are often used as adjuncts to the thiazides or loop diuretics to counteract potassium depletion.

ACE inhibitors and angiotensin II receptor blockers

The renin-angiotensin-aldosterone system participates in the pathophysiology of hypertension. This system can be blocked by renin inhibitors; by ACE inhibitors, which inhibit the conversion of angiotensin I to angiotensin II; by angiotensin II receptor blockers, which block angiotensin II activity at the receptor site; or by aldosterone inhibitors. ACE

Table 2-4   Oral Antihypertensive Drugs

Drug	Trade Name	Usual Dose Range, Total mg/day* (Frequency per Day)	Selected Side Effects and Comments*
Diuretics *(partial list)*			*Short term:* increases cholesterol and glucose levels; *biochemical abnormalities:* decreases potassium, sodium, and magnesium levels, increases uric acid and calcium levels; *rare:* blood dyscrasias, photosensitivity, pancreatitis, hyponatremia
Chlorthalidone (G)[†]	Hygroton	12.5–50 (1)	
Hydrochlorothiazide (G)	Hydrodiuril, Microzide, Esidrix	12.5–50 (1)	
Indapamide	Lozol	1.25–5 (1)	(Less or no hypercholesterolemia)
Metolazone	Mykrox	0.5–1.0 (1)	
	Zaroxolyn	2.5–10 (1)	
Loop diuretics			
Bumetanide (G)	Bumex	0.5–4 (2–3)	(Short duration of action, no hypercalcemia)
Ethacrynic acid	Edecrin	25–100 (1)	(Only nonsulfonamide diuretic, ototoxicity)
Furosemide (G)	Lasix	40–240 (2–3)	(Short duration of action, no hypercalcemia)
Torsemide	Demadex	5–100 (1)	
Potassium-sparing agents			
Amiloride hydrochloride (G)	Midamor	5–10 (1)	
Spironolactone (G)	Aldactone	25–100 (1)	(Gynecomastia)
Triamterene (G)	Dyrenium	25–100 (1)	
Adrenergic inhibitors			
Peripheral agents			
Guanadrel sulfate	Hylorel	1–75 (2)	(Postural hypotension, diarrhea)
Guanethidine monosulfate	Ismelin	10–150 (1)	(Postural hypotension, diarrhea)
Reserpine (G)[‡]	Serpasil	0.05–0.25 (1)	(Nasal congestion, sedation, depression, activation of peptic ulcer)

* These dosages may vary from those listed in the *Physicians' Desk Reference, 51st edition,* which may be consulted for additional information. The list of side effects is not all-inclusive, and side effects are for the class of drugs except where noted for individual drug (in parentheses); clinicians are urged to refer to the package insert for a more detailed listing.
[†] G indicates generic available.
[‡] Also acts centrally.

Table 2-4 Oral Antihypertensive Drugs (Continued)

Drug	Trade Name	Usual Dose Range, Total mg/day* (Frequency per Day)	Selected Side Effects and Comments*
Central α-antagonists			Sedation, dry mouth, bradycardia, withdrawal hypertension
Clonidine hydrochloride (G)	Catapres	0.2–1.2 (2–3)	(More withdrawal)
Guanabenz acetate (G)	Wytensin	8–32 (2)	
Guanfacine hydrochloride (G)	Tenex	1–3 (1)	(Less withdrawal)
Methyldopa (G)	Aldomet	500–3000 (2)	(Hepatic and "autoimmune" disorders)
α-Blockers			Postural hypotension
Doxazosin mesylate	Cardura	1–16 (1)	
Prazosin hydrochloride (G)	Minipress	2–30 (2–3)	
Terazosin hydrochloride	Hytrin	1–20(1)	
β-Blockers			Bronchospasm, bradycardia, heart failure, may mask insulin-induced hypoglycemia; *less serious:* impaired peripheral circulation, insomnia, fatigue, decreased exercise tolerance, hypertriglyceridemia (except agents with intrinsic sympathomimetic activity)
Acebutolol[§Π]	Sectral	200–800 (1)	
Atenolol (G)[§]	Tenormin	25–100 (1–2)	
Betaxolol hydrochloride[§]	Kerlone	5–20 (1)	
Bisoprolol fumarate[§]	Zebeta	2.5–10 (1)	
Carteolol hydrochloride[Π]	Cartrol	2.5–10 (1)	
Metoprolol tartrate (G)[§]	Lopressor	50–300 (2)	
Metoprolol succinate[§]	Toprol-XL	50–300 (1)	
Nadolol (G)	Corgard	40–320	

* These dosages may vary from those listed in the *Physicians' Desk Reference, 51st edition,* which may be consulted for additional information. The list of side effects is not all-inclusive, and side effects are for the class of drugs except where noted for individual drug (in parentheses); clinicians are urged to refer to the package insert for a more detailed listing.

[§] Cardioselective.

[Π] Has intrinsic sympathomimetic activity.

Table 2-4 Oral Antihypertensive Drugs (Continued)

Drug	Trade Name	Usual Dose Range, Total mg/day* (Frequency per Day)	Selected Side Effects and Comments*
Penbutolol sulfate[Π]	Levatol	10–20 (1)	
Pindolol (G)[Π]	Visken	10–60 (2)	
Propranolol hydrochloride (G)	Inderal	40–480 (2)	
	Inderal LA	40–480 (1)	
Timolol maleate (G)	Blocadren	20–60 (2) 0	Postural hypotension, bronchospasm
Combined α- and β-blockers			
Carvedilol	Coreg	12.5–50 (2)	
Labetalol hydrochloride (G)	Normodyne, Trandate	200–1200 (2)	
Direct vasodilators			Headaches, fluid retention, tachycardia
Hydralazine hydrochloride (G)	Apresoline	50–300 (2)	(Lupus syndrome)
Minoxidil (G)	Loniten	5–100 (1)	(Hirsutism)
Calcium antagonists			
Nondihydropyridines			Conduction defects, worsening of systolic dysfunction, gingival hyperplasia
Diltiazem hydrochloride	Cardizem SR	120–360 (2)	(Nausea, headache)
	Cardizem CD, Dilacor XR, Tiazac	120–360 (1)	
Mibefradil dihydrochloride (T-channel calcium antagonist)	Posicor	50–100 (1)	(No worsening of systolic dysfunction; contraindicated with terfenadine [Seldane], astemizole [Hismanal], and cisapride [Propulsid])
Verapamil hydrochloride	Isoptin SR, Calan SR	90–480 (2)	(Constipation)
	Verelan, Covera HS	120–480 (1)	
Dihydropyridines			Edema of the ankle, flushing, headache, gingival hypertrophy
Amlodipine besylate	Norvasc	2.5–10 (1)	

* These dosages may vary from those listed in the *Physicians' Desk Reference, 51st edition,* which may be consulted for additional information. The list of side effects is not all-inclusive, and side effects are for the class of drugs except where noted for individual drug (in parentheses); clinicians are urged to refer to the package insert for a more detailed listing.
[Π] Has intrinsic sympathomimetic activity.

Table 2-4 Oral Antihypertensive Drugs (Continued)

Drug	Trade Name	Usual Dose Range, Total mg/day* (Frequency per Day)	Selected Side Effects and Comments*
Felodipine	Plendil	2.5–20 (1)	
Isradipine	DynaCirc	5–20 (2)	
Nicardipine hydrochloride	Cardene SR	60–90 (2)	
Nifedipine	Procardia XL, Adalat CC	30–120 (1)	
Nisoldipine	Sular	20–60 (1)	
Angiotensin-converting enzyme inhibitors			*Common:* cough; *rare:* angioedema, hyperkalemia, rash, loss of taste, leukopenia
Benazepril hydrochloride	Lotensin	5–40 (1–2)	
Captopril (G)	Capoten	25–150 (2–3)	
Enalapril maleate	Vasotec	5–40 (1–2)	
Fosinopril sodium	Monopril	10–40 (1–2)	
Lisinopril	Prinivil, Zestril	5–40 (1)	
Moexipril	Univasc	7.5–15 (2)	
Quinapril hydrochloride	Accupril	5–80 (1–2)	
Ramipril	Altace	1.25–20 (1–2)	
Trandolapril	Mavik	1–4 (1)	
Angiotensin II receptor blockers			Angioedema (very rare), hyperkalemia
Losartan potassium	Cozaar	25–100 (1–2)	
Valsartan	Diovan	80–320 (1)	
Irbesartan	Avapro	150–300 (1)	

* These dosages may vary from those listed in the *Physicians' Desk Reference, 51st edition,* which may be consulted for additional information. The list of side effects is not all-inclusive, and side effects are for the class of drugs except where noted for individual drug (in parentheses); clinicians are urged to refer to the package insert for a more detailed listing.

(Reprinted from: Sixth report of the Joint National Committee on Prevention, Detection, Evaluation, and Treatment of High Blood Pressure. *Arch Intern Med.* 1997;157:2418. ©1997 American Medical Association.)

Table 2-5 Combination Drugs for Hypertension

Drug	Trade Name
β-Adrenergic blockers and diuretics	
Atenolol, 50 or 100 mg + chlorthalidone, 25 mg	Tenoretic
Bisoprolol fumarate, 2.5, 5, or 10 mg + hydrochlorothiazide, 6.25 mg	Ziac*
Metoprolol tartrate, 50 or 100 mg + hydrochlorothiazide, 25 or 50 mg	Lopressor HCT
Nadolol, 40 or 80 mg + bendroflumethiazide, 5 mg	Corzide
Propranolol hydrochloride, 40 or 80 mg + hydrochlorothiazide, 25 mg	Inderide
Propranolol hydrochloride (extended release), 80, 120, or 160 mg + hydrochlorothiazide, 50 mg	Inderide LA
Timolol maleate, 10 mg + hydrochlorothiazide, 25 mg	Timolide
Angiotensin-converting enzyme (ACE) inhibitors and diuretics	
Benazepril hydrochloride, 5, 10, or 20 mg + hydrochlorothiazide, 6.25, 12.5, or 25 mg	Lotensin HCT
Captopril, 25 or 50 mg + hydrochlorothiazide, 15 or 25 mg	Capozide*
Enalapril maleate, 5 or 10 mg + hydrochlorothiazide, 12.5 or 25 mg	Vaseretic
Lisinopril, 10 or 20 mg + hydrochlorothiazide, 12.5 or 25 mg	Prinzide, Zestoretic
Angiotensin II receptor antagonists and diuretics	
Losartan potassium, 50 mg + hydrochlorothiazide, 12.5 mg	Hyzaar
Calcium antagonists and ACE inhibitors	
Amlodipine besylate, 2.5 or 5 mg + benazepril hydrochloride, 10 or 20 mg	Lotrel
Diltiazem hydrochloride, 180 mg + enalapril maleate, 5 mg	Teczem
Verapamil hydrochloride (extended release), 180 or 240 mg + trandolapril, 1, 2, or 4 mg	Tarka
Felodipine, 5 mg + enalapril maleate, 5 mg	Lexxel
Other combinations	
Triamterene, 37.5, 50, or 75 mg + hydrochlorothiazide, 25 or 50 mg	Dyazide, Maxide
Spironolactone, 25 or 50 mg + hydrochlorothiazide, 25 or 50 mg	Aldactazide
Amiloride hydrochloride, 5 mg + hydrochlorothiazide, 50 mg	Moduretic
Guanethidine monosulfate, 10 mg + hydrochlorothiazide, 25 mg	Esimil
Hydralazine hydrochloride, 25, 50, or 100 mg + hydrochlorothiazide, 25 or 50 mg	Apresazide
Methyldopa, 250 or 500 mg + hydrochlorothiazide, 15, 25, 30, or 50 mg	Aldoril
Reserpine, 0.125 mg + hydrochlorothiazide, 25 or 50 mg	Hydropres
Reserpine, 0.10 mg + hydralazine hydrochloride, 25 mg + hydrochlorothiazide, 15 mg	Ser-Ap-Es
Clonidine hydrochloride, 0.1, 0.2, or 0.3 mg + chlorthalidone, 15 mg	Combipres
Methyldopa, 250 mg + chlorothiazide, 150 or 250 mg	Aldochlor
Reserpine, 0.125 or 0.25 mg + chlorthalidone, 25 or 50 mg	Demi-Regroton
Reserpine, 0.125 or 0.25 mg + chlorothiazide, 250 or 500 mg	Diupres
Prazosin hydrochloride, 1, 2, or 5 mg + polythiazide, 0.5 mg	Minizide

* Approved for initial therapy.

(Reprinted from: Sixth report of the Joint National Committee on Prevention, Detection, Evaluation, and Treatment of High Blood Pressure. *Arch Intern Med.* 1997;157:2417. ©1997 American Medical Association.)

Table 2-6 Considerations for Individualizing Antihypertensive Drug Therapy*

Indication	Drug Therapy
Compelling Indications Unless Contraindicated	
Diabetes mellitus (type 1) with proteinuria	ACE 1
Heart failure	ACE 1, diuretics
Isolated systolic hypertension (older patients)	Diuretics (preferred), CA (long-acting DHP)
Myocardial infarction	β-Blockers (non-ISA), ACE 1 (with systolic dysfunction)
May Have Favorable Effects on Comorbid Conditions[†]	
Angina	β-Blockers, CA
Atrial tachycardia and fibrillation	β-Blockers, CA (non-DHP)
Cyclosporine-induced hypertension (caution with the dose of cyclosporine)	CA
Diabetes mellitus (types 1 and 2) with proteinuria	ACE 1 (preferred), CA
Diabetes mellitus (type 2)	Low-dose diuretics
Dyslipidemia	α-Blockers
Essential tremor	β-Blockers (non-CS)
Heart failure	Carvedilol, losartan potassium
Hyperthyroidism	β-Blockers
Migraine	β-Blockers (non-CS), CA (non-DHP)
Myocardial infarction	Diltiazem hydrochloride, verapamil hydrochloride
Osteoporosis	Thiazides
Preoperative hypertension	β-Blockers
Prostatism (BPH)	α-Blockers
Renal insufficiency (caution in renovascular hypertension and creatinine level ≥265.2 μmol/L [≥3 mg/dL])	ACE I
May Have Unfavorable Effects on Comorbid Conditions[†‡]	
Bronchospastic disease	β-Blockers[§]
Depression	β-Blockers, central α-antagonists, reserpine[§]
Diabetes mellitus (types 1 and 2)	β-Blockers, high-dose diuretics
Dyslipidemia	β-Blockers (non-ISA), diuretics (high-dose)
Gout	Diuretics
2° or 3° heart block	β-Blockers,[§] CA (non-DHP)[§]
Heart failure	β-Blockers (except carvedilol), CA (except amlodipine besylate; felodipine)
Liver disease	Labetalol hydrochloride, methyldopa[§]
Peripheral vascular disease	β-Blockers
Pregnancy	ACE I,[§] angiotensin II receptor blockers[§]
Renal insufficiency	Potassium-sparing agents
Renovascular disease	ACE I, angiotensin II receptor blockers

* ACE I = angiotensin-converting enzyme inhibitors; BPH = benign prostatic hyperplasia; CA = calcium antagonists; DHP = dihydropyridine; ISA = intrinsic sympathomimetic activity; MI = myocardial infarction; non-CS = noncardioselective.

[†] Conditions and drugs are listed in alphabetical order.

[‡] These drugs may be used with special monitoring unless contraindicated.

[§] Contraindicated.

(Adapted from: Sixth report of the Joint National Committee on Prevention, Detection, Evaluation, and Treatment of High Blood Pressure. *Arch Intern Med.* 1997;157:2417. ©1997 American Medical Association.)

inhibitors are vasodilators that decrease vascular resistance while having less effect on plasma volume. Thus, left-ventricular hypertrophy may regress. The efficacy of ACE inhibitors is enhanced when they are used together with diuretics. Angiotensin II receptor blockers are more effective in high-renin types of hypertension. These drugs have been shown to be equipotent to ACE inhibitors, hydrochlorothiazide, beta blockers, and calcium channel blockers. The most common adverse effect of ACE inhibitors is a dry, nonproductive cough in 5%–20% of patients; the angiotensin II receptor blockers do not provoke cough. In general, angiotensin II receptor blockers are better tolerated (and more costly) than ACE inhibitors and are a useful alternative in patients who experience adverse effects from ACE inhibitors.

β-blockers

Circulating or locally released catecholamines stimulate β-adrenergic receptor sites, resulting in vasoconstriction, bronchodilation, tachycardia, and increased myocardial contractility. β-blockers reverse these effects. There are two types of β sites: $β_1$ is present on vascular and cardiac tissue, and $β_2$ is in the bronchial tree. In addition, β-blockers inhibit the release of renin, which is part of the angiotensin pathway.

The β-blockers can be divided into several groups: *nonselective* ($β_1$ and $β_2$), *cardioselective* (greater $β_1$ than $β_2$), and those with intrinsic sympathomimetic activity. Cardioselective agents cause the fewest asthmatic reactions and are less likely to delay recovery from hypoglycemia in diabetics. β-blockers with intrinsic sympathomimetic activity minimize the bradycardiac response of the other types of β-blockers.

$α_1$-blockers

When the postsynaptic $α_1$ receptors for catecholamines are blocked, both arterial and venous dilation occur, lowering peripheral vascular resistance. Although $α_1$-blockers cause less tachycardia than direct vasodilators, they produce more postural hypotension.

Direct vasodilators

Direct vasodilators lower peripheral vascular resistance. They frequently produce reflex tachycardia and, less often, cause orthostatic hypotension. These drugs are usually combined with a β-blocker or a central sympatholytic agent to minimize their effect on heart rate or cardiac output.

Calcium channel blockers

Calcium channel blockers inhibit the entry of calcium into smooth muscle cells. This effect reduces vascular contractility and decreases peripheral vascular resistance. However, they can partially block the SA and AV node as well as cause a negative inotropic effect in the heart. The three types of calcium channel blockers are phenylalkylamines (verapamil), dihydropyridines (eg, nifedipine, felodipine), and benzodiazepines (diltiazem).

Phenylalkylamines decrease cardiac output more than systemic vascular resistance. *Dihydropyridines* decrease vascular resistance more than cardiac output, and *benzodiazepines* reduce cardiac output and systemic vascular resistance equally. All types reduce renal afferent tone and cause an increase in salt and water excretion, lowering plasma volume.

Sympatholytics

The central sympatholytics affect the brain's vasomotor center, decreasing sympathetic output. This in turn reduces peripheral vascular resistance, cardiac output, and blood pressure.

Antihypertensive drugs are listed by brand name for convenient reference in Table 2-7. Selected drug interactions with antihypertensive therapy are listed in Table 2-8.

Moser M. National recommendations for the pharmacologic treatment of hypertension and should they be revised? *Arch Intern Med.* 1999;159:1403–1406.

The sixth report of the Joint National Committee on Prevention, Detection, Evaluation, and Treatment of High Blood Pressure. *Arch Intern Med.* 1997;157:2413–2446.

Table 2-7 Antihypertensive Drugs (by Brand Name)

Accupril—quinapril (**ACE**)
Aceon—perindopril (**ACE**)
Adalat—nifedipine (**Ca^{+2}**)
Aldactazide—HCTZ/spironolactone (**Dcomb**)
Aldactone—spironolactone (**K$^+$**)
Aldomet—methyldopa (**Symp**)
Aldoril—methyldopa/HCTZ (**Other**)
Altace—ramipril (**ACE**)
Apresoline—hydralazine (**Vaso**)
Atacand—candesartan (**ARB**)
Avapro—irbesartan (**ARB**)
Blocadren—timolol (**Beta**)
Bumex—bumetanide (**Loop**)
Calan—verapamil (**Ca^{+2}**)
Capoten—captopril (**ACE**)
Capozide—captopril/HCTZ (**ACE + D**)
Cardene—nicardipine (**Ca^{+2}**)
Cardizem—diltiazem (**Ca^{+2}**)
Cardura—doxazosin (**Alpha**)
Cartrol—carteolol (**Beta+**)
Catapres—clonidine (**Symp**)
Corgard—nadolol (**Beta**)
Corzide—nadolol/bendrof1umethiazide (**B + D**)
Cozaar—losartan (**AT-2**)
Demadex—torsemide (**Loop**)
Dilacor—diltiazem (**Ca^{+2}**)
Diuril—chlorothiazide (**TZ**)
Dyazide—HCTZ/triamterene (**Dcomb**)
DynaCirc—isradipine (**Ca^{+2}**)
Dyrenium—triamterene (**K$^+$**)
Enduron—methyclothiazide (**TZ**)
Esidrix—hydrochlorothiazide (**TZ**)
Hydropres—reserpine/HCTZ (**Other**)
Hygroton—chlorthalidone (**TZ**)
Hytrin—terazosin (**Alpha**)
Hyzaar—losartan/HCTZ (**AT-2 + D**)
Inderal—propranolol (**Beta**)
Inderide—propranolol/HCTZ (**B + D**)
Ismelin—guanethidine (**Periph**)
Isoptin—verapamil (**Ca^{+2}**)
Kerlone—betaxolol (**Beta**)

Lasix—furosemide (**Loop**)
Loniten—minoxidil (**Vaso**)
Lopressor—metoprolol (**Beta**)
Lopressor HCT—metoprolol/HCTZ (**B + D**)
Lotensin—benazepril (**ACE**)
Lotensin HCT—benazepril/HCTZ (**ACE + D**)
Lozol—indapamide (**TZ**)
Mavik—trandolapril (**ACE**)
Maxzide—HCTZ/triamterene (**Dcomb**)
Micardis—telmisartan (**ARB**)
Midamor—amiloride (**K+**)
Minipress—prazosin (**Alpha**)
Minizide—polythiazide (**TZ**)
Moduretic—HCTZ/amiloride (**Dcomb**)
Monopril—fosinopril (**ACE**)
Mykrox—metolazone (**TZ**)
Naqua—trichlormethiazide (**TZ**)
Normodyne—labetalol (**Beta+**)
Norvasc—amlodipine (**Ca^{+2}**)
Plendil—felodipine (**Ca^{+2}**)
Prinivil—lisinopril (**ACE**)
Prinizide—lisinopril/HCTZ (**ACE + D**)
Procardia—nifedipine (**Ca^{+2}**)
Sectral—acebutolol (**Beta+**)
Tenex—guanfacine (**Symp**)
Tenoretic—atenolol/chlorthalidone (**B + D**)
Tenormin—atenolol (**Beta**)
Teveten—eprosartan (**ARB**)
Timolide—timolol/HCTZ (**B + D**)
Toprol—metoprolol (**Beta**)
Trandate—labetalol (**Beta+**)
Univasc—moexipril (**ACE**)
Vaseretic—enalapril/HCTZ (**ACE + D**)
Vasotec—enalapril (**ACE**)
Verelan—verapamil (**Ca^{+2}**)
Visken—pindolol (**Beta+**)
Wytensin—guanabenz (**Symp**)
Zaroxolyn—metolazone (**TZ**)
Zebeta—bisoprolol (**Beta**)
Zestoretic—lisinopril/HCTZ (**ACE + D**)
Zestril—lisinopril (**ACE**)
Ziac—bisoprolol/HCTZ (**B + D**)

KEY

ACE = angiotensin-converting enzyme inhibitor
ACE + D = ACE inhibitor and diuretic
Alpha = α-adrenergic inhibitor
ARB = angiotensin II receptor blocker
AT-2 = angiotensin II receptor antagonist
AT-2 + D = angiotensin II receptor antagonist and diuretic
B + D = β-adrenergic blocker and diuretic
Beta = β-adrenergic blocker
Beta+ = β-adrenergic blocker with intrinsic sympathomimetic activity

Ca^{+2} = calcium channel blocker
Dcomb = diuretic combination
HCTZ = hydrochlorothiazide
K$^+$ = potassium-sparing diuretic
Loop = loop diuretic
Other = miscellaneous combination
Periph = peripheral adrenergic neuron antagonist
Symp = central sympatholytic
TZ = thiazide-type diuretic
Vaso = direct vasodilator

(Adapted from: Sixth report of the Joint National Committee on Prevention, Detection, Evaluation, and Treatment of High Blood Pressure. *Arch Intern Med.* 1997;157:2417. ©1997 American Medical Association.)

Table 2-8 Selected Drug Interactions with Antihypertensive Therapy*

Class of Agent	Increase Efficacy	Decrease Efficacy	Effect on Other Drugs
Diuretics	Diuretics that act at different sites in the nephron (eg, furosemide + thiazides)	Resin-binding agents NSAIDs Steroids	Diuretics raise serum lithium levels Potassium-sparing agents may exacerbate hyperkalemia due to ACE inhibitors
β-Blockers	Cimetidine (hepatically metabolized β-blockers) Quinidine (hepatically metabolized β-blockers) Food (hepatically metabolized β-blockers)	NSAIDs Withdrawal of clonidine Agents that induce hepatic enzymes, including rifampin and phenobarbital	Propranolol hydrochloride induces hepatic enzymes to increase clearance of drugs with similar metabolic pathways β-Blockers may mask and prolong insulin-induced hypoglycemia Heart block may occur with nondihydropyridine calcium antagonists Sympathomimetics cause unopposed α-adrenoceptor-mediated vasoconstriction β-Blockers increase angina-inducing potential of cocaine
ACE inhibitors	Chlorpromazine or clozapine	NSAIDs Antacids Food decreases absorption (moexipril)	ACE inhibitors may raise serum lithium levels ACE inhibitors may exacerbate hyperkalemic effect of potassium-sparing diuretics

* For initial drug therapy recommendations, see *Physicians' Desk Reference, 51st edition,* and *Cardiovascular Pharmacotherapeutics* (New York: McGraw-Hill; 1997). NSAIDs = nonsteroidal anti-inflammatory agents; ACE = angiotensin-converting enzyme.

Table 2-8 Selected Drug Interactions with Antihypertensive Therapy* (Continued)

Class of Agent	Increase Efficacy	Decrease Efficacy	Effect on Other Drugs
Calcium antagonists	Grapefruit juice (some dihydropyridines) Cimetidine or ranitidine (hepatically metabolized calcium antagonists)	Agents that induce hepatic enzymes, including rifampin and phenobarbital	Cyclosporine levels increase[†] with diltiazem hydrochloride, verapamil hydrochloride, mibefradil dihydrochloride, or nicardipine hydrochloride (but not felodipine, isradipine, or nifedipine) Nondihydropyridines increase levels of other drugs metabolized by the same hepatic enzyme system, including digoxin, quinidine, sulfonylureas, and theophylline Verapamil hydrochloride may lower serum lithium levels
α-Blockers			Prazosin hydrochloride may decrease clearance of verapamil hydrochloride
Central α_2-agonists and peripheral neuronal blockers		Tricyclic antidepressants (and probably phenothiazines) Monoamine oxidase inhibitors Sympathomimetics or phenothiazines antagonize guanethidine monosulfate or guanadrel sulfate Iron salts may reduce methyldopa absorption	Methyldopa may increase serum lithium levels Severity of clonidine hydrochloride withdrawal may be increased by β-blockers Many agents used in anesthesia are potentiated by clonidine hydrochloride

[†] This is a clinically and economically beneficial drug-drug interaction because it both retards progression of accelerated atherosclerosis in heart transplant recipients and reduces the required daily dose of cyclosporine.

CHAPTER 3

Cerebrovascular Disease

Recent Developments

- Intravenous thrombolysis with tissue plasminogen activator is safe and improves outcome if treatment is initiated within 3 hours after the onset of symptoms.
- Carotid endarterectomy is highly beneficial in reducing stroke in symptomatic patients with severe carotid stenosis (>70%).
- Aspirin offers a moderate benefit in preventing recurrent stroke.

Introduction

Vascular stroke is the third leading cause of death in developed countries, ranking behind heart disease and cancer. In the United States, approximately 750,000 strokes occur annually with a mortality rate exceeding 20%. Stroke is the leading cause of long-term disability in America today. Vascular stroke results from two major causes: cerebral ischemia and intracranial hemorrhage. For extensive discussion of the ophthalmologic manifestations of cerebrovascular disease, see BCSC Section 5, *Neuro-Ophthalmology.*

Cerebral Ischemia and Infarction

Cerebral ischemia results from interference with the circulation to the brain. The reduction in blood flow may be generalized or localized. Ischemia must be distinguished from hypoxemia due to such causes as carbon monoxide poisoning, chronic obstructive pulmonary disease, and pulmonary emboli. Other conditions that may mimic strokes include encephalitis, hypoglycemia, seizures, brain tumor, hypertension encephalopathy, and migraine.

Clinical manifestations of cerebral ischemia are paresis, paresthesia, amaurosis fugax, and facial paresthesias. Vertebrobasilar symptoms include vertigo, diplopia, binocular visual loss, ataxia, paresis, paresthesia, dysarthria, headache, nausea, and vomiting. Cardiac emboli can produce symptoms similar to insufficiency of the internal carotid or vertebrobasilar arteries; thus, transient symptoms do not constitute definitive evidence of an arterial abnormality in the carotid or vertebrobasilar territory. There are varying degrees of ischemia, which may be classified by severity and duration.

Transient ischemic attacks (TIAs) are a loss of neurologic function caused by ischemia. They are abrupt in onset, persist for less than 24 hours, and clear without residual signs. Most TIAs last only a few minutes. *Reversible ischemic neurologic disability* is a loss of neurologic function persisting for more than 24 hours but less than 7 days that leaves no lasting symptoms or signs. A *partial nonprogressive stroke* is an ischemic event that leaves a persistent disability but is short of a calamitous stroke. A *completed stroke* is an ischemic event that produces a major degree of permanent neurologic disability. Most ischemic strokes consist of small regions of complete ischemia in conjunction with a large area of incomplete ischemia. This ischemic but not infarcted area has been termed the *penumbra.* Recent studies have demonstrated that the penumbra is dynamic and have changed the once passive approach to treating patients with acute cerebral ischemia.

Medium- and small-artery disease caused by hypertension, diabetes, and atherosclerosis accounts for the majority of strokes. The most common site for obstructive disease of the carotid artery is in the region of the carotid sinus, followed by the portion within the cavernous sinus. Strokes caused by emboli of cardiac origin account for 20% of the total. Mural thrombi forming on the endocardium in conjunction with myocardial infarction account for 8%–10%. Atrial fibrillation, mitral stenosis, mitral valve prolapse, and atrial myxoma are other cardiac conditions associated with intracranial embolism.

Nonarteriosclerotic angiopathies capable of causing TIA and stroke include aortic dissection and inflammatory arteritis (eg, collagen vascular disease, giant cell arteritis, meningovascular syphilis, and moyamoya disease). Moyamoya disease is a rare vaso-occlusive disease of the carotid and cerebral arteries that causes TIA symptoms or hemorrhagic strokes in children and young adults. Moyamoya disease was originally described in Japanese patients in the 1960s but has been reported more recently in the United States and Europe as well.

Other conditions with potential for altering blood coagulation and leading to cerebral ischemia include pregnancy and the postpartum period, use of oral contraceptives, postoperative and posttraumatic states, hyperviscosity syndromes, polycythemia, and sickle cell disease.

Diagnostic Studies

Investigation of the systemic arteries and the heart is essential in determining the cause of cerebral ischemia. Differences in upper limb pulses and blood pressure may indicate serious subclavian disease. Multiple bruits may suggest widespread arterial disease but may be present without significant occlusion. Evidence for a cardiac embolic source should be pursued aggressively, especially in younger normotensive persons with cerebral ischemia. *Electrocardiography* should be routine to exclude cardiac dysrhythmia and occult myocardial infarction.

Echocardiography is often helpful in excluding intracardiac emboli. *Transesophageal Doppler echocardiography* is most sensitive in this regard. *Lumbar puncture* is required in rare cases of stroke or TIA, particularly if meningovascular syphilis is a serious consideration. *Duplex ultrasonography* is a noninvasive technique to detect obstructive or stenotic carotid artery disease; *transcranial Doppler* continues arterial examination to the intracranial branches of the internal carotid artery.

Ideally, all suspected cases of stroke and threatened stroke should prompt *computerized tomography (CT)* of the brain. *Magnetic resonance imaging (MRI)* is often more sensitive in detecting early cerebral infarction, whereas CT is very sensitive to the presence of intracranial hemorrhage. These techniques can distinguish among cerebral hemorrhage, old and recent infarction, and hemorrhagic infarction; such techniques can also exclude unsuspected space-occupying lesions. *Magnetic resonance cerebral angiography* may be needed if the neurologic event cannot be differentiated by clinical criteria from an arteriovenous malformation, cerebrovascular malformation, or giant aneurysm. *Diffusion-weighted* and *perfusion-weighted MRI* are new techniques that are useful in the evaluation of early cerebral ischemia and regional blood flow. They may help to open an early window of opportunity during which treatment is beneficial in salvaging tissue at risk. Cerebral arteriography is required if intra-arterial thrombolysis is being strongly considered.

Treatment

Treatment of threatened stroke includes reduction of risk factors when possible. Hypertension should be controlled, although blood pressure reduction during acute ischemic stroke may cause harmful decreases in local perfusion. Control of both hyperlipidemia and diabetes is indicated. Cigarette smoking and excessive alcohol consumption should be eliminated. The use of anticoagulant drugs, such as heparin and warfarin sodium, is widely accepted in threatened stroke from emboli arising in mural thrombi following myocardial infarction and in nonvalvular atrial fibrillation.

Controlled studies have not demonstrated the effectiveness of anticoagulants in the treatment of TIAs in the carotid and vertebrobasilar territory. Heparin is not helpful in patients with completed stroke but can be useful in ischemic stroke to prevent deep venous thrombosis. Because of the associated risk of hemorrhage in the ischemic area, there is no consensus on the best time to start anticoagulant therapy.

Antiplatelet therapy with aspirin is beneficial in patients with cardiac cerebral emboli who cannot tolerate long-term use of anticoagulant drugs. Recent clinical trials indicate that aspirin offers a moderate benefit in the prevention of recurrent stroke. Low doses of aspirin (160–300 mg daily) cause less gastrointestinal discomfort than higher doses and reduce the incidence of stroke in patients with unstable angina or acute myocardial infarction. Ticlopidine (Ticlid) is a platelet-inhibiting drug proven beneficial in clinical trials. It alters platelet membrane fibrinogen interaction but does not affect the cyclooxygenase pathway. Side effects include bone-marrow suppression, rash, and commonly (22% of cases) diarrhea. Clopidogrel (Plavix) prevents clot formation in a similar fashion as ticlopidine and initially appears to have a more promising side effect profile. Clopidogrel was more likely to cause rash and diarrhea than aspirin.

Recent studies have further investigated the role of thrombolytic agents for acute ischemic stroke. The National Institute of Neurologic Disorders and Stroke Recombinant Tissue Plasminogen Activator Stroke study supports the use of tissue plasminogen activator for the treatment of acute ischemic stroke in patients who meet certain eligibility requirements, if treatment is initiated within 3 hours after the onset of symptoms. Tissue plasminogen activator is administered intravenously. However, use of this agent incurred a 6.4% risk of symptomatic intracerebral hemorrhage. The risk of intracerebral hemorrhage was unacceptably high in trials utilizing intravenous streptokinase. Another thrombolytic agent in the treatment of acute ischemic stroke is urokinase, which has been used intra-arterially up to 6 hours after symptom onset. Urokinase may play a role in patients with occlusion of the middle cerebral artery and possibly in basilar artery occlusion. Ancrod is a fibrinogenolytic agent that may increase the chance of total or near-total recovery in patients with stroke.

Intracranial Hemorrhage

Intracranial hemorrhage constitutes approximately 15% of acute cerebrovascular disorders. Bleeding from aneurysms of arteries composing the circle of Willis, bleeding from arterioles damaged by hypertension or arteriosclerosis, and trauma are the most common causes of intracranial hemorrhage. Although there are many causes of intracranial hemorrhage, the anatomic location of the bleeding greatly influences the clinical picture. By location, hemorrhages can be grouped into the following general categories:

- Subarachnoid hemorrhage
- Intracerebral hemorrhage
- Surface bleeding that extends into the brain
- Intraventricular hemorrhage

Aneurysms that rupture entirely into the subarachnoid space present with features of meningeal irritation or a transient increase in intracranial pressure. The most common symptom of subarachnoid hemorrhage is the sudden development of a violent, usually localized, headache. This headache is at first frontal or temporal, later becoming occipital and then spreading to involve the entire head and neck. In an adult not prone to headaches, a moderately intense headache (with or without associated neck stiffness) that disappears in 2–3 days may be a sign of a warning leak. Brief loss of consciousness or a seizure preceded by an awareness of dizziness or vertigo and by vomiting are common at the onset. Common physical signs include neck rigidity, fundus or preretinal hemorrhages, and cranial nerve palsies.

Vascular malformations within and on the surface of the brain parenchyma commonly present with seizures and headaches, less often with hemorrhage. Arteriovenous malformations produce symptoms more commonly than other types of cerebrovascular malformations.

Hypertensive-arteriosclerotic intracerebral hemorrhages are often catastrophic events. Headache is a predominant feature at the onset in at least one half of hemorrhages and, by contrast, in less than one fourth of thromboembolisms. Vomiting is prominent as an early symptom. Restlessness and vomiting are more common with hemorrhage than with infarction. Generalized seizures are common with intracerebral hemorrhage, are less frequent with subarachnoid hemorrhage, and are uncommon (<10% of cases) with cerebral infarction.

Arterial "berry" aneurysms are round or saccular dilatations characteristically found at arteriole bifurcations on the circle of Willis and its major branches or connections. Intracranial aneurysms occur in all age groups but most commonly rupture in the fifth, sixth, and seventh decades of life. Approximately 85% of congenital berry aneurysms develop in the anterior part of the circle of Willis derived from the internal carotid artery in its major branches. The most common site is at the origin of the posterior communicating artery from the internal carotid artery. Such an aneurysm typically presents with headache and third nerve palsy involving the pupil. Vascular malformations within and on the surface of the brain parenchyma constitute about 7% of cases with subarachnoid hemorrhage. Four varieties are recognized:

- Capillary telangiectasia
- Cavernous angioma
- Venous angioma
- Arteriovenous malformation (AVM)

Capillary telangiectasias are most commonly discovered as incidental postmortem findings in the brain stem. Venous angiomas are cerebrovascular abnormalities often associated with the Sturge-Weber syndrome. These lesions are best identified by MRI.

The most important clues in the diagnosis of hypertensive intracranial hemorrhage are explosive onset, history of high blood pressure, early decline of the level of consciousness, and detection of meningeal irritation and blood in the spinal fluid (preferably by CT) with evidence of a focal lesion. Little other than the past history clinically distinguishes the symptoms of subarachnoid hemorrhage resulting from the rupture of an AVM from those caused by a ruptured aneurysm. Focal neurologic signs and evidence of the sudden development of a mass lesion frequently accompany a rupture.

Findings that suggest an AVM as the cause of subarachnoid hemorrhage include a history of previous focal seizures, slow stepwise progression of focal neurologic signs, and occasionally recurrent unilateral throbbing headache resembling migraine. In addition to meningeal irritation and focal neurologic signs reflecting bleeding, a bruit is present over the orbit or skull in approximately 40% of patients.

Immediate CT examination demonstrates blood in the subarachnoid space in about 95% of the cases of ruptured aneurysm or AVM. CT identifies the size and location of intracerebral hemorrhages, as well as the degree of surrounding edema and the amount and location of any distortion of the brain. CT can identify blood in the subarachnoid space or brain and ventricles in 95% of patients with subarachnoid hemorrhage.

If subarachnoid hemorrhage is suspected and CT results are negative, lumbar puncture is indicated. CT should always be carried out first to rule out a mass lesion. Arteriography remains the definitive procedure to identify an aneurysm or AVM. Angiography is essential to identify areas of local or general vasospasm and should be performed in all cases of subarachnoid hemorrhage that are considered reasonable operative risks or when the diagnosis is in doubt.

Initial restoration of normal blood pressure and its maintenance at normal levels is mandatory in the treatment of ruptured aneurysms. Surgical intervention is best accomplished by placing a small clip or ligature across the neck of the sac. If the aneurysm cannot be directly obliterated, surgical ligation of a proximal vessel may be necessary. Symptomatic AVMs can sometimes be dissected and removed, depending on location. Proton-beam irradiation remains controversial. Ligation of the feeding vessels coupled with balloon catheter embolization may be carried out. Treatment of intracerebral hemorrhage is mostly unsatisfactory.

Carotid Artery Disease

Asymptomatic carotid bruits occur in 4% of the population over age 40. The annual stroke rate in patients with an asymptomatic bruit is 1.5%. This same population has an annual mortality rate of 4%, primarily from complications of heart disease. Bruit is more a marker for the presence of arteriosclerotic disease than a predictor of stroke. Patients with asymptomatic carotid bruits should be screened for risk factors related to atherosclerosis: hypertension, smoking, and hypercholesterolemia. The degree and severity of stenosis should be determined by noninvasive studies. Patients with asymptomatic carotid stenosis have a 2% annual risk of ipsilateral stroke.

In the Asymptomatic Carotid Atherosclerosis Study, patients with asymptomatic stenosis of greater than 60% were randomized to either carotid endarterectomy (CEA) or medical treatment. Although the estimated 5-year risk of stroke was 53% lower (5.1% vs. 11.0%) for the CEA group, the only significant difference was in the frequency of TIA or minor stroke ipsilateral to the CEA. No significant differences were discerned between the medical and surgical groups with regard to major ipsilateral stroke or death, and the benefits disappear with operative risk of greater than 3%. Therefore, patients with asymptomatic carotid stenosis of greater than 60% may be considered for elective CEA; patients with less than 60% stenosis should be retested at intervals of 6–12 months and followed for disease progression. Aspirin (325 mg daily) and risk factor reduction are also employed in this patient group.

Ocular and cerebral conditions associated with carotid stenosis include amaurosis fugax, ocular ischemic syndromes, TIAs, and stroke. The ophthalmologist is often the first physician to see a patient with amaurosis fugax or ocular ischemia. Amaurosis is usually embolic, having either a carotid or a cardiac source. The annual stroke rate among patients with isolated amaurosis fugax is thought to be approximately 2%. A cardiac source of embolization should be excluded for all patients presenting with isolated amaurosis fugax or transient visual loss. The best procedure for this is transesophageal cardiac ultrasonography. Untreated patients with amaurosis fugax, retinal plaques, retinal infarcts, or any combination thereof share with TIA patients not only an equal prevalence of carotid stenosis but also a 30% 5-year expectancy rate for myocardial infarction and an 18% death rate during the same interval.

If evidence suggests that a carotid lesion is the cause of the amaurosis fugax, or if venous stasis retinopathy is present, duplex scanning should be performed to determine the presence of vessel wall disease or carotid stenosis.

No hard data are currently available from which to make a clear recommendation about an appropriate course of therapy. It appears that a trial of aspirin (325 mg/day) should be the initial approach for all patients. Ticlopidine or clopidogrel therapy may be considered for patients unable to take aspirin. CEA with electroencephalographic monitoring should be considered only if the surgeon has a perioperative morbidity rate of less than 3% and if any of the following conditions exist:

- Antiplatelet therapy proves to be ineffective
- Stenosis appears to be progressive
- The patient has no operative risk factors

Patients with TIA or previous stroke in the territory of carotid stenosis are judged to be symptomatic. The risk of stroke within a year of symptom onset is 10% in patients with TIA; the risk thereafter is about 6% per year with a 5-year risk of 35%–50%.

In the North American Symptomatic Carotid Endarterectomy Trial, CEA was evaluated in patients with a recent (within 120 days) hemispheric or retinal TIA or a recent nondisabling stroke, who had high-grade (70%–99%) stenosis in the ipsilateral carotid artery. All of the patients received optimal medical care, including antiplatelet therapy with aspirin, as well as treatment for hypertension, hyperlipidemia, or diabetes, when appropriate. The surgical group experienced lower rates of ipsilateral stroke (9.0% vs. 26.0%), any stroke (12.6% vs. 27.6%), major or fatal stroke (3.7% vs. 13.1%), and death from all causes (4.6% vs. 6.3%). The perioperative mortality rate was only 0.6%, and the perioperative rate of major stroke or death was 2.1%. The benefit of surgery for reducing the risk of ipsilateral stroke increased with higher degrees of stenosis: 12% risk reduction for 70%–79% stenosis; 18% risk reduction for 80%–89% stenosis; and 26% risk reduction for 90%–99% stenosis. The European Carotid Surgery Trial also demonstrated a statistically significant benefit for CEA in selected patients with greater than 70% stenosis. Uncertainty continues regarding CEA for symptomatic stenosis in the range of 30%–69%.

The risks of major morbidity and mortality with CEA are proportional to the severity of neurologic illness and comorbid factors such as ischemic heart disease. The risks for patients with symptomatic unilateral high-grade stenosis and favorable comorbidity are 1%–3% in the hands of capable surgeons. The long-term restenosis rate following CEA is about 10% at 5 years.

It is feasible to reopen the internal carotid artery after acute (<8 hours) occlusion. The risks are high with emergency CEA, however, and the success rate is less than 50%. Patients with carotid occlusion are usually placed on warfarin therapy for several months in the hope of decreasing distal thrombus progression and subsequent embolic stroke.

In summary, patients with symptomatic carotid stenosis exceeding 70% should be considered for CEA unless there is acute stroke, maximal neurologic defect, or other medical contraindication to surgery. The major perioperative morbidity and mortality rates for the surgical team should not exceed 5% for patients with TIA, 7% for patients with minor stroke, or 10% for patients with recurrent stenosis.

The following approach to a patient presenting with a cerebral or retinal TIA should be considered:

- The patient should be evaluated for the presence of risk factors associated with atherogenesis: hypertension, diabetes mellitus, obesity, hyperlipidemia, and smoking.
- Appropriate medical therapy should be instituted.
- The presence of coronary artery disease and a cardiac source of emboli should be excluded by appropriate testing.
- The patency of the extracranial carotid artery system should be determined using duplex ultrasonography.

If ipsilateral carotid stenosis exceeds 70%, if bilateral carotid stenosis greater than 50% is present, or if long-term evidence indicates progressive disease, CEA should be considered—but only if the surgeon's perioperative stroke and death rate is less than 3%. Otherwise, antiplatelet therapy with aspirin (325 mg/day), clopidogrel, or ticlopidine should be initiated. A patient presenting with TIA symptoms who has previously undergone CEA should be evaluated and treated similarly. Special attention should be paid to the evaluation of early restenosis and thrombosis.

As an additional note, elevated plasma homocysteine levels have been linked to extracranial carotid stenosis and directly to an increased risk of stroke and occlusive vascular disease. Folic acid reduces this risk by lowering plasma homocysteine levels. Folates naturally occur in green vegetables and are supplemented in bread and breakfast cereals in the United States. Therefore, increasing dietary folic acid intake can be recommended to all patients with carotid stenosis and generalized cardiovascular disease. Dietary antioxidants (ie, vitamin C and vitamin E) may also play a role in the pathophysiology of stroke. Because of the low cost and low risk of these supplements, physicians may choose to recommend them for patients at risk.

Barnett HJ, Eliasziw M, Meldrum HE, et al. Drugs and surgery in the prevention of ischemic stroke. *N Engl J Med.* 1995;332:238–246.

Beauchamp NJ, Bryan RN. Acute cerebral ischemic infarction: a pathophysiologic review and radiologic perspective. *AJR Am J Roentgenol.* 1998;171:73–84.

Brott T, Bogousslavsky J. Treatment of acute ischemic stroke. *N Engl J Med.* 2000;343:710–722.

Moore WS, Barnett HJ, Beebe HG, et al. Guidelines for carotid endarterectomy: a multidisciplinary consensus statement from the ad hoc Committee, American Heart Association. *Stroke.* 1995;26:188–201.

Selhub J, Jacques PF, Bostrom AG, et al. Association between plasma homocysteine concentration and extracranial carotid artery stenosis. *N Engl J Med.* 1995;332:286–291.

CHAPTER 4

Acquired Heart Disease

Recent Developments

- Cardiac-specific troponins gain acceptance as the primary biochemical marker of cardiac injury in acute coronary syndromes.
- Potential new coronary artery disease (CAD) risk factors include homocysteine, fibrinogen, and C-reactive protein.
- Implantable cardioverter-defibrillator (ICDs) are the preferred first-line therapy for patients who have survived a cardiac arrest or an episode of hemodynamically unstable ventricular tachycardia.
- New pharmacologic adjuncts for the management of acute coronary syndromes include low-molecular-weight heparin and glycoprotein IIb/IIIa inhibitors.
- Use of coronary stents continues to grow. Indications now include the revascularization of an acute coronary syndrome.

Ischemic Heart Disease

Pathophysiology

Ischemia is defined as a local, temporary oxygen deprivation associated with inadequate removal of metabolites caused by reduced tissue perfusion. *Ischemic heart disease (IHD)* is typically caused by decreased perfusion of the myocardium secondary to stenotic or obstructed coronary arteries. The balance between arterial supply and myocardial demand for oxygen determines whether ischemia occurs. Significant coronary stenosis, thrombosis, occlusion, reduced arterial pressure, hypoxemia, or severe anemia can impede the supply of oxygen to the myocardium. On the demand side, an increase in heart rate, ventricular contractility, or wall tension (which is determined by systolic arterial pressure, ventricular volume, and ventricular wall thickness) may each cause increased utilization of oxygen. When the demand for oxygen exceeds the supply, ischemia occurs. If this ischemia becomes prolonged, infarction and myocardial necrosis result. The necrotic process begins in the subendocardium, usually after about 20 minutes of coronary obstruction, and progresses to transmural and complete infarction in 4–6 hours.

Atherosclerosis

Coronary artery atherosclerosis is by far the most common cause of cardiac ischemia. Other disorders that may also result in regional or generalized ischemia include coronary artery spasm, coronary arteritis, intercoronary shunting, severe anemia, hypoxemia, or reduced arterial perfusion pressure.

Atherosclerosis is a thickening and hardening of medium-size and larger arteries. Progressive changes in the arteries take the form of intimal fatty streaks, followed by fibrous plaques, then atherosclerotic plaques. Atherosclerotic plaques narrow the arterial lumen by the focal accumulation of lipids, fibrous tissue, and blood products in the intima of the arteries. Atherosclerotic lesions in the heart primarily involve the vessels on the epicardial surface of the heart and not the small arterioles within the myocardium itself. Small-vessel CAD appears to be distinct from atherosclerosis and is more common in patients with diabetes, hypertension, collagen vascular diseases, amyloidosis, and cardiomyopathies. Atherosclerosis also occurs in arteries outside the heart. Therefore, patients with IHD are at increased risk for peripheral vascular disease and cerebrovascular disease, and vice versa.

The major cause of morbidity and mortality associated with coronary atherosclerosis is plaque rupture, which often results in one of the *acute coronary syndromes*: unstable angina, non–Q wave myocardial infarction (MI), or Q wave MI.

Risk Factors

The most widely accepted risk factors for atherosclerosis and IHD are cigarette smoking, elevated serum cholesterol, hypertension, a family history of IHD, and diabetes mellitus. Obesity, sedentary lifestyle, stress, personality type, use of oral contraceptive drugs, and menopause are of less clear significance. Lipids other than cholesterol are also important in assessing the risk of CAD. However, our understanding of the causes of CAD is incomplete. Half of patients with CAD do not have these traditional risk factors. This finding has prompted a search for new biological markers. New potential risk factors include elevated levels of homocysteine, fibrinogen, and C-reactive protein. However, these substances have not been studied enough to support routine testing for them.

Clinical Syndromes

Clinical presentations of IHD include:

- Angina pectoris: stable angina, variant (Prinzmetal) angina
- Acute coronary syndromes: unstable angina, non–Q wave MI, Q wave MI
- Congestive heart failure
- Sudden cardiac death
- Asymptomatic IHD

Angina pectoris

The cardinal symptom in patients with IHD is *angina pectoris,* usually manifested as a substernal pressure–like pain or tightness that is often triggered by physical exertion, emotional distress, or eating. Angina typically lasts 5–10 minutes and is usually relieved by rest, nitroglycerin, or both. Patients may present with pain radiating into other areas, including the jaw, arm, neck, shoulder, back, chest wall, or abdomen. Occasionally, angina may be misinterpreted as indigestion or musculoskeletal pain. The level of physical activity that results in angina pectoris is clinically significant, and it is useful in determining the severity of CAD, treatment, and prognosis. Myocardial ischemia may be painless in diabetic patients, often delaying the diagnosis until the disease is more advanced. The pain associated with MI is similar to angina, but classically it is usually more severe and more prolonged.

Stable angina pectoris Angina is considered stable if it responds to rest or nitroglycerin and if the patterns of frequency, ease of onset, duration, and response to medication have not changed substantially over 3 months.

Variant (Prinzmetal) angina Variant angina occurs at rest and is not related to physical exertion. The ST segment is elevated on electrocardiography during the anginal episodes, which are caused by coronary artery spasm. Underlying atherosclerosis is present in 60%–80% of cases, and thrombosis and occlusion may result during the episodes of coronary spasm.

Acute coronary syndrome (ACS)

Advances in our understanding of the pathophysiology of IHD have led to a reorganization of the clinical presentations into what is now called the *acute coronary syndromes.* The ACSs represent the pathological continuum of unstable angina, non–Q wave infarction, and Q wave infarction. Plaque rupture is considered to be the common underlying event.

Unstable angina and non–Q wave myocardial infarction The presentations of unstable angina and non–Q wave MI are similar. They may be characterized by a significant increase in the frequency or duration of chest pain (with or without a decrease in the level of physical activity required to provoke angina) or as angina at rest. These presentations differ primarily in whether the ischemia is severe enough to cause myocardial necrosis. The electrocardiogram typically demonstrates ST segment depression, T wave inversion, or both. If it is established that no biochemical marker of myocardial necrosis has been released, the patient may be considered to have experienced unstable angina. When clinical evidence of necrosis is detected by cardiac enzyme testing and no pathological Q waves evolve on the electrocardiogram, the diagnosis is non–Q wave MI, a condition midway between unstable angina and Q-wave infarction. Plaque rupture in unstable angina and non–Q wave MI is typically accompanied by a less obstructive thrombus or lesser amounts of fibrin formation compared with what occurs in Q wave MI.

Q wave myocardial infarction Q wave MI usually occurs when plaque rupture results in a completely occlusive thrombus. Typically, ST segment elevation is apparent on the ECG. Necrosis involving the full or nearly full thickness of the ventricular wall in the distribution of the affected artery ultimately occurs, leading to Q waves on the ECG.

Myocardial infarction: general considerations MI may occur suddenly, without warning, in a previously asymptomatic patient or in a patient with stable or variant angina; MI may also follow a period of unstable angina. Patients commonly experience chest pain, nausea, vomiting, diaphoresis, weakness, anxiety, dyspnea, lightheadedness, and palpitations. Nearly 25% of myocardial infarcts are painless; painless MI is more common in diabetics and with increasing age. These patients may present with congestive heart failure or syncope. Symptoms may begin during or after exertion or at rest.

The clinical findings in IHD vary and depend on the location and severity of myocardial ischemia or injury. Approximately half of all infarctions involve the inferior myocardial wall, and most of the remaining half involve the anterior regions. Examination may reveal pallor, coolness of the extremities, low-grade fever, signs of pulmonary congestion and increased central venous pressure (if left-ventricular dysfunction is present), an S_3 or S_4 gallop, an apical systolic murmur (caused by papillary muscle dysfunction), hypertension, or hypotension. The ECG may demonstrate a variety of ST segment and T wave changes and arrhythmias.

Subendocardial (non–Q wave, nontransmural) infarcts usually result in a smaller region of myocardial injury and cause less ventricular dysfunction and heart failure. However, the patient with a non–Q wave infarction may be considered to have an incomplete infarction, with potential for reocclusion of the affected artery. Not surprisingly, these patients experience a greater incidence of post-MI angina and reinfarction during the initial hospitalization and during the first 6 months following the infarction. Approximately 20% experience an acute Q wave infarction within 3 months. Although the in-hospital prognosis for patients with non–Q wave infarction is better than that for patients with Q wave infarction, the prognosis at 6–12 months tends to equalize. As such, patients with non–Q wave infarction constitute a specific subgroup requiring aggressive diagnostic evaluation and treatment. Detection and dilation or bypass of a high-grade coronary stenosis may prevent subsequent reinfarction.

About 60% of patients who die of cardiac disease expire suddenly before reaching the hospital. The prognosis for those hospitalized with MI, on the other hand, has become remarkably good. In some recent studies using thrombolytic therapy, the mortality rate has been in the range of 5%–8%. Mortality is affected by a wide variety of factors, such as the degree of heart failure, myocardial damage, severity of the underlying atherosclerotic process, heart size, and previous ischemia.

The complications of MI depend on its severity. Regional and global ventricular contractile dysfunction may result in congestive heart failure or pulmonary edema. Mild to moderate heart failure occurs in nearly 50% of patients following MI, and severe heart failure in about 15%. Cardiogenic shock, which results in a dramatic fall in systemic blood pressure, is observed in 10% of patients with MI and carries a mortality rate of over 75%. Rupture of the ventricular septum or a papillary muscle is uncommon, with each occurring in about 5% of patients. Rupture of the left ventricular wall, which may occur at any time within 2 weeks, has been found to be the cause of sudden death in about 9% of autopsies after acute MI. Some patients experience post-MI pericarditis, characterized by a pericardial friction rub 2–3 days after infarction. When accompanied by fever, arthralgia, and pleuropericardial pain, the diagnosis is most likely *post-MI, or Dressler, syndrome.* This condition is treated with aspirin, nonsteroidal anti-inflammatory agents, or corticosteroids. Injury along the conduction pathways of the atria or ventricles may result in bradycardia, heart block, supraventricular tachycardias, or ventricular arrhythmias. Arrhythmias often exacerbate ischemic injury by reducing the perfusion pressure in the coronary arteries. Most acute deaths from MI result from arrhythmia.

An important aim of a good cardiac program is to enable patients to return to their usual jobs after discharge from the hospital. About 80%–90% of patients with uncomplicated MI can return to work within 2–3 months. Patients are advised to modify or eliminate their risk factors for atherosclerosis. Dietary programs, reduction of physiologic and psychological stress, and a cardiac rehabilitation program benefit many patients.

Congestive heart failure secondary to IHD

Congestive heart failure is discussed later in this chapter.

Sudden cardiac death

Sudden cardiac death is usually caused by a severe arrhythmia, such as ventricular tachycardia, ventricular fibrillation, profound bradycardia, or asystole. Sudden cardiac death may result from MI, occur during an episode of angina, or occur without warning in a patient with frequent arrhythmias secondary to underlying IHD or ventricular dysfunction. Other causes for sudden cardiac death are Wolff-Parkinson-White syndrome, long QT syndrome, torsades de pointes, atrioventricular block, aortic stenosis, myocarditis, cardiomyopathy, ruptured or dissecting aortic aneurysm, and pulmonary embolism.

Asymptomatic IHD

Asymptomatic patients with IHD are at particular risk for unexpected MI, life-threatening arrhythmias, and sudden cardiac death. These patients may develop advanced CAD and experience multiple infarcts before the correct diagnosis is made and appropriate treatment is initiated. Diabetics and elderly patients are more likely to have painless ischemia. Approximately 25% of MIs may be asymptomatic and detected on a subsequent ECG. A patient who has unexplained dyspnea, weakness, arrhythmias, or poor exercise tolerance requires cardiac testing to evaluate for the presence of undiagnosed IHD.

Noninvasive Cardiac Diagnostic Procedures

Noninvasive diagnostic testing in IHD includes electrocardiography, serum enzyme measurements, echocardiography, various types of stress testing, and newer imaging studies, such as positron emission tomography and magnetic resonance cardiac imaging.

The *electrocardiogram (ECG)* may appear normal between episodes of ischemia in patients with angina. During *angina*, the ST segments often become elevated or depressed by up to 4–5 mm. T waves may be inverted; they may become tall and peaked; or inverted T waves may normalize. These ECG findings, when associated with characteristic anginal pain, are virtually diagnostic of IHD. However, absence of ECG changes does not exclude myocardial ischemia with certainty.

During *MI*, QT interval prolongation and peaked T waves may appear. The ST segments may be depressed or elevated. ST segment elevation may persist for several days to weeks, then return to normal. T wave inversion appears in the leads corresponding to the site of the infarct. Q waves or a reduction in the QRS amplitude appear with the onset of myocardial necrosis. Q waves are typically absent in a subendocardial (nontransmural) infarction. ST segment elevation, T wave inversion, and Q waves (if present) usually occur in the ECG leads related to the site of the infarct and may be accompanied by reciprocal ST depression in the opposite leads. Tachycardia and ventricular arrhythmias are most common within the first few hours after the onset of infarction. Bradyarrhythmias such as heart block are more common with inferior infarction; ventricular tachycardia and fibrillation are more common with anteroseptal infarction.

Cardiac enzymes are released into the blood stream when myocardial necrosis occurs and are therefore valuable in differentiating MI from unstable angina and noncardiac causes of chest pain. With the advent of assays for cardiac-specific troponins, serum enzyme testing has also proved useful in identifying those patients with ACS at greatest risk for adverse outcomes.

Cardiac-specific troponins are gaining acceptance as the primary biochemical cardiac marker in ACS. Cardiac isoforms of *troponins (troponins T and I)* are important regulatory elements in myocardial cells and, unlike creatine kinase MB (CK-MB), are not normally present in the serum of healthy persons. Troponins T and I have been shown to be more cardiac specific and sensitive than CK-MB, allowing for more accurate diagnosis of cardiac injury. Moreover, unlike CK-MB, troponins T and I are not elevated in patients with skeletal muscle injury. Troponin levels remain elevated from 3 hours to 14 days after MI (long after CK-MB levels have normalized). Therefore, in patients who delay seeking medical attention for MI, troponin assays are the test of choice. However, troponin T is a less sensitive marker than CK-MB in the early stages of infarction (6–12 hours). The greater sensitivity of cardiac troponin assay allows for the detection of lesser amounts of myocardial damage. In fact, mildly elevated troponin levels may be observed in patients with unstable angina as a result of "microinfarctions."

Apart from their diagnostic value, troponin levels also confer prognostic information. It has been demonstrated that patients with an ACS who present with normal CK-MB and elevated troponin T levels have an increased risk of death, recurrent nonfatal infarction, and need for revascularization with *percutaneous transluminal coronary angioplasty (PTCA)* or *coronary artery bypass graft (CABG)*. Similarly, studies have shown that patients with elevated troponin levels at the time of hospital admission are at increased risk for death, cardiogenic shock, or congestive heart failure. Finally, a quantitative relationship between the amount of troponin I measured and the risk of death in patients who present with ACS has been demonstrated (Fig 4-1). Therefore, patients who are at greatest risk for adverse outcomes can be identified in the emergency room setting, allowing for more appropriate medical decisions and therapeutic triage.

Until recently, CK-MB isoenzyme has been the principal serum cardiac marker used in the evaluation of ACS. Although not quite as sensitive or specific as the troponins, CK-MB by mass assay remains a useful marker for the detection of more than minor myocardial damage. Serial plasma samples should be drawn for CK and CK isoenzymes after the onset of chest pain. CK levels begin to rise approximately 4 hours after MI, peaking between 12 and 24 hours after the event. CK is nonspecific and can also be elevated following injury to skeletal muscles or the brain. Three isoenzymes of CK can be identified. The MB isoenzyme is relatively specific for myocardium, although it constitutes only about 15% of the total CK released after infarction, the remainder being

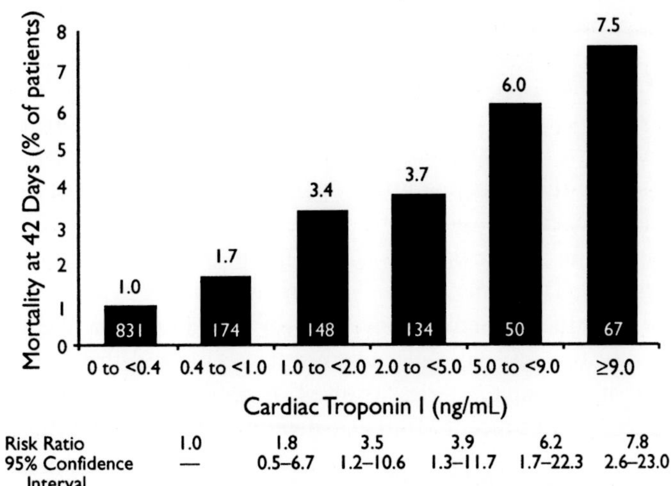

Figure 4-1 Relationship between cardiac troponin levels and risk of death in patients with ACS. *(From Antman EM, Tanasijevic MJ, Thompson B, et al. Cardiac-specific troponin I levels to predict the risk of mortality in patients with acute coronary syndromes. N Engl J Med. 1996;335:1342–1349.)*

MM or skeletal muscle isoenzyme. The third isoenzyme is *BB* and is found primarily in the brain and kidneys. An abnormally elevated CK-MB isoenzyme level is the hallmark for diagnosis of MI; however, elevations also occur in patients with severe skeletal muscle injury (perioperative or traumatic). CK-MB returns to normal within 36–48 hours after an initial MI. Therefore, in patients who arrive at the hospital more than 36 hours after the onset of chest pain, elevated CK-MB levels will be missed unless a reinfarction occurs.

Serum *myoglobin* is the first marker to rise following myocardial damage and can be elevated between 1 and 20 hours after infarction. Although myoglobin might appear to be ideal for early detection of MI, its performance is not consistent and its specificity for cardiac events is poor. Therefore, myoglobin should not be used as the *only* diagnostic marker for the identification of patients with MI, but its early appearance with myocardial injury makes its absence useful in ruling out myocardial necrosis.

Routine *lactate dehydrogenase* analysis is no longer advocated.

Echocardiography employs one- and two-dimensional ultrasound and color flow Doppler techniques to image the ventricles and atria, the heart valves, left-ventricular contraction and wall-motion abnormalities, left-ventricular ejection fraction, and the pericardium. Patients with IHD, particularly following infarction, commonly have regional wall-motion abnormalities that correspond to the areas of myocardial injury. Other less frequent complications of infarction, such as mitral regurgitation from papillary muscle injury, ventricular septal defect, ventricular aneurysm, ventricular thrombus, and pericardial effusion, can also be detected with echocardiography. Color flow Doppler provides information on the flow of blood across abnormal valves, pressure differences within the chambers, intracardiac shunts, and cardiac output.

Exercise echocardiography (stress echocardiography) is useful for imaging cardiac valve and wall-motion abnormalities and ventricular dysfunction induced by ischemia during exercise. Predischarge exercise stress echocardiography provides useful prognostic information following acute MI.

Exercise stress testing

Patients with angina may have normal findings on clinical examination, ECG, and echocardiography between episodes of ischemia. Standardized exercise tests have been developed to induce myocardial ischemia under controlled conditions. The ECG, heart rate, blood pressure, and general physical status of the patient are monitored during the procedure. The endpoint in angina patients is a symptom or sign of cardiac ischemia, such as chest pain, dyspnea, ST segment depression, arrhythmia, or hypotension. The level of exercise required to induce ischemia is inversely correlated with the likelihood of significant CAD. False-positive and false-negative results occur, and the sensitivity increases with the number of coronary arteries involved. A modified exercise stress test is also performed in patients with a recent MI to help determine functional status and prognosis.

Radionuclide scintigraphy and scans

The sensitivity of exercise testing can be increased via radionuclide techniques. A relatively new agent, *technetium-99m Sesta-MIBI (Cardiolite)*, has higher energy than prior substances and thus may provide better image resolution and less soft tissue attenuation. Other techniques include *thallium-201 myocardial* and *technetium-99 pyrophosphate (Tc-99) scintigraphy*, or *blood-pool isotope scans.*

Thallium accumulates in normal myocardium and reveals a perfusion defect in areas of myocardial ischemia. Thallium scans have a high sensitivity and specificity for CAD. Reversible thallium/technetium-99m Sesta-MIBI defects consist of a defect that is present during exercise but resolves during rest. This correlates with myocardial ischemia. In contrast, a fixed thallium/Cardiolite defect is present during both exercise and rest and represents a region of prior infarction/nonviable tissue. For those patients unable to exercise vigorously enough to reach the required heart rates, a thallium scan or echocardiogram in conjunction with a pharmacologic stress test using intravenous adenosine, dipyridamole, or dobutamine may provide information similar to that of an actual exercise examination. *Tomographic imaging* of myocardial perfusion is possible with thallium-201 via a technique called *single-photon emission computed tomography*. This technique provides better imaging of infarcts and improved detection of multivessel disease.

Technetium-99 pyrophosphate (Tc-99) is an infarct-avid imaging agent. Tc-99 accumulates in necrotic myocardial cells rather than normal myocardium, creating a "hot spot" on imaging. A new infarct is visualized best between 24 and 48 hours after onset with Tc-99 scintigraphy. Other imaging tests that are being evaluated in the detection and management of IHD are *positron emission tomography, ultrafast computed tomography, cardiac magnetic resonance imaging*, and *magnetic resonance fluoroscopy.*

Invasive Cardiac Diagnostic Procedures

Intravascular ultrasound imaging is an evolving invasive modality for studying the intraluminal coronary anatomy. Technologic limitations and uncertainty about long-term safety are a concern. However, as the technology matures, this technique might assume an expanding role in interventional cardiology.

Coronary arteriography and *ventriculography* provide valuable information about the presence and severity of CAD and about ventricular function. These techniques can indicate the specific areas of coronary artery stenosis or occlusion, the number of involved vessels, the ventricular systolic and diastolic volumes, the ejection fraction, and regional wall-motion abnormalities. This information assists the cardiologist and cardiac surgeon in planning appropriate management of the patient.

Coronary artery stenosis is hemodynamically significant when the arterial lumen diameter is narrowed by more than 50% or the cross-sectional area is reduced by more than 75%. Common indications for coronary arteriography are:

- ACS
- Post-MI angina
- Stable angina unresponsive to medical therapy
- A markedly positive exercise stress test result
- Recent MI in a patient under age 40
- Valvular heart disease
- Ventricular septal defect or papillary muscle dysfunction
- Cardiomyopathy of unknown cause
- Unexplained ventricular arrhythmias

Management of Ischemic Heart Disease

The goals of management for the patient with CAD are to reduce or eliminate angina, prevent myocardial damage, and prolong life. The first line of attack should include eliminating or reducing risk factors for atherosclerosis. Recent studies have reported actual regression of atherosclerotic lesions following intensive lipid-lowering therapy. Antiplatelet therapy with daily aspirin has also been advocated for all patients with CAD because of the significant reduction in risk of MI.

Treatment of stable angina pectoris

Medical management of angina pectoris is designed to deliver as much oxygen as possible to the potentially ischemic myocardium, to reduce the oxygen demand to a level where symptoms are eliminated or reduced to a comfortable level, or both. Oxygen delivery through the coronary arteries may be maximized via coronary vasodilators. *Nitroglycerin* or other *nitrates* may be given sublingually for acute episodes of angina. Long-acting orally administered nitrates or topically applied nitroglycerin ointments or transdermal patches may be administered for prevention and long-term control of angina. The systemic effects of nitrates include venous dilation and a decline in arterial pressure; these physiologic effects contribute to the therapeutic effects. Oxygen demands can be reduced by decreasing the heart rate and contractility.

The best agents for reducing heart rate and contractility are the *β-adrenergic blockers*. Their favorable properties have made them the first line and mainstay of treatment for these patients. β-Blockers are useful in the management of stable and unstable angina.

The *slow-channel calcium-blocking agents* (such as *diltiazem, nifedipine, verapamil, nicardipine,* and *amlodipine*) are effective in chronic angina and may be useful in preventing episodes of coronary spasm. However, β-adrenergic blockers and calcium channel blockers (particularly verapamil) must be used with caution when left-ventricular dysfunction is present. Myocardial oxygen requirements can also be reduced by decreasing ventricular wall tension through controlling systemic hypertension and by reducing the ventricular volume with venous dilators such as nitrates. In addition, routine administration of aspirin reduces the likelihood of thrombus formation. Improving the oxygen-carrying capacity of the blood by treating anemia or coexisting pulmonary disease provides some additional benefit. Patients in whom medical therapy is unsuccessful may be candidates for revascularization with either PTCA or CABG.

Revascularization provides the opportunity to improve coronary blood flow, control of angina, and exercise tolerance. In high-risk patients (Table 4-1), risk of infarction is reduced and long-term survival is enhanced.

PTCA was developed as an alternative to surgical revascularization. Angioplasty involves passing a balloon catheter into a stenosed vessel and inflating the balloon at the site of the narrowing to widen the lumen. A high-grade proximal stenosis (70%) that is smooth, concentric, less than 0.5 cm in length, and noncalcified is considered the lesion most amenable to PTCA. The immediate success rate for PTCA for patients with favorable lesions exceeds 85%. However, the risk of restenosis is considerable, approximately 25%–40% at 6 months. The insertion of a wire-mesh *stent* with PTCA improves patency and reduces the risk of restenosis by nearly 50%. Because stent placement can trigger *acute thrombosis* (heralded by angina) or *subacute thrombosis* (manifested by acute infarction or death), the procedure is followed immediately by 2–4 weeks of potent antiplatelet therapy. Although PTCA with stenting has become commonplace, its cost effectiveness and long-term impact on cardiovascular morbidity and mortality remain to be established. Indications for revascularization with PTCA (with or without stent) include those anginal patients who have unacceptably symptomatic *single- or two-vessel disease without leftventricular dysfunction despite medical therapy.* PTCA may also be offered as the initial treatment to moderate-risk patients with considerable symptoms because it can be more effective than medical therapy.

Table 4-1 Risk Stratification for Patients with Stable Angina

Low risk	No angina currently or minimal angina
	Normal left-ventricular function (normal ejection fraction)
	Small amount of myocardium at risk (probable single-vessel disease)
Moderate risk	Moderate angina
	Normal left-ventricular function (normal ejection fraction)
	Moderate amount of myocardium at risk (probable two-vessel or proximal left anterior descending artery disease)
High risk	Severe angina
	Impaired left-ventricular function (ejection fraction <0.40)
	Extensive amount of myocardium at risk (probable three-vessel, left main, or "left main equivalent" disease)

When angioplasty is inappropriate or ineffective and medical therapy has failed to control symptoms in severe multivessel disease, CABG may be considered. CABG is the treatment of choice in persons with *high-risk disease* (ie, those with significant *left-main, proximal left-anterior descending,* or *three-vessel disease,* especially if accompanied by left-ventricular dysfunction) because CABG is superior to medical therapy for prevention of infarction and prolongation of survival. The bypass graft provides a shunt from the aorta to the diseased coronary artery beyond the area of obstruction in order to increase blood flow, thereby eliminating angina and often preventing or reducing the risk of infarction and cardiac death. Coronary artery bypass grafting has also been shown to increase left-ventricular function, improve quality of life, and increase life expectancy compared with medical treatment for patients with significant high-risk disease. Saphenous veins are most commonly used as the bypass material, but use of the internal mammary artery has become the standard for the left anterior descending artery because of its improved long-term patency rate. Some patients now receive "off the pump bypass surgery" in which the grafts are sewn onto a beating heart. This technique avoids the adverse effects of cardiopulmonary bypass, which include memory, cognitive, and other neurologic deficits. The technique is technically more difficult, and its outcomes are still being studied.

Newer methods of revascularization currently under investigation include atherectomy devices employing *excimer* and *argon lasers, atheroma-cutting blades,* and *high-speed rotary devices and water-jets.* Thus far, outcomes remain disappointing because of unacceptably high complication rates due to debris and endothelial damage associated with these procedures.

Treatment of acute coronary syndromes

Patients with a definite ACS are admitted to the hospital for monitoring and treatment. Patients are initially treated aggressively with anti-ischemic pharmacotherapy. Once these initial measures are instituted, further management and triage of patients with an ACS is based on the presence or absence of ST segment elevation. Patients with ST segment elevation ACS are given reperfusion therapy with either thrombolysis or catheter-based interventions; patients with a non–ST segment elevation ACS may be appropriately followed with either medical treatment alone or a more aggressive interventional approach.

Management of non–ST segment elevation ACS In general, myocardial oxygen demands are managed with medications and supplemental oxygen. Patients are given 160–325 mg of aspirin, which has been demonstrated to be effective in reducing the mortality of MI. The first dose of aspirin should be chewed rather than swallowed to achieve rapid blood levels. As long as the patient is not hypotensive or bradycardic, nitroglycerin is given. Nitroglycerin may be administered sublingually or intravenously. Intravenous administration of nitrates permits careful titration, allowing control of anginal symptoms without causing excessive hypotension. When nitroglycerin does not provide pain relief, morphine sulfate may be administered. β-Blocker therapy reduces myocardial oxygen demands and should be considered for all patients with evolving MI if no contraindication exists.

For patients who do not receive reperfusion therapy, β-blocker therapy provides a survival benefit, particularly for the high-risk subset of patients, which includes elderly patients and patients with previous MI and mild pulmonary venous congestion. When β-blockers cannot be used, heart rate-slowing calcium antagonists (eg, verapamil or diltiazem) offer an alternative; however, rapid-release, short-acting dihydropyridine-type calcium channel blockers (eg, nifedipine) should be avoided in the absence of adequate concurrent beta blockade in ACS, because controlled trials suggest increased risk of MI and cardiac death. Moreover, risk of cardiac death is significantly increased when calcium channel blockers are used in the setting of left-ventricular failure.

Angiotensin-converting enzyme (ACE) inhibitors such as captopril (Capoten), lisinopril (Prinivil), and ramipril (Altace), given orally during the acute phase of MI, can potentially decrease the risk of immediate mortality when initiated within the first 24 hours of acute MI. ACE inhibitors confer benefit with or without concomitant reperfusion therapy. Patients receiving the greatest benefit are those in high-risk groups, including those with anterior infarctions, evidence of left-ventricular systolic dysfunction, mild congestive heart failure, and previous MI. ACE inhibitors are contraindicated in patients with hypotension and should be used with caution in patients with renal insufficiency. If congestive heart failure or pulmonary edema are present, they are managed with vasodilators, diuretics, digoxin, or other inotropic agents. Patients with an ACS are also commonly given an antithrombin agent. A glycoprotein IIb/IIIa inhibitor should also be considered.

Unfractionated heparin is the antithrombin usually used, largely because of clinical experience. However, there is evidence that the newer antithrombin class, the low-molecular-weight heparins (LMWHs—eg, enoxaparin), are superior. Antithrombin therapy with unfractionated heparin has several important disadvantages, such as a variable anticoagulant effect, an inability to inhibit clot-bound thrombin, and the potential to cause thrombocytopenia. LMWHs have increased anti–factor Xa activity and improved bioavailability, and LMWHs can be administered by subcutaneous injection. The ESSENCE and TIMI 11B trials have demonstrated that for patients with unstable angina/non–Q wave MI, LMWHs are superior to traditional unfractionated heparin. Whether LMWHs are a useful adjunct to thrombolysis in patients with ST segment elevation ACS is currently under investigation.

The glycoprotein IIb/IIIa receptor is present on the surface of platelets. When platelets are activated, this receptor increases its affinity for fibrinogen and other ligands, which results in platelet aggregation. This mechanism constitutes the final and obligatory pathway for platelet aggregation. The platelet GP IIb/IIIa receptor antagonists *tirofiban* (Aggrastat), *abciximab* (ReoPro), and *eptifibatide* (Integrilin) act by preventing fibrinogen binding and thereby preventing platelet aggregation. Platelets are involved in the development of both ACS and complications after percutaneous coronary interventions. Glycoprotein IIb/IIIa inhibitors have been shown to reduce the risk of death and MI in patients with non–ST segment elevation ACS and after coronary angioplasty and stenting. Aside from percutaneous interventions, the glycoprotein IIb/IIIa inhibitors are also indicated in the treatment of non–ST segment elevation ACS. However, the benefit in these patients is less than that observed with percutaneous interventions. Patients with a non–ST segment elevation ACS and an elevated troponin level may constitute a subset of patients who are particularly likely to receive a treatment benefit from platelet GP IIb/IIIa inhibitors and LMWH. The use of glycoprotein IIb/IIIa inhibitors in ST segment elevation MI is currently under investigation.

Once unstable angina and non–ST segment elevation MI have been managed as described above, patients may be evaluated with either an early invasive (angiographic) strategy or a conservative noninvasive approach, depending on their level of risk for adverse outcome. In the early conservative strategy, coronary angiography is reserved for patients with evidence of recurrent ischemia (angina or ST segment changes at rest or with minimal activity) or a strongly positive stress test result despite vigorous medical therapy. In the early invasive strategy, patients without clinically obvious contraindications to coronary revascularization are routinely recommended for coronary angiography and angiographically directed revascularization, if possible. The decision to proceed from diagnostic angiography to revascularization is influenced not only by the coronary anatomy but by a number of additional factors, including anticipated life expectancy, ventricular function, comorbidity, functional capacity, severity of symptoms, and quantity of viable myocardium at risk.

Management of ST segment elevation ACS Modern therapy for evolving Q wave MI involves rapid and effective reperfusion because necrosis is a time-dependent process. Not surprisingly, optimal myocardial salvage requires that nearly complete reperfusion be achieved as soon as possible. Benefit is maximized if reperfusion therapy can be instituted within 1 hour of symptom onset; a significant benefit is retained if reperfusion therapy is instituted within 6 hours of symptom onset, and some benefit is still obtained if reperfusion therapy is instituted 6–12 hours after symptom onset. The benefit of reperfusion therapy after 12 hours of symptom onset has not been established.

Methods of reperfusion include thrombolysis and catheter-based percutaneous interventions (balloon angioplasty with or without stent placement). Newer adjuncts to therapy may include LMWH and glycoprotein IIb/IIIa inhibitors.

Percutaneous interventions require the availability of a cardiac catheterization laboratory and an experienced interventional cardiologist. Such facilities are available in fewer than 20% of hospitals worldwide. Even when these resources are available, a considerable delay (>90 minutes) may be encountered in transferring patients to the cardiac catheterization laboratory. Given the limited worldwide ability to perform timely catheterization, most patients with evolving ST segment elevation MI are considered for intravenous thrombolytic therapy as soon as the diagnosis is made.

Thrombolysis Indications for thrombolysis include patients with ischemic chest pain lasting 30 minutes to 12 hours with ST segment elevation of greater than 1 mm in two contiguous leads. Currently, several intravenous thrombolytic agents are available, which effectively lyse coronary thrombi and restore coronary blood flow in most patients. The most frequently used agents are *streptokinase* (1.5 million units over 30–60 minutes), the recombinant tissue plasminogen activator (t-PA) *reteplase* (Retavase), *t-PA* (Activase), and *anisoylated plasminogen streptokinase activator complex* (30 units given as a bolus). The "front-loaded" t-PA regimen is most frequently used in the United States. It consists of a 15 mg bolus followed by 0.75 mg/kg every 30 minutes (maximum, 50 mg) and then 0.50 mg/kg every 60 minutes (maximum, 35 mg). The efficacy of reteplase is similar to that of t-PA, but reteplase's administration (two bolus injections of 10 IU at 30 minute intervals) is easier than that of t-PA. When either t-PA or reteplase is used, intravenous heparin should be used concurrently.

The disadvantage of streptokinase therapy is that the rate of recanalization of the infarct-related artery is significantly lower than when t-PA is used. With front-loaded t-PA and heparin therapy, approximately 50% of infarct-related arteries recanalize, providing normal flow to the ischemic myocardium. The major disadvantage of t-PA is a slightly greater risk of intracranial hemorrhage compared with streptokinase. The other disadvantage is that t-PA therapy is more expensive than streptokinase. Although most studies have restricted the use of these drugs to patients age 75 or younger, older patients experience distinctly more infarction mortality and may benefit from thrombolytic therapy. Contraindications include known sites of potential bleeding, a history of prior cerebrovascular accident, recent surgery, or prolonged cardiopulmonary resuscitation efforts.

Catheter-based reperfusion Instead of thrombolysis, the infarct-related artery can be recanalized via mechanical means using balloon angioplasty (PTCA) with or without a stent. Mechanical reperfusion of a thrombotic coronary occlusion with normal arterial flow can be achieved in at least 90% of patients with ST elevation and acute MI, a significantly greater percentage than is achieved with thrombolysis. Primary angioplasty compared with thrombolysis has a greater potential to reduce the risk of 30-day mortality for patients with acute MI. Better survival is observed, particularly in high-risk patients with anterior MI, patients with previous MI, and patients with evidence of left-ventricular dysfunction. A delay in the institution of reperfusion therapy significantly reduces the magnitude of the treatment's benefits, which apart from decreasing the risk of mortality include preserving left-ventricular function and decreasing the risk of congestive heart failure.

Therefore, if a considerable delay (>90 minutes) is anticipated before primary angioplasty can be performed, thrombolysis is preferable. Primary PTCA is the preferred reperfusion strategy for patients with contraindications to thrombolytic therapy and for those in cardiogenic shock. Primary PTCA may also be preferable for patients with increased risk of intracranial hemorrhage and in patients who have undergone previous CABG. PTCA is also indicated for patients in whom thrombolytic reperfusion has apparently failed (ie, those with persistent chest pain and ST segment elevation). Although recent trials suggest that primary angioplasty may be at least as beneficial as thrombolytic therapy for treatment of acute MI, additional questions surrounding the respective roles of these two treatments remain. Randomized trials comparing primary angioplasty and thrombolytic therapy are still relatively small, and no trial to date has compared immediate angioplasty with accelerated reteplase plus IV heparin or with newer thrombolytic regimens. The cost-effectiveness of primary angioplasty has not been fully evaluated.

Antman EM, Cohen M. Newer antithrombin agents in acute coronary artery syndromes. *Am Heart J.* 1999;138:S563–S569.

Bhatt DL, Topol EJ. Current role of platelet glycoprotein IIb/IIIa inhibitors in acute coronary syndromes. *JAMA.* 2000;284:1549–1558.

Braunwald E, Antman EM, Beasley JW, et al. ACC/AHA guidelines for the management of patients with unstable angina and non-ST segment elevation myocardial infarction: executive summary and recommendations. *Circulation.* 2000;102:1193.

Braunwald E, Zipes DP, Libby P, eds. *Heart Disease: A Textbook of Cardiovascular Medicine.* 6th ed. Philadelphia: Saunders; 2001.

Gore JM, Dalen JE. Cardiovascular disease. *JAMA*. 1997;277:1845–1846.

Goroll AH, Mulley AG. *Goroll: Primary Care Medicine*. 4th ed. Philadelphia: Lippincott Williams & Wilkins; 2000.

Goy JJ, Eeckhout E. Intracoronary stenting. *Lancet*. 1998;351:1943–1949.

Hamm CW, Katus HA. New biochemical markers for myocardial cell injury. *Curr Opin Cardiol*. 1995;10:355–360.

Hennekens CH, O'Donnell CJ, Ridker PM, et al. Current issues concerning thrombolytic therapy for acute myocardial infarction. *J Am Coll Cardiol*. 1995;25(suppl 17):18S–22S.

Massie BM. The safety of calcium channel blockers. *Clin Cardiol*. 1998;21(12 suppl 2):12–17.

Morey SS. ACC/AHA guidelines on the management of acute myocardial infarction. American College of Cardiology and the American Heart Association. *Am Fam Physician*. 2000; 61:1901–1902.

Congestive Heart Failure

Congestive heart failure (CHF) is a general term that applies to a clinical state in which a patient manifests subjective or objective features indicative of impaired function of the left or right ventricle (or both). Symptoms and signs of CHF may occur when the heart is not able to pump a sufficient amount of blood for a prolonged period to meet the body's requirements. Compensated CHF refers to patients whose clinical manifestations of CHF have been controlled by treatment. *Decompensated CHF* represents heart failure with symptoms that are not under control. *Refractory CHF* exists when previous therapeutic measures have failed to control the clinical manifestations of the syndrome. Pulmonary edema usually results from severe left-ventricular failure with increased pulmonary capillary pressure, causing parenchymal and intra-alveolar fluid accumulation in the lung. Table 4-2 shows the New York Heart Association classification scheme for heart failure symptoms.

Symptoms

Heart failure causes a variety of symptoms, depending on the severity of ventricular dysfunction. Symptoms may result from inadequate tissue perfusion caused by pump failure or from the failing heart's inability to empty adequately, leading to edema and fluid accumulation in the lungs, extremities, and other sites. The most frequent symptoms of left-ventricular failure are dyspnea with exertion or at rest, orthopnea, paroxysmal nocturnal dyspnea, diaphoresis, generalized weakness, fatigue, anxiety, and lightheadedness. With more severe CHF, the patient may also experience a productive cough;

Table 4-2 New York Heart Association Classification for Heart Failure Symptoms

Symptom Class	Symptom
I	No symptoms
II	Comfortable at rest; symptoms with ordinary activity
III	Comfortable at rest; symptoms with less than ordinary activity
IV	Symptoms at rest

copious pink, frothy sputum; and mental confusion. Angina may also occur if the CHF results from IHD. Right-sided heart failure may occur separately from or secondary to chronic left-sided heart failure. Patients with right-sided heart failure typically develop peripheral edema.

Clinical Signs

Examination findings in acute left-ventricular failure may include respiratory distress, use of the respiratory accessory muscles, pinkish sputum or frank hemoptysis, coarse rales on pulmonary auscultation, expiratory wheezes, a rapid heart rate, an S gallop, diaphoresis, and deterioration in mental status. Blood pressure is often markedly elevated but may be reduced during MI. Long-standing cases of CHF show signs of right-ventricular failure, especially elevated central venous pressure, pedal edema, hepatomegaly, and cyanosis. In some patients, pleural effusion or ascites may be detected.

Diagnostic Evaluation

The history and clinical examination are the most important components in the diagnostic assessment of CHF. Helpful diagnostic studies in the evaluation of CHF and its underlying causes include chest radiograph, ECG, blood gases, hemoglobin level, serum electrolytes, and urinalysis. If the primary mechanism of heart failure is unclear, additional tests may prove useful in selected patients. Such tests may include echocardiography, exercise stress testing, cardiac nuclear-imaging studies, coronary arteriography, right- and left-sided heart catheterization, Holter monitoring, pulmonary function tests, and thyroid function tests.

The ECG may reveal acute ischemic changes, acute or old MI, ventricular hypertrophy, chamber enlargement, atrial fibrillation, or other arrhythmias. Typical chest radiographic findings are prominent pulmonary vessels, interstitial or alveolar pulmonary edema, cardiomegaly, and pleural effusions. Patients with severe pump failure may have abnormal serum electrolytes owing to poor renal perfusion. Abnormalities in the blood or urine may help detect severe anemia or renal failure as a precipitating factor in CHF. Abnormal liver enzymes are common if venous congestion is present as a result of right-ventricular failure. Echocardiography and other cardiac studies can help differentiate the many cardiac causes of CHF, including IHD, valvular heart disease, cardiomyopathies, and cardiac arrhythmias. Pure right-ventricular failure may result from chronic pulmonary disease, pulmonary hypertension, tricuspid or pulmonary valve disease, right-ventricular infarction, or constrictive pericarditis.

Ejection fraction (EF) is the calculated percentage of blood ejected by the ventricle during a single or average contraction. In normal patients, the EF is over 50%. An EF of 40%–50% indicates mild impairment; 25%–40%, moderate impairment; and less than 25%, severe impairment. EF can be measured using echocardiography, radionuclide ventriculography, and contrast ventriculography. Echocardiography is the most useful and least invasive method of determining and sequentially following EF and the systolic state of the ventricles.

Epidemiology

In a large percentage of patients with CHF, the epidemiology parallels that of IHD because IHD is currently the primary cause of heart failure. Accordingly, the same risk factors for atherosclerosis apply to ischemic CHF. Patients with CHF are more sensitive to a high intake of sodium and should receive dietary instructions to achieve a low-sodium diet. When CHF is not the result of IHD, other causes must be investigated. A history of rheumatic fever, atrial fibrillation, pernicious anemia, hyperthyroidism, or other disorders may suggest one of the less common causes of CHF. Although CHF is most common in adults, it can also occur in children with congenital heart or valve defects, cardiomyopathy, myocarditis, or, in rare instances, following infarction from Kawasaki disease.

The prognosis for patients with CHF depends directly on the degree of ventricular impairment. The New York Heart Association classification system of CHF by symptoms (see Table 4-2) correlates well with survival. In a study from Duke University, patients with class IV CHF had 1- and 3-year mortality rates of 55% and 82%, respectively. In the Framingham study, the overall 5-year mortality rate was 62% in men with CHF and 42% in women.

Etiology

As noted above, IHD is the most common cause of CHF. Cumulative injury to the ventricular myocardium from ischemia and infarction can lead to impaired ventricular systolic and diastolic function, and, ultimately, pump failure. Additional causes of systolic dysfunction are:

- Valvular heart disease (primarily aortic stenosis and aortic or mitral regurgitation)
- Cardiomyopathies (which may have metabolic, infectious, toxic, connective tissue, or idiopathic causes)
- Myocarditis (from viral or inflammatory diseases)

Diseases that impair the relaxation and filling properties of the left ventricle can result in diastolic dysfunction. Such disorders include:

- Infiltrative diseases (amyloidosis, sarcoidosis, metastatic disease, and others)
- Left-ventricular hypertrophy (which can be caused by arterial hypertension, idiopathic hypertrophic subaortic stenosis, and coarctation of the aorta)

Actually, both systolic and diastolic dysfunction often occur simultaneously in the common causes of CHF, namely IHD, valvular disease, and the congestive cardiomyopathies. Some of the causes of high–cardiac output heart failure are:

- Severe anemia
- Hyperthyroidism
- Arteriovenous fistulas
- Beriberi
- Paget disease

In high-output failure, the demand for oxygen is so great that the heart eventually fails because it cannot maintain the excessive cardiac output indefinitely. Some patients may have more than one mechanism for heart failure, such as a patient with IHD who develops CHF after becoming severely anemic. The specific causes for right-ventricular failure were mentioned earlier.

Pathophysiology and Clinical Course

The left and right ventricles function as pumping chambers, and their action can be subdivided into a *systolic,* or contraction, phase and a *diastolic,* or relaxation, phase. During *systole,* the ventricular muscle actively contracts, developing pressure and ejecting blood into the aorta or pulmonary artery for forward perfusion. During *diastole,* the ventricular muscle actively and passively relaxes and allows a refilling of the ventricle from the corresponding atrium. Either or both of these phases may become impaired, leading to dysfunction of systole, diastole, or both. Some of the symptoms and clinical signs of CHF can be distinguished as being attributable to systolic or diastolic impairment. Treatment varies, depending on which type of dysfunction predominates.

Systolic dysfunction

The ability of the heart to contract and eject blood is determined by preload, afterload, and contractility. *Preload* refers to the amount of stretch to which muscle fibers are subjected at the end of diastole, or refilling. Preload is determined by blood volume and venous return. Excessive preload is often called *volume overload.* Up to a point, as the preload increases, the force of contraction also increases, allowing adequate emptying of the ventricle.

Afterload is the amount of tension or force in the ventricular muscle mass just after onset of contraction, as the ventricle begins emptying. Clinically, afterload represents the pressure that the ventricle must withstand during contraction. Thus, the aortic pressure determines afterload for the left ventricle, whereas the pulmonary artery pressure determines afterload for the right. Even a normal ventricle may fail with extremely high preload or afterload.

Contractility refers to the intrinsic ability of the myocardial fibers to contract, independent of the preload or afterload conditions. Contractility can be adversely affected by metabolic, ischemic, or other structural derangement of the myocardial cells. Abnormal intracellular modulation of calcium ions is a key component in heart failure. Clinical disorders that affect preload, afterload, or contractility result in systolic dysfunction. Likewise, therapy directed toward improvements in these parameters can be used to treat systolic dysfunction.

Diastolic dysfunction

Several of the disorders that impair the diastolic, or relaxation, properties of the ventricle were listed above among the causes of CHF. Diastolic dysfunction causes elevated filling pressures in the ventricles and atria. In the left ventricle, diastolic dysfunction causes pulmonary venous hypertension and its clinical manifestations, such as dyspnea on exertion, orthopnea, and paroxysmal nocturnal dyspnea. Clinical signs of diastolic dysfunction are pulmonary edema with rales, lung congestion visible on chest radiograph, and hypoxemia.

The clinical course of CHF may follow a downward spiral of left-ventricular systolic and diastolic dysfunction, ventricular dilation, and a decline in the EF, followed by right-sided heart failure. A continuous reduction in cardiac output and tissue perfusion may be accompanied by increasing pulmonary and systemic venous congestion. Appropriate treatment may slow or even halt progression in some patients.

Medical and Nonsurgical Management

In the management of heart failure, treatment strategies can be directed at systolic or diastolic ventricular dysfunction. Specific treatment for some causes of right-sided heart failure is also available.

Systolic dysfunction

If the preload is reduced, systolic function can occasionally be improved by carefully increasing preload by volume infusion. This increase in preload dilates the ventricle and is one of the mechanisms by which the heart intrinsically attempts to compensate for poor systolic function. However, this mechanism fails and systolic function is impaired when the ventricle becomes overly dilated.

Reducing afterload is the most effective way to manage systolic dysfunction in most clinical situations. Reducing vascular resistance and lowering arterial blood pressure decreases the burden on the left ventricle and enhances contraction and ejection. Regardless of the baseline values, lowering blood pressure (while maintaining adequate tissue perfusion) is the mainstay of treatment of systolic dysfunction. The most effective drugs for reducing afterload in current clinical practice are the *ACE inhibitors,* which include *captopril, enalapril, lisinopril,* and *ramipril.* These drugs effectively decrease the clinical manifestations of CHF and have been demonstrated in clinical trials to lower both mortality and morbidity rates among patients with CHF, morbidity being defined as hospitalization (or therapy) for worsening heart failure. These beneficial effects can be seen in patients with idiopathic dilated cardiomyopathy as well as in those with diminished left-ventricular function after an MI. *Angiotensin-receptor antagonists* have been developed for the therapy of CHF, and many physicians have used them as alternative therapy for the management of the ACE-intolerant patient. However, the potential benefits of angiotensin-receptor antagonists have not been assessed in large multicenter randomized studies, and thus their use cannot be recommended at present.

Other drugs that reduce afterload by lowering blood pressure and peripheral vascular resistance are *hydralazine, clonidine,* and *calcium channel blockers.* However, calcium channel blockers have generally been found to be of little benefit in patients with CHF. In fact, diltiazem (Cardizem) was associated with increased mortality when used in patients with CHF. Amlodipine (Norvasc) is the only calcium channel blocker that has been shown to be safe in patients with CHF and is therefore the calcium channel blocker of choice in patients with CHF and ongoing IHD not controlled by other means. The α-*adrenergic blockers* such as *prazosin* or *doxazosin* can also be considered for patients who cannot tolerate ACE inhibitors because of renal dysfunction or other relative contraindications. Hospitalized patients with more severe CHF, particularly pulmonary edema, may require more aggressive afterload reduction with intravenous agents such as *nitroprusside, nitroglycerin,* or *enalapril.*

For patients with systolic dysfunction, the contractility of the left ventricle can be enhanced with inotropic agents. *Digitalis,* the time-honored drug for increasing contractility, is a mainstay of treatment, especially for long-term outpatient maintenance therapy. With the exception of digoxin, oral inotropic agents have not proved safe or effective in patients with chronic CHF. However, intravenous inotropic agents play a key role in the therapy of patients hospitalized for worsening heart failure. Three intravenous inotropic agents are FDA approved for the therapy of acute exacerbations of CHF: the adrenergic agonist *dobutamine* (Dobutrex), the phosphodiesterase inhibitor *milrinone* (Primacor), and the dopaminergic/adrenergic agonist *dopamine* (Intropin). For patients with disease refractory to either dobutamine or milrinone, both drugs can be used together to take advantage of synergistic actions. Patients on these potent drugs require close monitoring of blood pressure, heart rate, cardiac output, and urine production.

Patients with CHF have an increased adrenergic drive that is associated with a worsened prognosis. High levels of norepinephrine are both arrhythmogenic and cardiotoxic. The use of β-blockers such as carvedilol (Coreg), bisoprolol (Zebeta), and metoprolol (Lopressor) has clearly been shown to improve heart failure symptoms and to reduce all-cause mortality and the risk of hospitalization in patients with CHF. These benefits are most obvious in patients with moderate to severe symptoms; however, several important caveats should be noted. First, β-blocker therapy has not been assessed in patients with bradycardia, hypotension, or class IV symptoms. Similarly, the effects of β-blockers have not been assessed in patients with left-ventricular dilatation but compensated function and the absence of symptoms. In addition, as many as 6% of patients may not tolerate even small amounts of a β-blocker. Therefore, the initial doses of β-blocker must be very low, with gradual and careful upward titration over a period of 3–6 months.

Diastolic dysfunction

Diastolic function can be improved by reducing preload, which in turn lowers filling pressures in the ventricle. Preload can be reduced by reducing circulating blood volume, by increasing the capacitance of the venous bed, and by improving systolic function to more effectively empty the ventricle. Diuretics are the most effective agents for reducing blood volume. *Oral thiazide* or *loop diuretics* are effective for long-term diuresis, but *intravenous loop diuretics* such as *furosemide* or *bumetanide* are more potent for severe CHF or pulmonary edema. Venous capacitance can be increased by administering venous dilators, particularly the nitrates. Intravenous *furosemide* and *morphine* also have some venodilation effects, partially explaining their effectiveness in treating pulmonary edema. Any of the measures previously discussed that improve systolic function also indirectly enhance diastolic function by reducing the residual blood volume in the ventricle following contraction.

Other approaches to CHF

Other strategies for managing CHF include seeking the underlying causes or contributing factors responsible for the failure and correcting them, if possible. Precipitating factors can include excessive salt or fluid intake, poor medication compliance, excessive activity, obesity, pulmonary infection or embolism, MI, renal disease, anemia, thyrotoxicosis, or arrhythmias.

Intermittent arrhythmias may seriously compromise ventricular function. Tachyarrhythmias may aggravate ischemia; bradyarrhythmias may decrease cardiac output and blood pressure further. However, antiarrhythmic therapy has been shown to have little benefit in the management of patients with CHF, inasmuch as most of these agents have significant proarrhythmic and negative inotropic properties. However, amiodarone (at low dosage) has proved useful in some patients with recalcitrant atrial fibrillation. In patients with documented *sustained* ventricular tachycardia or fibrillation, implantable cardiac defibrillators (ICDs) are beneficial. However, the role of ICDs in the therapy for patients with *nonsustained* ventricular tachycardia is still under investigation (see later discussion, Disorders of Cardiac Rhythm). Patients with heart block and other severe bradyarrhythmias may require cardiac pacing.

Patients with a dilated cardiomyopathy and atrial fibrillation should be treated with warfarin (Coumadin) unless specific contraindications exist. Many physicians also place patients with a dilated cardiomyopathy, low ejection, and normal sinus rhythm on warfarin if no contraindications exist.

Other measures that can assist in the management of CHF are restricting dietary sodium, avoiding fluid overload by carefully monitoring oral and intravenous fluid intake, controlling pain and anxiety, treating concomitant metabolic or pulmonary diseases, and providing supplemental oxygen to hypoxemic patients. Finally, all patients with CHF should receive an influenza vaccination and the pneumococcal vaccine. New agents and devices currently under investigation for the treatment of CHF include etanercept, a recombinant-produced soluble receptor for tumor necrosis factor; angiotensin-receptor antagonists; tezosentan and bosentan, which are endothelin-receptor antagonists; novel inotropic agents; and biventricular pacing devices, which attempt to "resynchronize" the electrical activity of the heart and thereby improve pump function.

Invasive or Surgical Management

Depending on the underlying causes, surgical procedures that may benefit patients with CHF include percutaneous balloon valvuloplasty, mitral commissurotomy, mitral or aortic valve replacement, coronary angioplasty, coronary artery bypass grafting, left-ventricular aneurysmectomy, or pericardectomy. Cardiac transplantation has become an effective surgical treatment for patients with refractory CHF. Many transplant centers have achieved a 5-year survival rate above 75%. The use of corticosteroids and immunosuppressive agents, such as cyclosporine and FK-506, has reduced transplant rejection and mortality.

Colucci S, Braunwald E. Pathophysiology of heart failure. In: Braunwald E, Zipes DP, Libby P, eds. *Heart Disease: A Textbook of Cardiovascular Medicine.* 6th ed. Philadelphia: WB Saunders; 2001:503–614.

Effect of enalapril on survival in patients with reduced left ventricular ejection fractions and congestive heart failure. The SOLVD Investigators. *N Engl J Med.* 1991;325:293–302.

Feldman AM, Schneider VM. Congestive heart failure. In: Rakel R, ed. *Conn's Current Therapy 2000.* 52nd ed. Philadelphia: WB Saunders; 2000:292–297.

Giuliani ER, Fuster V, Gersh B, et al., eds. *Cardiology: Fundamentals and Practice.* 2nd ed. St Louis: Mosby; 1991:651–687, 791–858.

Goldberger E. *Essentials of Clinical Cardiology.* Philadelphia: Lippincott; 1990:148–160, 180–200.

Disorders of Cardiac Rhythm

Abnormalities of cardiac rhythm can vary widely from asymptomatic premature atrial complexes or mild sinus bradycardia to life-threatening ventricular tachycardia or fibrillation. Disorders of cardiac rhythm can be categorized into several groups.

These include:

- Bradyarrhythmias and conduction disturbances
- Ectopic or premature contractions
- Tachyarrhythmias

Although many rhythm and conduction disturbances are caused by underlying IHD, other causes include valvular heart disease, myocarditis, cardiomyopathy, congenital aberrant conduction pathways, pulmonary disease, toxic or metabolic disorders, neurogenic causes, and cardiac trauma.

The electrical impulse that initiates each heartbeat normally begins in the *sinoatrial (SA) node* and is conducted down through the atria and ventricles, resulting in a coordinated series of contractions of these chambers. The SA node is the primary pacemaker of the heart. It controls the heart rate and is influenced by neural, biochemical, and pharmacologic factors. If the SA node function is depressed or absent, secondary pacemakers in the *atrioventricular (AV) junction, the bundle of His,* or the *ventricular muscle* can generate stimuli and maintain the heartbeat. Normally, stimulus formation in these other secondary pacemaker sites is slower than that of the SA node. However, abnormal stimuli can also be generated at any of these sites at a rapid pace, resulting in tachycardia.

Bradyarrhythmias and Conduction Disturbances

A bradyarrhythmia is any rhythm resulting in a ventricular rate of less than 60 beats per minute (bpm).

Sinus bradycardia

A sinus rhythm (initiated by the SA node) slower than 60 bpm is called *sinus bradycardia.* It is usually innocuous and can occur in normal persons. Other typical causes include increased vagal tone, antiarrhythmic drug effect, ischemia, and primary sinus node disease. Affected patients may be asymptomatic or may complain of fatigue, angina, or syncope. Treatment is almost never indicated.

Sinus arrest

Also called *sinus block* or *SA block,* sinus arrest involves an absence of the entire complex for one or more beats. Single or multiple beats may be dropped. If the period of sinus arrest is prolonged, an AV nodal or ventricular escape beat may occur. Sinus arrest may be caused by increased vagal tone, sick sinus syndrome, carotid artery sinus hypersensitivity, hypokalemia, or the same medications that can cause sinus bradycardia. Patients may be asymptomatic if the pause is brief, or they may experience lightheadedness or syncope. If the condition is unstable or syncope develops from a long pause, emergency treatment with intravenous atropine usually increases the heart rate temporarily while definitive treatment is planned. In some cases, a pacemaker may be necessary.

Atrioventricular junctional rhythm

When the sinus node is depressed or nonfunctional, the AV node may take over the pacemaking function. During AV nodal pacing, the atria and ventricles contract independently. The heart rate in an AV junctional rhythm is usually about 30–60 bpm. Periodic prominent pulsations in the neck veins, occurring during systole, are noted. On the ECG, the QRS complex appears normal; however, the P waves are abnormal in shape and may follow the QRS in some leads. No treatment is usually necessary, but evaluating the patient for underlying cardiac disease may be appropriate.

Atrioventricular block

AV block is caused by a delay or block in conduction through the AV junction. In first-degree AV block, the PR interval seen on ECG may only be prolonged; in second- or third-degree AV block, ventricular beats may be dropped. Causes of AV block include vagal stimulation, medications, and heart disease.

First-degree AV block is asymptomatic and is diagnosed by the prolongation of the PR interval beyond 0.2 seconds on ECG. There are two types of *second-degree AV block*. In the *Wenckebach type*, the ECG reveals progressive PR prolongation prior to a nonconducted P wave, resulting in QRS complexes in regular groupings (grouped beating). In *Mobitz type II* AV block, the QRS complex is dropped at regular intervals and the QRS complex is usually widened. Patients with second-degree AV block may experience palpitations. The pulse rate is irregular in Wenckebach block and slow and regular in Mobitz type II block. The prognosis is usually worse with Mobitz type II block because it more often heralds underlying cardiac disease and may progress to complete heart block.

Complete, or *third-degree, AV block* is more ominous and usually causes more symptoms. All of the atrial stimuli are blocked at the AV node, so the P waves from the atria and the QRS complexes are completely asynchronous. The rate and width of the QRS complexes depend on whether they originate in the AV node, the bundle of His, or the ventricles. When the stimuli arise in the ventricles, the QRS complex is very wide and aberrant; this is called an *idioventricular escape rhythm.* Patients may be asymptomatic or may become lightheaded if the rate is very slow. If the ventricular rate is profoundly slow or if the beats cease for an interval, syncope may occur. This is known as *Stokes-Adams syndrome.* Atropine or isoproterenol can be given intravenously for immediate management of profound bradycardia or symptomatic heart block. A temporary transvenous pacemaker may be inserted to pace the heart until a permanent programmable pacemaker is implanted.

Intraventricular or fascicular blocks

The bundle of His has two main branches, the right and the left. The right branch is composed of a single fascicle, and the left is composed of at least two. *Left anterior hemiblock (fascicular block)* is characterized by marked left axis deviation on ECG and may result from MI, pulmonary embolism, cardiac surgery, or cardiac catheterization. This condition is insignificant unless it occurs concomitantly with right bundle branch block. *Left posterior hemiblock (fascicular block)* results in right axis deviation on ECG and may be caused by IHD, myocarditis, or valvular heart disease. This type of block is nearly always associated with right bundle branch block, resulting in a bifascicular block. No treatment is required for fascicular blocks.

Complete left bundle branch block (LBBB) LBBB results in a delay in conduction to the left ventricle, causing some asynchrony between the contraction of the two ventricles. This condition may be transient or permanent. It is usually secondary to various types of heart disease, but occasionally it is seen in normal hearts. LBBB is asymptomatic; however, it may interfere with the electrocardiographic diagnosis of MI by obscuring the Q wave and its secondary ST segment and T wave changes. Most clinicians think that the prognosis is excellent in young patients with LBBB. Older patients with LBBB appear to have a higher risk of cardiac disease and 10-year mortality compared with patients who do not have LBBB. Treatment is not necessary, but an evaluation for underlying heart disease is advised.

Right bundle branch block (RBBB) RBBB delays conduction to the right ventricle but does not cause symptoms. RBBB occurs in normal persons, but it can also be associated with pulmonary embolism, heart disease, cardiac surgery, chest trauma, cor pulmonale, and congenital heart defects. The ECG shows wide QRS complexes. When RBBB is not associated with pulmonary embolism or MI, prognosis is good. However, significant CAD has been reported in as many as 20% of asymptomatic patients with RBBB.

Premature Contractions

The principal types of premature contractions are:

- Premature atrial complexes
- Premature junctional complexes
- Premature ventricular complexes

Premature atrial complexes (PACs)

PACs result from ectopic atrial depolarizations occurring prior to the next depolarization from the sinus node. The resultant P waves usually differ in contour and axis from the normal sinus P wave. PACs may occur in the absence of structural heart disease but are common in the clinical settings of infection, inflammation, myocardial ischemia, drug toxicity, catecholamine excess, electrolyte imbalance, or excessive use of tobacco, alcohol, or caffeine. Symptoms range from none to feelings of "skipped" beats. PACs typically require no therapy. If symptoms are present, therapy should be directed toward correction of underlying abnormalities. β-Adrenergic antagonists or calcium channel antagonists may be useful.

Premature junctional complexes (PJCs)

PJCs are premature depolarizations from the AV node or the proximal portion of the His-Purkinje system. PJCs usually occur in the absence of structural heart disease but may be seen in clinical settings similar to those surrounding PACs. PJCs typically result in a premature, normally conducted QRS. An inverted P wave occurs during or just after the QRS complex, when retrograde AV nodal conduction occurs. The next, normally timed sinus P wave may be delayed or blocked in the AV node because of the retrograde conduction of the PJC. Symptoms and therapy are similar to those pertinent to PACs.

Premature ventricular complexes (PVCs)

PVCs are premature depolarizations that originate from the ventricles and occur prior to the next normally conducted sinus beat. PVCs often occur in the absence of structural heart disease and are increasingly frequent with age. Potential causes are similar to those for PACs. The ECG reveals a premature QRS complex of bizarre morphology with a T wave polarity opposite to that of the QRS complex. Patients may be asymptomatic or feel "skipped" beats. PVCs typically require no therapy. When patients are symptomatic, therapy should be directed toward correction of underlying abnormalities. Frequent or complex PVCs in the presence of cardiac disease are markers of an increased risk of sudden cardiac death. However, a direct causal link between PVCs and the onset of malignant ventricular tachyarrhythmias has never been established. The Cardiac Arrhythmia Suppression Trial showed that suppression of asymptomatic ventricular premature beats with class I antiarrhythmic drugs does not improve mortality in patients who have experienced infarction. In fact, this study showed that class IC drugs (flecainide and encainide) were associated with excessive mortality compared with placebo. The results of other studies also support the conclusion that class I antiarrhythmic drugs should not be used for treatment of PVCs, either asymptomatic or symptomatic, in patients with underlying structural heart disease and IHD.

Tachyarrhythmias

Tachyarrhythmias are defined as a heart rate in excess of 100 bpm. Tachycardias are distinguished as being supraventricular or ventricular, depending on the mechanism and site of origin.

Narrow complex tachycardias are almost exclusively supraventricular in origin.

Sinus tachycardia occurs when the sinus mechanism is accelerated. The pattern of atrial and ventricular activation is normal. Sinus tachycardia may occur in the setting of increased sympathetic or diminished vagal tone, catecholamine excess, pain, hypovolemia, hypoxemia, myocardial ischemia or infarction, pulmonary embolism, fever, and inflammation. The atrial rate is typically between 100 and 160 bpm. The ECG demonstrates P waves with a normal configuration and axis, a normal or slightly shortened PR interval, and a normal QRS pattern. Therapy should be targeted at the underlying pathophysiologic process. β-Blockers may be used to slow the sinus rate, particularly in the setting of myocardial ischemia.

Supraventricular tachycardias

This category includes paroxysmal atrial tachycardia, AV junctional tachycardia, atrial flutter, and atrial fibrillation. The exact site of the pacing focus may be difficult to determine when the heart rate is very rapid. The prognosis for supraventricular tachycardias is usually better than that associated with ventricular tachycardia. These tachycardias may be paroxysmal or chronic, as with chronic atrial fibrillation. Causes include emotional stress, caffeine, alcohol, drugs, thyrotoxicosis, lung disease, and cardiac disease.

Paroxysmal atrial tachycardia (PAT) The heart rate in PAT is often higher than 140 bpm. The P waves have an abnormal configuration and axis, the PR interval depends on the atrial rate, and the QRS pattern is either normal or reflects aberrant conduction secondary to the increased rate. If AV block and PAT are observed together, digitalis toxicity should be suspected. Multifocal PAT often is associated with chronic obstructive pulmonary disease and CHF. Clinical manifestations of PAT include palpitations, sensation of a rapid heart rate, lightheadedness, and rarely syncope. Patients with IHD may experience angina or dyspnea. Currently, the treatment of choice for PAT is *intravenous adenosine*. It has a very short half-life and has approximately a 90% success rate in yielding normal sinus rhythm. Other therapeutic measures include Valsalva maneuvers, carotid sinus pressure or massage, intravenous verapamil (except in Wolff-Parkinson-White syndrome), digitalis, and β-blockers. Patients with hemodynamic instability may require DC cardioversion. Precipitating factors should be reduced or eliminated, and any underlying disease should be treated. Unifocal or reentrant atrial tachycardias often can be eliminated permanently via radiofrequency catheter or surgical ablation.

Junctional tachycardia Junctional tachycardia is a rare rhythm disorder due to increased automaticity of the AV node. Junctional tachycardia typically produces heart rates of 60–130 bpm. It occurs in such clinical settings as ischemia, the postoperative state, and myocarditis. If retrograde AV conduction occurs, P waves are inverted and may appear during or immediately after the QRS. Also possible is competitive AV dissociation, wherein normal-appearing nonconducted P waves occur at a rate slower than the ventricular rate. The QRS pattern is either normal or reflects rate-related aberrant conduction. Treatment consists of correcting the underlying pathophysiologic process and discontinuing potentially offending agents. If required, lidocaine or β-blockers may be effective. For patients with competitive AV dissociation and hemodynamic compromise, atrial overdrive pacing may restore AV synchrony.

Wolff-Parkinson-White (WPW) syndrome The diagnosis of WPW syndrome should be considered in patients who present with tachycardia characterized by a widened QRS with an initial up-sloping (delta wave). WPW syndrome is characterized by pre-excitation (short PR interval and a delta wave slurring the upstroke of the QRS complex) and supraventricular tachycardia. In this syndrome, the ventricles are stimulated early by pre-excitation through accessory fibers. PAT, atrial flutter, or atrial fibrillation may occur with a very rapid rate in WPW syndrome because of a circus movement involving the accessory conduction pathways. The wide QRS complex that accompanies PAT and the WPW syndrome can resemble ventricular tachycardia.

Atrial flutter Atrial flutter is associated with a rapid atrial rate of 200–380 bpm. The ventricular rate is slower, usually with 2:1, 3:1, or 4:1 conduction. Atrial flutter is caused by a macro reentrant circuit isolated in the right atrium. Atrial flutter occurs in some normal patients, but it is also associated with MI, hyperthyroidism, mitral stenosis, and underlying lung disease. If the ventricular rate is slow, atrial flutter may occur without symptoms. If the rate is very rapid (>200 bpm), the symptoms are similar to those of PAT. The regular, rapid P waves of atrial flutter are called *F (flutter) waves* and have a sawtooth appearance. Some degree of AV block is usually present, resulting in QRS complexes at regular intervals. Atrial flutter may be paroxysmal or persistent. This arrhythmia can be fatal if the ventricular rate is very rapid in the setting of ischemia or heart failure. Conversion of atrial flutter to sinus rhythm should be attempted. Acute treatment measures include both controlling the ventricular response with β-blockers, calcium channel blockers, and digitalis and an attempt at restoring sinus rhythm with electrical cardioversion and antiarrhythmic drugs. *Ibutilide (Corvert)* is a relatively new agent that rapidly converts recent-onset atrial flutter or fibrillation. Adenosine can be used to confirm the diagnosis of atrial flutter, but its utility as a rate-slowing agent is limited by its very short half-life.

Atrial fibrillation Atrial fibrillation is caused by multiple simultaneous wavelets occurring in both the right and the left atria. This results in a chaotic electrical rhythm with ineffective atrial contraction. The causes and symptoms are similar to those of atrial flutter. The pulse rate is usually irregular, and characteristic changes—irregular (fibrillation) waves and an irregular ventricular rate—are common on ECG. Occasionally, aberrantly conducted beats result in a wide QRS that can resemble a PVC.

Because atrial contractions are ineffective in atrial fibrillation, cardiac output can be reduced markedly when the ventricular rate is very rapid. This may result in CHF. Atrial thrombi may accumulate from stagnation of blood in the atrial appendages. These thrombi may embolize to the lungs, brain, or other organs. Anticoagulation is indicated for patients with chronic atrial fibrillation associated with valvular disease, cardiomyopathy, or cardiomegaly and before conversion to sinus rhythm is attempted.

Conversion of atrial fibrillation can be attempted with quinidine, procainamide, ibutilide, or DC cardioversion. In many patients with chronic atrial fibrillation, maintenance therapy is often directed toward controlling the ventricular rate. This can usually be accomplished with digitalis, verapamil, or β-blockers.

Newer curative approaches have been developed for both atrial fibrillation and atrial flutter. These treatments include radiofrequency catheter ablation and the surgical Maze procedure. The Maze procedure interrupts all of the possible reentry circuits to the atrium with multiple incisions. A single uninterrupted pathway is left intact to allow normal conduction from the sinus node to the AV node. Of the 178 patients who underwent the Maze procedure, 93% were free of arrhythmia; the rest were converted to sinus rhythm with medical therapy.

Wide-complex tachycardias Wide-complex tachycardias may be either supraventricular or ventricular in origin, and correct identification of the origin and mechanism of the tachycardia is critical to the selection of appropriate treatment.

Ventricular tachyarrhythmias

Ventricular tachycardia (VT) VT is defined as a series of three or more ventricular complexes occurring at a rate of 100–250 bpm; the origin of activation is within the ventricle. The QRS is wide (usually >120 msec), with T wave polarity opposite to that of the major QRS deflection. Sustained VT is defined as tachycardia lasting longer than 30 seconds or associated with hemodynamic collapse. Monomorphic VT has a single QRS morphology throughout the arrhythmia, whereas polymorphic VT is characterized by ever-changing QRS morphology. Underlying causes include CAD, hypokalemia, hypomagnesemia, digitalis, quinidine, and other drugs that are potentially proarrhythmic. A recent study suggests that hearts with low EFs receive markedly increased reflex cardiac sympathetic stimulation, which may play a role in initiating and sustaining ventricular arrhythmias.

VT occurs infrequently in young patients with no organic heart disease. Brief episodes of VT cause palpitations; prolonged attacks in patients with organic cardiac disease can lead to heart failure or cardiac shock. If the rate is not very high and there is no significant underlying heart disease, VT may be well tolerated; however, VT may degenerate into ventricular fibrillation, resulting in hemodynamic collapse and death.

Treatment with immediate synchronized DC cardioversion is indicated for sustained VT associated with hemodynamic compromise, severe CHF, or ongoing ischemia or infarction. Pharmacologic cardioversion with IV procainamide or lidocaine and amiodarone may be attempted in patients with clinically stable VT. Amiodarone is probably the agent of choice for recurrent VT if its side effects are tolerated.

Electrophysiologic testing is often performed on patients with suspected or documented ventricular arrhythmias. In this procedure, direct transcatheter electrical stimulation of various sites in the ventricle induces arrhythmias. Given the efficacy and low risk associated with implantation, ICD therapy (often in conjunction with antiarrhythmic drugs) has become the treatment of choice for patients with life-threatening ventricular arrhythmias. Less common therapies include ventricular aneurysmectomy, ventricular electrical mapping and resection of the arrhythmogenic focus, and radiofrequency catheter ablation.

Implantable cardioverter-defibrillator ICDs are devices that monitor the heart rhythm and, when a tachyarrhythmia is identified, deliver therapy. Their evolution has been impressive. Initially, a thoracotomy was necessary to implant an epicardial patch or patches. Currently, the overwhelming majority of patients receive a transvenous system, which significantly reduces the morbidity and mortality associated with the implantation of these devices. Current-generation ICDs are generally implanted in the prepectoral region (similar to pacemaker implantation). Although first-generation ICDs delivered only high-energy "defibrillating" shocks, current-generation devices provide tiered therapy, including:

- Antitachycardia pacing algorithms
- Low-energy cardioversion for stable VT
- High-energy cardioversion for VT or ventricular fibrillation
- Single- or dual-chamber bradycardic pacing support
- Stored diagnostic information for rhythm discrimination

ICDs treat arrhythmias when they occur and do not prevent them. Many patients require concomitant antiarrhythmic therapy to reduce the frequency of device discharges or facilitate antitachycardia pacing by slowing the tachycardia rate. The development of an effective and safe antiarrhythmic prescription may be complex and requires the skills of a trained electrophysiologist. Generally, the acute management of life-threatening ventricular arrhythmias in these patients does not differ from that of other patients with similar rhythm disturbances. If the device fails to terminate an arrhythmia, cardiopulmonary resuscitation and external defibrillation should proceed normally. Three randomized prospective studies have demonstrated that automated ICDs are the preferred first-line therapy for patients who have survived a cardiac arrest or an episode of hemodynamically unstable VT. At 2-year follow-up, the automated ICD was associated with a 20%–30% relative reduction in the risk of death. Recent studies have also proved the benefit of ICDs used for primary prevention of sudden death in patients with CAD, reduced EFs, nonsustained VT, and inducible ventricular arrhythmias during electrophysiologic testing. Ongoing trials may expand the role of ICDs in the primary prevention of sudden death.

Torsades de pointes Torsades de pointes is a variant of VT. Specifically, it is a polymorphic VT characterized by QRS complexes that progressively oscillate in amplitude and morphology, giving the appearance of a twisting axis of depolarization. Torsades de pointes is often associated with a prolonged QT interval and may be caused by antiarrhythmic drugs, phenothiazines, tricyclic antidepressants, nonsedating antihistamines (terfenadine or astemizole), hypokalemia, hypocalcemia, or hypomagnesemia. Treatment involves replacement of potassium or magnesium and overdrive pacing, if necessary. Therapy for sustained arrhythmia should be immediate DC cardioversion. Quinidine and similar drugs should not be used because they may increase the abnormal QT interval and worsen the arrhythmia. All potentially offending agents should be discontinued.

Ventricular fibrillation (VF) VF is the most ominous of all the cardiac arrhythmias because it is fatal when untreated or when refractory to treatment. It is a major cause of sudden cardiac death outside the hospital. The ventricular contractions are rapid and uncoordinated, resulting in absence of effective ventricular pumping that soon leads to syncope, convulsions, and death if the VF is not interrupted. VF often occurs as a terminal rhythm in a dying patient, during or after MI, in patients with complete heart block, and as a result of electrocution, anesthesia, or drug toxicity from digitalis, quinidine, or other antiarrhythmic agents. VF rarely occurs spontaneously in an otherwise healthy person. The prognosis is generally poor because each episode can be fatal. However, some patients with complete heart block have recurrent self-limiting episodes of VF for years.

The ECG reveals irregular and rapid oscillations (250–400 bpm) of highly variable amplitude without identifiable QRS complexes or T waves. Emergency cardiopulmonary resuscitation efforts must be initiated right away. Immediate unsynchronized DC cardioversion is the primary therapy. After successful cardioversion, continuous intravenous infusion of effective antiarrhythmic therapy should be maintained until any reversible causes have been corrected. The choice of chronic antiarrhythmic therapy depends on the nature of the conditions responsible for the initial VF episode. Primary VF occurring within the first 72 hours of an acute MI is not associated with an elevated risk of recurrence and does not require chronic antiarrhythmic therapy. However, VF without an identifiable and reversible cause requires chronic therapy in the form of either prophylactic antiarrhythmic drug therapy (eg, amiodarone, sotalol) or implantation of an automatic defibrillator.

Block M, Breithardt G. The implantable cardioverter defibrillator and primary prevention of sudden death: the multicenter automatic defibrillator implantation trial and the coronary artery bypass graft (CABG)-patch trial. *Am J Cardiol.* 1999;83:74D–78D.

Botteron GW, Smith JM. Cardiac arrhythmias. In: Carey CF, Lee HH, Woeltje KF, eds. *Washington Manual of Medical Therapeutics.* 29th ed. Philadelphia: Lippincott-Raven; 1998:130–156.

Braunwald E, Zipes DP, Libby P, eds. *Heart Disease: A Textbook of Cardiovascular Medicine.* 6th ed. Philadelphia: WB Saunders; 2001.

Cox JL, Schuessler RB, Lappas DG, et al. An 8½-year clinical experience with surgery for atrial fibrillation. *Ann Surg.* 1996;224:267–273.

Higgins SL. Impact of the multicenter automatic defibrillator implantation trial on implantable cardioverter defibrillator indication trends. *Am J Cardiol.* 1999;83:79D–82D.

Hohnloser SH. Implantable devices versus antiarrhythmic drug therapy in recurrent ventricular tachycardia and ventricular fibrillation. *Am J Cardiol.* 1999;84:56R–62R.

Wagner GS. *Marriott's Practical Electrocardiography.* 10th ed. Philadelphia: Lippincott Williams & Wilkins; 2001.

Ophthalmologic Considerations

Many of the adult patients seen and treated by ophthalmologists are in the age group at risk for IHD and its many complications. These patients often undergo stressful eye surgery under local or general anesthesia. Ophthalmologists need to be cognizant of the risks of myocardial ischemia, infarction, CHF, and arrhythmias in these patients. Similarly, ophthalmologists need to be aware of the association between proliferative diabetic retinopathy and IHD. This information should be given to the patient's primary medical care provider so that appropriate screening tests can be considered.

A preoperative history and physical examination are important for all patients undergoing surgery. See Chapter 15 for a detailed discussion of preoperative testing. Cardiovascular contraindications to elective surgery include MI within the last 6 months, unstable angina, symptoms or clinical findings of severe CHF, and frequent or poorly controlled arrhythmias.

We would like to acknowledge Brian H. Sarter, MD, for his contributions to this chapter.

CHAPTER 5

Hypercholesterolemia

Recent Developments

- The association of low cholesterol with increased noncardiac death rates has been challenged.
- Lipid-lowering therapy with atorvastatin (Lipitor) reduces recurrent ischemic events in the first 16 weeks in patients with acute coronary syndrome.
- In patients with low pretreatment high-density lipoprotein (HDL)-C levels, coronary heart disease events were significantly reduced when levels of HDL-C were increased by gemfibrozil (Lopid) treatment.
- The National Cholesterol Education Program releases Adult Treatment Panel (ATP) III report.
- Researchers report that "statins" reduce (by at least one third) the chance of a heart attack, a stroke, or the need for a major procedure to clear obstructed coronary arteries for all high-risk patients (with previous myocardial infarction, existing heart disease, previous stroke, history of arterial obstructions, or diabetes), even patients whose cholesterol is below recommended levels.

Ahsun CH, Shah A, Ezekowitz M. Acute statin treatment in reducing risk after acute coronary symdrome: the MIRACL (Myocardial Ischemia Reduction with Aggressive Cholesterol Lowering) Trial. *Curr Opin Cardiol.* 2001;16:390–393.

Winslow R. Study shows statins help wider range of patients. *Wall Street Journal.* November14, 2001:B, 7.

Highlights

- Dietary therapy should be the first line of treatment in reducing serum cholesterol.
- Regular aerobic exercise and small amounts of alcohol intake have a beneficial effect on serum cholesterol by increasing HDL cholesterol.
- The 3-hydroxy-3-methyl glutaryl coenzyme A (HMG-CoA) reductase inhibitors lovastatin (Mevacor), pravastatin (Pravachol), simvastatin (Zocor), fluvastatin (Lescol), and atorvastatin significantly reduce serum low-density lipoprotein (LDL) cholesterol and total cholesterol.

Introduction

Coronary heart disease (CHD) is the leading cause of death in the United States, accounting for more deaths than all forms of cancer combined. Several major studies have confirmed earlier reports that lowering of elevated LDL cholesterol reduces the risk of CHD. The National Cholesterol Education Program has provided three updates for treatment of elevated blood cholesterol in adults (ATP I, II, III). ATP I proposed a strategy for primary prevention of CHD in persons with high levels of LDL cholesterol (>160 mg/dL) or borderline high levels of LDL (130–159 mg/dL) and multiple (at least two) risk factors (discussed below). ATP II added intensive management of LDL cholesterol in persons with established CHD (target cholesterol <100 mg/dL). Table 5-1 lists the new guidelines of ATP III.

Risk Assessment

About half of the United States population has a cholesterol level that puts them at significant risk. To determine an individual's risk status, a fasting lipoprotein profile (total cholesterol, LDL cholesterol, HDL cholesterol, and triglyceride levels) should be obtained in all adults over age 20 at least once every 5 years. Table 5-1 shows the ATP III classification of cholesterol levels:

- According to American Heart Association guidelines, the HDL ratio (ratio of total serum cholesterol to HDL cholesterol) should be less than 5.
- Along with cholesterol testing, other CHD risk factors should be assessed and managed appropriately in all adults (Table 5-2).

Management

In its simplest terms, the management of hypercholesterolemia consists of matching the intensity of LDL-lowering therapy with absolute risk; the higher the risk, the lower the target level. Multiple risk factors influence management recommendations as outlined in Table 5-3.

The clinical evaluation should include a complete history, physical examination, and basic laboratory tests. This workup attempts to determine whether the high LDL cholesterol level is secondary to another disease (such as diabetes, hypothyroidism, obstructive liver disease, or chronic renal failure) or to a drug (such as progestins, anabolic steroids, or corticosteroids) or whether a familial lipid disorder is present. The patient's total coronary risk and clinical status, as well as age and sex, should be considered in developing a cholesterol-lowering treatment program.

Some meta-analyses of cholesterol-lowering trials revealed an increase in mortality from nonatherosclerotic causes (cancer, suicide, accidental and violent death) associated with *low* levels of cholesterol (especially <160 mg/dL). On further review, some authorities think these apparent associations may be invalid for the following reasons:

Table 5-1 Adult Treatment Panel III Classification of LDL, Total, and HDL Cholesterol (mg/dL)

LDL cholesterol		
	<100	Optimal
	100–129	Near or above optimal
	130–159	Borderline high
	160–189	High
	≥190	Very high
Total cholesterol		
	<200	Desirable
	200–239	Borderline high
	≥240	High
HDL cholesterol		
	<40	Low
	≥60	High

(Modified from Executive Summary of the Third Report of the National Cholesterol Education Program (NCEP) Expert Panel on Detection, Evaluation, and Treatment of High Blood Cholesterol in Adults (Adult Treatment Panel III). *JAMA.* 2001;285:2486–2497.)

Table 5-2 Major Risk Factors (Exclusive of LDL Cholesterol) That Modify LDL Goals*

Cigarette smoking
Hypertension (blood pressure ≥140/90 mm Hg or on antihypertensive medication)
Low HDL cholesterol (<40 mg/dL)[†]
Family history of premature CHD (CHD in male first-degree relative <55 yr; CHD in female first-degree relative <65 yr)
Age (men ≥45 yr; women ≥55 yr)

* Diabetes is regarded as a CHD risk equivalent.
[†] HDL cholesterol ≥60 mg/dL counts as a "negative" risk factor; its presence removes one risk factor from the total count.

(Modified from Executive Summary of the Third Report of the National Cholesterol Education Program (NCEP) Expert Panel on Detection, Evaluation, and Treatment of High Blood Cholesterol in Adults (Adult Treatment Panel III). *JAMA.* 2001;285:2486–2497.)

Table 5-3 Three Categories of Risk That Modify LDL Cholesterol Goals

Risk Category	LDL Goal (mg/dL)
CHD and CHD risk equivalents	<100
Multiple (2+) risk factors*	<130
0–1 risk factor	<160

* Risk factors that modify the LDL goal are listed in Table 5-2.

(Modified from Executive Summary of the Third Report of the National Cholesterol Education Program (NCEP) Expert Panel on Detection, Evaluation, and Treatment of High Blood Cholesterol in Adults (Adult Treatment Panel III). *JAMA.* 2001;285:2486–2497.)

- The meta-analyses were flawed because some of the studies were not similar enough to allow meta-analysis.
- Preexisting disease can lower serum cholesterol.
- Low cholesterol is likely a marker for poor health and nutrition.
- The number of violent deaths were few in both the treated and the control groups.

The two major modalities of LDL-lowering therapy are therapeutic lifestyle changes (TLCs) and drug therapy. All persons with elevated LDL cholesterol may benefit from dietary therapy (reduced intake of saturated fat and cholesterol), increased physical activity, and weight control. Table 5-4 defines LDL cholesterol goals and cutpoints for initiation of TLCs and for consideration of initiating medication.

The essential features of TLCs are:

- Reduced intake of saturated fats (<7% of total calories) and cholesterol (<200 mg/dL) (see Table 5-5 for overall composition of diet)
- Use of plant stanols/sterols (2 g/day) and increased viscous (soluble) fiber (10–25 g/day) in the diet
- Weight reduction
- Increased physical activity

Figure 5-1 presents a model of steps in instituting TLCs.

Some patients in whom the short-term or long-term risk of CHD is high require LDL-lowering drugs *in addition to TLCs* to reach target cholesterol levels. Currently available drugs (and their characteristics) for this purpose are listed in Table 5-6. Figure 5-2 provides an outline for planning drug therapy.

Historically, the drugs of first choice were the *bile acid sequestrants (cholestyramine, colestipol)* and *nicotinic acid* (see Table 5-6). Both cholestyramine and nicotinic acid have

---

Table 5-4 LDL Cholesterol Goals and Cutpoints for Therapeutic Lifestyle Changes and Drug Therapy in Different Risk Categories

Risk Category	LDL Goal (mg/dL)	LDL Level at Which to Initiate TLCS (mg/dL)	LDL Level at Which to Consider Drug Therapy (mg/dL)
CHD or CHD risk equivalents (10-yr risk >20%)	<100	≥100	≥130 (100–129: drug optional)*
2+ risk factors (10-yr risk ≤20%)	<130	≥130	10-yr risk 10%–20%: ≥130 10-yr risk <10%: ≥160
0–1 risk factor[†]	<160	≥160	≥190 (160–189: LDL-lowering drug optional)

* Some authorities recommend use of LDL-lowering drugs in this category if an LDL cholesterol level of <100 mg/dL cannot be achieved by TLCs. Other authorities prefer use of drugs that primarily modify triglycerides and HDL (eg, nicotinic acid or fibrate). Clinical judgment also may call for deferring drug therapy in this subcategory.

[†] Almost all persons with 0–1 risk factor have a 10-yr risk that is <10%; thus, 10-yr risk assessment is not needed in persons with 0–1 risk factor.

(Modified from Executive Summary of the Third Report of the National Cholesterol Education Program (NCEP) Expert Panel on Detection, Evaluation, and Treatment of High Blood Cholesterol in Adults (Adult Treatment Panel III). *JAMA.* 2001;285:2486–2497.)

Table 5-5 Nutrient Composition of the Therapeutic Lifestyle Changes Diet

Nutrient	Recommended Intake
Saturated fat*	<7% of total calories
Polyunsaturated fat	Up to 10% of total calories
Monounsaturated fat	Up to 20% of total calories
Total fat	25%–35% of total calories
Carbohydrate[†]	50%–60% of total calories
Fiber	20–30 g/d
Protein	Approximately 15% of total calories
Cholesterol	<200 mg/dL
Total calories[‡]	Balance energy intake and expenditure to maintain desirable body weight/prevent weight gain

* *Trans* fatty acids are another LDL-raising fat that should be kept at a low intake.
[†] Carbohydrates should be derived predominantly from foods rich in complex carbohydrates including grains (especially whole grains), fruits, and vegetables.
[‡] Daily energy expenditure should include at least moderate physical activity (contributing approximately 200 kcal/d).

(Modified from Executive Summary of the Third Report of the National Cholesterol Education Program (NCEP) Expert Panel on Detection, Evaluation, and Treatment of High Blood Cholesterol in Adults (Adult Treatment Panel III). *JAMA.* 2001;285:2486–2497.)

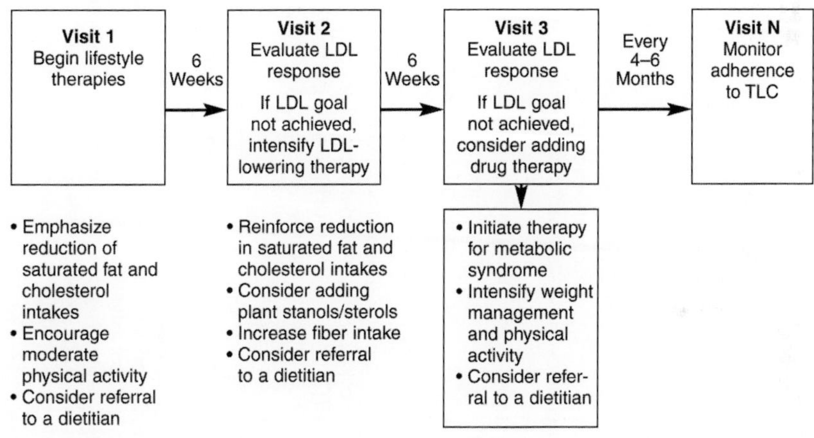

Figure 5-1 Model of steps in therapeutic lifestyle changes (TLC). LDL, low-density lipoprotein.

been shown to lower CHD risk in clinical trials, and their long-term safety has been established. However, these drugs require considerable patient education to achieve compliance because they are associated with poor patient tolerance. Nicotinic acid is preferred in patients with concurrent hypertriglyceridemia (triglyceride levels >250 mg/dL) because bile acid sequestrants tend to increase triglyceride levels.

The newer drugs that have begun to replace older medications as first-line therapy are the HMG-CoA reductase inhibitors (also known as *statins*, which include lovastatin, pravastatin, and simvastatin). Newer agents in this class include fluvastatin and atorvastatin. These drugs effectively lower LDL cholesterol levels and have been shown to reduce

Table 5-6 Drugs Affecting Lipoprotein Metabolism*

Drug Class, Agents, and Daily Doses	Lipid/Lipoprotein Effects	Side Effects	Contraindications	Clinical Trial Results
HMG-CoA reductase inhibitors[†]	LDL ↓ 18%–55% HDL ↑ 5%–15% TG ↓ 7%–30%	Myopathy; increased liver enzymes	*Absolute:* active or chronic liver disease *Relative:* concomitant use of certain drugs[§]	Reduced major coronary events, CHD deaths, need for coronary procedures, stroke, and total mortality
Bile acid sequestrants[‡]	LDL ↓ 15%–30% HDL ↑ 3%–5% TG no change or increase	Gastrointestinal distress; constipation; decreased absorption of other drugs	*Absolute:* dysbetalipoproteinemia; TG > 400 mg/dL *Relative:* TG > 200 mg/dL	Reduced major coronary events, CHD deaths
Nicotinic acid[¥]	LDL ↓ 5%–25% HDL ↑ 15%–35% TG ↓ 20%–50%	Flushing; hyperglycemia; hyperuricemia (or gout); upper gastrointestinal distress; hepatotoxicity	*Absolute:* chronic liver disease; severe gout *Relative:* diabetes; hyperuricemia; peptic ulcer disease	Reduced major coronary events and possible total mortality
Fibric acids[¶]	LDL ↓ 5%–20% (may be increased in patients with high TG) HDL ↑ 10%–20% TG ↓ 20%–50%	Dyspepsia; gallstones; myopathy; unexplained non-CHD deaths in WHO study	*Absolute:* severe renal disease; severe hepatic disease	Reduced major coronary events

* HMG-CoA indicates 3-hydroxy-3-methylglutrayl coenzyme A; LDL, low-density lipoprotein; HDL, high-density lipoprotein; TG, triglycerides; ↓, decrease; ↑, increase; CHD, coronary heart disease.

[†] Lovastatin (20–80 mg), pravastatin (20–40 mg), simvastatin (20–80 mg), fluvastatin (20–80 mg), atorvastatin (10–80 mg), and cerivastatin (0.4–0.8 mg). *Note:* Cerivastatin (Baycol) was withdrawn from the U.S. market in 2001 because of liver-related complications.

[‡] Cholestyramine (4–16 g), colestipol (5–20 g), and colesevelam (2.6–3.8 g).

[§] Cyclosporine, macrolide antibiotics, various antifungal agents, and cytochrome P-450 inhibitors (fibrates and niacin should be used with appropriate caution).

[¥] Immediate-release (crystalline) nicotinic acid (1.5–3 g), extended-release nicotinic acid (1–2 g), and sustained-release nicotinic acid (1–2 g).

[¶] Gemfibrozil (600 mg twice daily), fenofibrate (200 mg daily max dose), and clofibrate (1000 mg twice daily)

(Modified from Executive Summary of the Third Report of the National Cholesterol Education Program (NCEP) Expert Panel on Detection on Detection, Evaluation, and Treatment of High Blood Cholesterol in Adults (Adult Treatment Panel III). *JAMA.* 2001;285:2486–2497.)

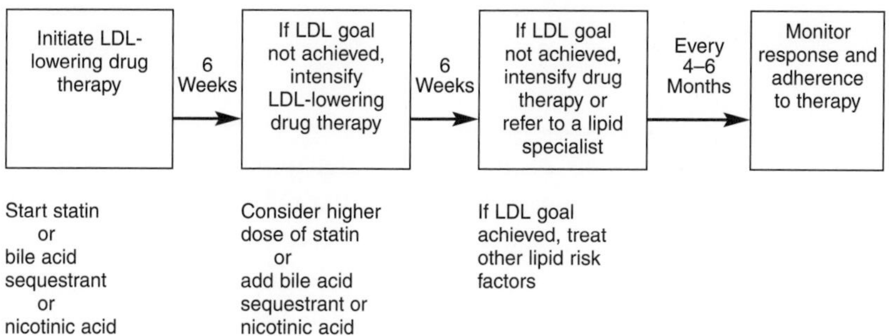

Figure 5-2 Progression of drug therapy in primary prevention. LDL, low-density lipoprotein.

mortality from ischemic heart disease. In a study of 8245 patients with moderate hypercholesterolemia, lovastatin was found to be well tolerated. The Myocardial Ischemia Reduction with Aggressive Cholesterol Lowering (MIRACL) study found that lowering lipids with atorvastatin, 80 mg/day, reduced recurrent ischemic events in patients with acute coronary syndrome in the first 16 weeks. Adverse drug effects requiring discontinuation ranged from 1.2% at 40 mg/day to 1.9% at 80 mg/day. The most common adverse reactions with this class of drugs are liver transaminase elevations and diarrhea.

Other available drugs include the *fibric acid derivatives gemfibrozil, clofibrate,* and *fenofibrate.* They are primarily used for lowering elevated triglyceride levels but also are effective in reducing total cholesterol and LDL cholesterol levels. Gemfibrozil also increases HDL cholesterol levels and may have beneficial effects on atherogenesis. In the Veterans Administration High-Density Lipoprotein Intervention Trial (VA-HIT), raising low HDL-C levels with gemfibrozil predicted significant reductions in CHD events.

In postmenopausal women with high serum cholesterol, *estrogen replacement therapy,* which lowers LDL cholesterol and raises HDL cholesterol levels, provides an additional treatment option, but the risks must be considered.

In hypertensive patients, *α-adrenergic blockers* provide modest reduction in cholesterol and triglyceride levels; thiazide diuretics and beta blockers may have an adverse effect.

Other Therapeutic Factors

Regular aerobic exercise provides a supplemental benefit in the management of hypercholesterolemia by increasing HDL cholesterol levels. Moderate alcohol consumption (1–2 drinks/day, up to 60 mL of alcohol/day) also increases HDL cholesterol levels. In patients with elevated LDL cholesterol levels, alcohol consumption was inversely related to risk of ischemic heart disease. This association was not observed in patients without elevated LDL cholesterol levels.

Special Issues

The Metabolic Syndrome

The so-called *metabolic syndrome* comprises a constellation of lipid and nonlipid risk factors of metabolic origin. Diagnosis is based on the presence of three or more risk determinants (Table 5-7).

The metabolic syndrome is closely linked to the disorder of insulin resistance. Excess body fat (particularly abdominal fat) and physical inactivity promote impaired responses to insulin, which may also occur as a genetic predisposition. The risk factors for metabolic syndrome are highly concordant; in aggregate, they increase the risk of CHD at any given LDL level. Management is as outlined previously, with emphasis on increased physical activity and weight reduction.

Comments on Specific Dyslipidemias

- *Very high LDL (>190 mg/dL).* This condition typically occurs in people with a genetic form of hypercholesterolemia (monogenic or polygenic hypercholesterolemia, familial defective apolipoprotein B). Screening of other family members is important for identification and treatment.
- *Elevated serum triglycerides* are an independent risk factor for CHD. Such elevation is most common in the metabolic syndrome. *Classification:* normal = <150 mg/dL; borderline high = 150–199 mg/dL; high = 200–499 mg/dL; very high = >500 mg/dL.
- *Low HDL level.* A low HDL level (<40 mg/dL) is a strong independent predictor of CHD.
- *Diabetic dyslipidemia.* Lowering LDL is the primary concern.

Table 5-7 Clinical Identification of the Metabolic Syndrome

Risk Factor	Defining Level
Abdominal obesity* (waist circumference)[†]	
Men	>102 cm (>40 in)
Women	>88 cm (>35 in)
Triglycerides	≥150 mg/dL
HDL cholesterol	
Men	<40 mg/dL
Women	<50 mg/dL
Blood pressure	≥130/≥85 mm Hg
Fasting glucose	≥110 mg/dL

* Overweight and obesity are associated with insulin resistance and the metabolic syndrome. However, the presence of abdominal obesity is more highly correlated with the metabolic risk factors than is an elevated body mass index (BMI). Therefore, the simple measure of waist circumference is recommended to identify the body weight component of the metabolic syndrome.

[†] Some male patients can develop multiple metabolic risk factors when the waist circumference is only marginally increased (eg, 94–102 cm [37–40 in]). Such patients may have strong genetic contribution to insulin resistance, and they should benefit from changes in life habits, similar to men with categorical increases in waist circumference.

Ophthalmologic Considerations

Hypercholesterolemia is a significant risk factor for ischemic heart disease, cerebrovascular disease, and peripheral vascular disease. The ophthalmologist may be the first physician to detect or recognize manifestations of atherosclerosis, particularly amaurosis fugax, retinal vascular emboli or occlusions, ischemic optic neuropathy, or cortical visual field deficits from a previous cerebral infarction. Detection of atherosclerosis may initiate a diagnostic evaluation that reveals significant carotid artery stenosis or coronary artery disease.

Because of early high-dose animal studies, cataract development was thought to be a possible adverse effect of lovastatin. However, clinical experience has revealed that lovastatin and other HMG-CoA reductase inhibitors do not significantly increase the risk of cataracts.

American College of Physicians Clinical Guideline, Part I—Guidelines for using serum cholesterol, high-density lipoprotein cholesterol, and triglyceride levels as screening tests for preventing coronary heart disease in adults. *Ann Intern Med.* 1996;124:515–517.

Binder EF, Williams DB, Schectman KB, et al. Effects of hormone replacement therapy on serum lipids in elderly women: a randomized, placebo-controlled trial. *Ann Intern Med.* 2001;134:754–760.

Eaton CB, Lapane KL, Garber CE, et al. Physical activity, physical fitness, and coronary heart disease risk factors. *Med Sci Sports Exerc.* 1995;27:340–346.

Executive Summary of the Third Report of the National Cholesterol Education Program (NCEP) Expert Panel on Detection, Evaluation, and Treatment of High Blood Cholesterol in Adults (Adult Treatment Panel III). *JAMA.* 2001;285:2486–2497. (Full text available online at www.nhlbi.nih.gov.)

Fortman SP, Maron DJ. Diagnosis and treatment of lipid disorders [CD-ROM]. *Sci Am Med.* March 1998.

Frick MH, Elo O, Haapa K, et al. Helsinki Heart Study: Primary prevention trial with gemfibrozil in middle-aged men with dyslipidemia. *N Engl J Med.* 1987;317:1237–1245.

Geurian KL. The cholesterol controversy. *Ann Pharmacother.* 1996;30:495–500.

Hamilton VH, Racicot FG, Zowall H, et al. The cost-effectiveness of HMG-CoA reductase inhibitors to prevent coronary heart disease. Estimating the benefits of increasing HDL-C. *JAMA.* 1995;273:1032–1038.

Hein HO, Suadicani P, Gyntelberg F. Alcohol consumption, serum low density lipoprotein cholesterol concentration, and risk of ischemic heart disease: six year follow up in the Copenhagen male study. *BMJ.* 1996;312:736–741.

Millay RH, Klein MI, Illingworth DR. Niacin maculopathy. *Ophthalmology.* 1988;95:930–936.

Ozsener S, Sendag F, Koc T, et al. A comparison of continuous combined hormone replacement therapy, HMG-CoA reductase inhibitor and combined treatment in the management of hypercholesterolemia in postmenopausal women. *J Obstet Gynaecol Res.* 2001;27:353–358.

Robins SJ, Collins D, Wittes JT, et al. Relation of gemfibrozil treatment and lipid levels with major coronary events—VA-HIT: a randomized controlled trial. *JAMA.* 2001;285:1585–1591.

Schwartz GG, Olsson AG, Ezekowitz MD, et al. Effects of atorvastatin on early recurrent ischemic events in acute coronary syndromes—the MIRACL study: a randomized controlled trial. *JAMA.* 2001;285:1711–1718.

Pulmonary Diseases

Recent Developments

- The National Asthma Education and Prevention Program has recommended that asthma treatment be tailored according to indicators of disease severity. The new approach also differentiates between medications that are used for long-term control of asthma versus medications that are to be used for rapid relief of acute symptoms.

Introduction

The lungs can be affected by numerous pathological processes, including inflammation (allergic, infectious, autoimmune, occupational exposure, toxic), vascular insults, fibrosis, carcinoma, and changes secondary to cardiac or musculoskeletal problems. The functional consequences of the pathological changes can be divided into *obstructive* and *restrictive* limitations on gas exchange.

Symptoms of lung disease include dyspnea, cough, and wheezing. *Dyspnea* develops when the demand for gas exchange exceeds the capacity of the respiratory response, as in hypoxemia or hypercapnia. *Cough* develops when mucus, inflammatory debris, or irritants affect the bronchi, causing reflex clearing expectoration. *Wheezing* occurs when bronchospasm narrows the large airways and exhaled air is forced through the narrowed passages.

Obstructive Lung Diseases

Chronic obstructive lung disease is the fourth leading cause of death in the United States. In obstructive lung diseases, the rate of exhalation is slowed, which prolongs the respiratory cycle. Changes in the bronchi and bronchioles and in the lung parenchyma can cause airway obstruction. Obstructive diseases can be separated into reversible and irreversible conditions, although a component of each is present in all obstructive diseases.

Reversible obstructive diseases are grouped under the term *asthma*, which denotes airway obstruction secondary to bronchospasm. In asthma, the airways are hyperresponsive and develop an inflammatory response to various stimuli, although the specific cause and duration of the bronchospasm vary. In some persons, allergic IgE-mediated reactions to defined antigens cause bronchospasm. In many other patients, the cause is unknown. Precipitating factors may include exercise, aspirin, sulfites, tartrazine dye, emotional stress, cold air, environmental pollutants, or viral infection. Bronchial smooth muscle constriction, mucosal edema, excess mucus accumulation, and epithelial cell shedding all contribute to airway obstruction. This obstruction may be reversible spontaneously or with treatment.

Irreversible obstructive disease (sometimes known as *chronic obstructive pulmonary disease*) comprises a group of conditions in which forced expiratory flow is reduced in either a constant or a slowly progressive manner over months or years. Some conditions, such as *cystic fibrosis*, an inherited defect in exocrine gland function, or *bronchiectasis*, either secondary to recurrent necrotizing bacterial infections or occurring as part of Kartagener syndrome, have an identifiable cause. However, most irreversible obstructive diseases, such as *emphysema, chronic bronchitis*, or *peripheral airway disease*, cannot be ascribed to specific conditions; rather, they represent an individual response to cigarette smoking and other airborne pollutants. For example, such responses occur in the setting of either α_1-antitrypsin deficiency (in certain forms of emphysema) or airway hyperactivity and mucus hypersecretion (as in bronchitis). The pathological consequences of the abnormal response result in specific damage to lung tissue. Emphysema is characterized by pathological enlargement of the terminal bronchiole air spaces by destruction of the alveolar connective tissue septa. Bronchitis is characterized by hypertrophied mucous glands in the bronchi; in peripheral airway disease, only the small airways demonstrate fibrosis, inflammation, and tortuosity.

Two clinical types of patients are seen in the advanced stages of chronic airway obstruction. The first type, known as *pink puffers*, tend to be thin, have hyperinflated lung fields, exhibit dyspnea without significant hypoxemia, and are free of the signs of right-sided heart failure. The second type, known as *blue bloaters*, demonstrate cyanosis, marked hypoxemia, and peripheral edema with right-sided heart failure *(cor pulmonale)*.

Restrictive Lung Diseases

The restrictive lung diseases encompass a diverse group of conditions that cause diffuse parenchymal damage. The physiologic consequences of this damage include a reduction in total lung volume, diffusing capacity, and vital capacity. Occasionally, patients without parenchymal involvement who have diseases of the chest wall, respiratory muscles, pleura, or spine may have similarly restricted lung volumes. A *fibrotic* parenchymal response can result from occupational exposure to various substances, including asbestos, silica dust, graphite, talc, coal, and tungsten. A *granulomatous* hypersensitivity reaction can develop in response to moldy hay, grains, birds, humidifiers and cooling systems, sawdust and wood pulp, or isocyanates and other noxious gases. Nonoccupational pulmonary disease can result from collagen vascular diseases, sarcoidosis, eosinophilic granuloma, Wegener granulomatosis, Goodpasture syndrome, alveolar proteinosis, idiopathic pulmonary hemosiderosis, idiopathic pulmonary fibrosis, and other idiopathic parenchymal diseases. Therapeutic agents such as dilantin, penicillin, gold, methotrexate, or radiation can also cause pulmonary disease.

Evaluation

Although all patients with respiratory problems should be under the care of a capable internist or pulmonologist, ophthalmologists and other physicians should also be aware of the methods used in the diagnosis and evaluation of breathing disorders. The following should be considered:

- *Symptoms:* Symptoms include dyspnea, orthopnea, chronic cough, and chronic sputum production.
- *History:* History may reveal occupational exposure, family history, cigarette use.
- *Signs:* Signs include audible wheezing, cyanosis, finger clubbing, forced expiratory time greater than 4 seconds, increased anteroposterior diameter of the chest.
- *Laboratory studies:* Results may reveal elevated hematocrit and hypoxia or hypercapnia on arterial blood gas measurement.
- *Chest radiography:* Radiographic findings include parenchymal disease, hyperinflation, diaphragmatic flattening, increased retrosternal lucency, and pleural abnormalities.
- *Computerized tomography of the chest* can detect minimal degrees of emphysema, obviating the need for tissue diagnosis.
- *Pulmonary function tests* measure the volume of air forcefully expelled over time. The forced expiratory volume over 1 second (FEV_1) represents the first second of exhalation; the total lung capacity represents the total volume exhaled. Both parameters and their serial rate of decline in a patient are objective measures of lung function as well as prognostic indicators of comorbidity and mortality from lung cancer and cardiovascular disease. FEV_1 less than 80% of predicted suggests obstructive disease; total lung capacity less than 70% of predicted suggests restrictive disease.
- *Bronchoscopy, transbronchial biopsy,* and *bronchial lavage* are used to obtain culture material, cytologic material, and pathological specimens for analysis.

Treatment

Treatment of pulmonary disease has two major goals: first, to favorably alter the natural history of the disease; and second, to improve the patient's symptoms and functional status and minimize associated problems.

Nonpharmacologic Approaches

In the case of chronic bronchitis and emphysema, *cessation of smoking* can favorably alter the course of the disease. Similarly, *avoidance of precipitants* of airway obstruction is important in ameliorating asthmatic conditions. In patients with severe pulmonary hypertension and cor pulmonale, use of supplemental oxygen to maintain an arterial oxygen pressure above 60 mm Hg confers a modest reduction in pulmonary hypertension and improved survival. However, a patient receiving supplemental oxygen must be carefully monitored because such treatment may decrease the respiratory drive to eliminate carbon dioxide, aggravating the respiratory acidosis that may lead to carbon dioxide narcosis. *Breathing exercises* and *postoperative chest physiotherapy* have demonstrable short-term effects in improving respiratory function.

Noninvasive pressure support ventilation can be used to deliver increased airway pressure. Continuous positive airway pressure (CPAP) provides continuous steady positive airway pressure throughout the ventilation cycle to improve alveolar oxygen exchange. During noninvasive pressure support ventilation, a tight, well-fitting mask is placed over the patient's mouth and nose or just over the nose. Noninvasive pressure support ventilation is best applied to patients with respiratory failure who are expected to quickly respond to medical therapy. Mask CPAP treatment of cardiogenic pulmonary edema was first described more than 50 years ago and has been shown to be a useful adjunct and reduces the need for intubation. Use of mask CPAP also aids in the treatment of respiratory failure due to pulmonary infections, trauma, and acute exacerbations of chronic obstructive pulmonary disease. Noninvasive pressure support ventilation for acute respiratory failure requires an alert patient capable of protecting the airway and handling secretions. Intubation and standard ventilation is preferred for patients who require total ventilatory support because the mask may slip and effective ventilation may cease. Nasal CPAP can be used in the management of obstructive sleep apnea. Ophthalmologists should be aware that nasal CPAP has been reported to modestly increase intraocular pressure in patients with glaucoma.

Pharmacologic Therapy

Pharmacologic approaches include medications that are specific for the particular pulmonary condition and medications that improve the patient's symptoms and functional status. *Specific medications* directly alter the pathophysiologic mechanisms underlying the patient's pulmonary disease. Some examples include cyclophosphamide for Wegener granulomatosis, steroids for sarcoidosis, and plasmapheresis with immunosuppressive drugs in Goodpasture syndrome.

Symptomatic medications are designed to reduce the obstructive or restrictive components affecting the patient's lung function. Medications used to treat symptomatic bronchospastic airway obstruction include bronchodilators, inhibitors of inflammation, and antibiotics during infection-precipitated airway closure (Table 6-1).

Bronchodilators, which include theophylline, β-adrenergic agonists, and anticholinergics, act primarily by relaxing the tracheobronchial smooth muscle. Although the bronchodilation produced by *theophylline* varies directly with the serum level, it is a weak phosphodiesterase inhibitor whose mechanism of action is unclear. Theophylline has a narrow therapeutic index: thus, serum levels should be measured (normally 10–20 mg/L) to avoid toxic effects such as nausea, tachycardia, headache, seizures, and ventricular arrhythmias while maintaining efficacy. Theophylline and its derivatives are administered either parenterally or orally.

β-Adrenergic agonists activate smooth muscle adenyl cyclase and cause a rise in intracellular cyclic adenosine monophosphate, resulting in bronchodilation. The selective β_2-adrenergics, which have greater bronchodilatory and less cardiostimulatory effects, are commonly used, often in metered-dose inhalers (they can also be administered orally or parenterally). These drugs have replaced the nonselective β-adrenergic agents such as

Table 6-1 Drugs for the Treatment of Asthma

β₂-selective adrenergic agents
  Albuterol (Proventil, Ventolin)
  Bitolterol mesylate (Tornalate)
  Pirbuterol acetate (Maxair)
  Salmeterol xinafoate (Serevent)*
  Terbutaline sulfate (Brethaire, Brethine, Bricanyl)
Anticholinergics
  Ipratropium bromide (Atrovent)
Xanthine derivatives and combinations
  Theophylline (Aerolate, Marax, Quibron, Respbid, Slo-Phyllin, Theo-Dur, Uniphyl)
Leukotriene modifiers
  Zafirlukast (Accolate)
  Zileuton (Zyflo)
  Montelukast (Singulair)
Mast cell stabilizers
  Cromolyn sodium (Intal)
  Nedocromil sodium (Tilade)
Corticosteroids
  Beclomethasone dipropionate (Beclovent, Vanceril)
  Budesonide (Pulmicort)
  Flunisolide (AeroBid)
  Triamcinolone acetonide (Azmacort)
  Fluticasone (Flovent)

* Only long-acting β₂-agonist.

isoproterenol. The selective β₂-agonists include albuterol, bitolterol, isoetharine, meta-proterenol, and terbutaline. These drugs differ in onset and duration of action. For example, isoetharine's onset is within 1–3 minutes and lasts for 60–90 minutes, whereas bitolterol's duration is 6–8 hours. Salmeterol, a particularly long-acting β₂-adrenergic, is helpful in maintenance treatment of asthma; it should not be used for acute exacerbations. Although epinephrine causes predominantly β-adrenergic stimulation in the lungs, it also causes peripheral α-adrenergic stimulation, resulting in vasoconstrictive hypertension and tachycardia. Epinephrine is most often administered subcutaneously to help control an acute asthma attack.

Anticholinergic agents directly relax smooth muscle by competing for acetylcholine at muscarinic nerve-ending receptors. Atropine and similar agents have been replaced by poorly absorbing atropinic congeners such as *ipratropium bromide* and *atropine methonitrate*. These newer inhalation agents have few systemic and minimal cardiac effects. They have an additive bronchodilator effect when combined with submaximal doses of β-adrenergic agonists.

Inhibitors of inflammation include corticosteroids, leukotriene inhibitors, and cromolyn sodium. *Corticosteroids* not only suppress inflammation of the bronchioles but also potentiate the bronchodilator response to β-adrenergic receptors. *Inhaled steroids* can be used chronically to reduce bronchial hyperreactivity; they are not used to manage acute attacks. *Systemic steroids*, however, are highly effective in managing acute episodes. Systemic steroids should be reserved for serious flare-ups to avoid adverse side effects.

Leukotriene inhibitors suppress the effects of inflammatory mediators. They are especially useful for prophylaxis and chronic maintenance therapy in asthma. *Cromolyn sodium* prevents the release of chemical mediators from mast cells in the presence of IgE antibody and the specific antigen. *Immunotherapy* has been shown to be helpful for asthma triggered by a defined antigen.

The National Asthma Education and Prevention Program has recommended that asthma treatment be tailored according to indicators of disease severity. This approach recommends that medication doses be adequate to rapidly control symptoms and later reduced to the minimal level required to maintain control. The new approach also differentiates between medications used for long-term control of asthma (maintenance medications that modify the asthmatic airway environment such that acute airway narrowing, requiring rescue treatments, occurs much less frequently) and medications used for rapid relief of acute symptoms. The goals of therapy should include prevention of symptoms, reduction in frequency and severity of exacerbations, maintenance of normal (or near-normal) pulmonary function, maintenance of normal activity levels, and minimization of medication side effects. Maintenance medications include inhaled corticosteroids, chromones, leukotriene modifiers, long-acting β_2-agonists such as albuterol and pirbuterol (Maxair), ipratropium bromide (Atrovent), and oral corticosteroids. Table 6-2 illustrates the stepwise approach for use of asthma medications. Figure 6-1 demonstrates a recommended approach to the management of reversible chronic obstructive pulmonary disease.

As mentioned above, appropriately used supplemental oxygen increases survival among patients with cor pulmonale. In addition, *diuretics* and *vasodilators* can improve the symptoms of cor pulmonale but they have not been proven to increase survival.

Preoperative and Postoperative Considerations

Before undertaking surgery in a patient with lung disease, the surgeon should consult with an internist or pulmonologist to carefully define the patient's functional respiratory status, especially with respect to the supine position. The patient's respiratory function should be maximized with medications and nonpharmacologic means as appropriate. The patient should be sedated only if necessary and, in that case, should be carefully monitored for arterial gas values.

Alvarez-Sala R, Diaz S, Prados C, et al. Increase of intraocular pressure during nasal CPAP. *Chest.* 1992;101:1477.

Baker WE, Lanoix R, Field DL, et al. Noninvasive assessment and support of oxygenation and ventilation. In: Roberts JR, Hedges JR, eds. *Clinical Procedures in Emergency Medicine.* 3rd ed. Philadelphia: Saunders; 1998:82–107.

Corren J. Asthma in adolescents and adults. In: Rakel R, ed. *Conn's Current Therapy 2000.* 52nd ed. Philadelphia: Saunders; 2000:730–740.

Niklas RA. National and international guidelines for the diagnosis and treatment of asthma. *Curr Opin Pulm Med.* 1997;3:51–55.

Petty TL, Weinmann GG. Building a national strategy for the prevention and management of and research in chronic obstructive pulmonary disease. National Heart, Lung, and Blood Institute Workshop Summary. *JAMA.* 1997;277:246–253.

Table 6-2 Asthma Severity and Treatment

	Mild Episodic	Mild Persistent	Moderate Persistent	Severe Persistent
Classification by:				
Symptoms	2 times a week	>2 times a week and <1 time a day	Daily	Continuous
		Flares may limit activity	Flares limit activity	Limited physical activity
Nighttime symptoms	2 times a month	>2 times a month	>1 time a week	Frequent
Lung function				
FEV_1 or PEF	80% predicted	80% predicted	>60% to <80% predicted	60% predicted
PEF variability	<20%	20%–30%	>30%	>30%
Treatment				
Asthma education	Yes	Yes	Yes	Yes
Trigger avoidance	Yes	Yes	Yes	Yes
Relievers (inhaled beta agonist such as albuterol, pirbuterol)*	1–2 puffs as needed	1–2 puffs as needed	2 puffs as needed	2 puffs as needed
Controllers				
Anti-inflammatory				
Inhaled corticosteroids	Not indicated	Low dose	Medium dose[†]	High dose w/ long-acting bronchodilator[†]
Cromolyn	Not indicated	Optional	Optional	Optional
Nedocromil	Not indicated	Optional	Optional	Optional
Systemic corticosteroid	Not indicated	Not indicated	Not indicated	If not controlled by topical
Immunotherapy	Optional in allergics	Optional in allergics	Optional in allergics	Optional in allergics

FEV_1 = forced expiratory volume in 1 sec; ICS = inhaled corticosteroids; PEF = peak expiratory flow
* With exacerbation, four puffs or 2.5–5 mg albuterol by nebulizer each 20 min × 3 doses, then each 1–4 h as needed; strongly consider short burst of oral steroid (ie, prednisone, 40 mg daily for 5 days).
[†] Preferred.

Table 6-2 Asthma Severity and Treatment (Continued)

	Mild Episodic	Mild Persistent	Moderate Persistent	Severe Persistent
Long-acting bronchodilators				
Sustained-release theophylline	Not indicated	Optional	Optional	Often w/ICS
Salmeterol (Serevent)	Not indicated	Optional	Optional w/anti-inflammatory	Often w/ICS
Long-acting β_2-agonist tablets	Not indicated	Optional	Optional w/anti-inflammatory	Often w/ICS
Leukotriene antagonists				
Zafirlukast (Accolate)	Not indicated	Optional	Optional w/ICS	Optional w/ICS
Montelukast (Singulair)	Not indicated	Optional	Optional w/ICS	Optional w/ICS
Leukotriene formation inhibitors				
Zileuton	Not indicated	Optional	Optional w/ICS	Optional w/ICS

(Adapted from Rakel R, ed. *Conn's Current Therapy 2001*. 53rd ed. Philadelphia: Saunders; 2001.)

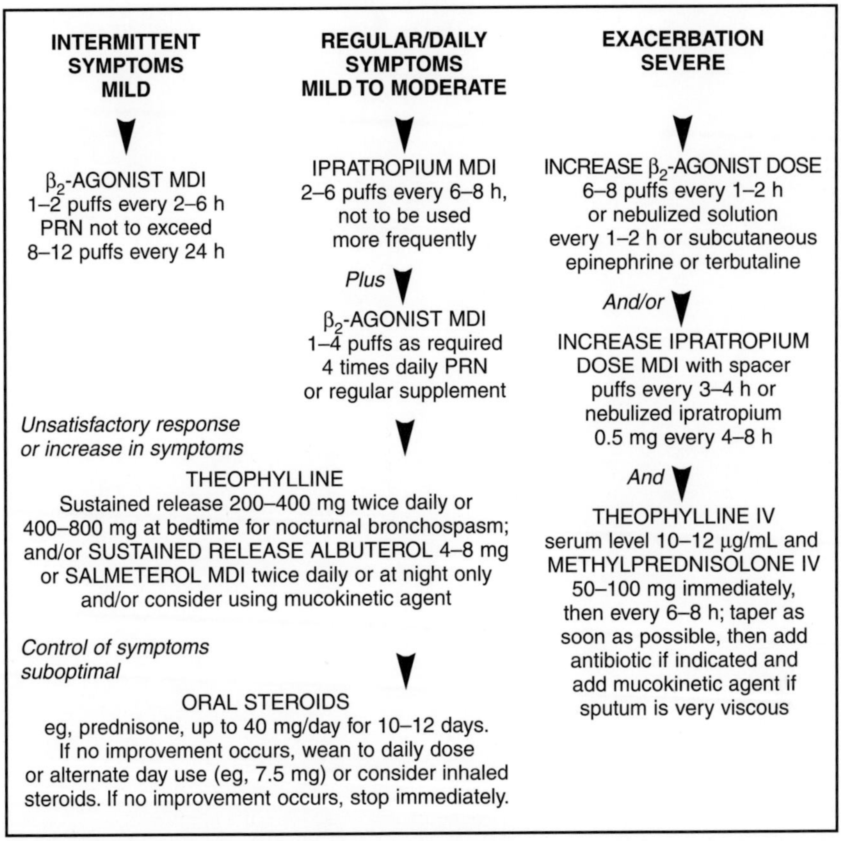

INTERMITTENT SYMPTOMS MILD	REGULAR/DAILY SYMPTOMS MILD TO MODERATE	EXACERBATION SEVERE

β₂-AGONIST MDI
1–2 puffs every 2–6 h
PRN not to exceed
8–12 puffs every 24 h

IPRATROPIUM MDI
2–6 puffs every 6–8 h,
not to be used
more frequently

INCREASE β₂-AGONIST DOSE
6–8 puffs every 1–2 h
or nebulized solution
every 1–2 h or subcutaneous
epinephrine or terbutaline

Plus 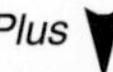

β₂-AGONIST MDI
1–4 puffs as required
4 times daily PRN
or regular supplement

And/or 

**INCREASE IPRATROPIUM
DOSE MDI with spacer**
puffs every 3–4 h or
nebulized ipratropium
0.5 mg every 4–8 h

*Unsatisfactory response
or increase in symptoms*

THEOPHYLLINE
Sustained release 200–400 mg twice daily or
400–800 mg at bedtime for nocturnal bronchospasm;
and/or SUSTAINED RELEASE ALBUTEROL 4–8 mg
or SALMETEROL MDI twice daily or at night only
and/or consider using mucokinetic agent

And 

THEOPHYLLINE IV
serum level 10–12 µg/mL and
METHYLPREDNISOLONE IV
50–100 mg immediately,
then every 6–8 h; taper as
soon as possible, then add
antibiotic if indicated and
add mucokinetic agent if
sputum is very viscous

*Control of symptoms
suboptimal*

ORAL STEROIDS
eg, prednisone, up to 40 mg/day for 10–12 days.
If no improvement occurs, wean to daily dose
or alternate day use (eg, 7.5 mg) or consider inhaled
steroids. If no improvement occurs, stop immediately.

Figure 6-1 Approach to the treatment of reversible chronic obstructive pulmonary disease (COPD). MDI = metered-dose inhaler. *(Adapted from American Thoracic Society. Standards for the diagnosis and care of patients with chronic obstructive pulmonary disease. American Thoracic Society. Am J Respir Crit Care Med. 1995;152(5 Pt 2):S77–S121.)*

Hematologic Disorders

Recent Developments

- Iron deficiency anemia can now be distinguished from anemia of chronic disease by using serum transferrin receptor assays.
- Additional thrombotic risk factors (eg, factor V and prothrombin gene mutations, hyperhomocystinemia) have been identified.
- Thrombophilia (the hypercoagulable state) is associated with recurrent fetal loss and preeclampsia.

Blood Composition

Formed elements—erythrocytes (red blood cells, or RBCs), white blood cells, and platelets—compose approximately 45% of the total blood volume. The fluid portion, plasma, is about 90% water. The remaining 10% of the plasma consists of proteins (albumin, globulin, fibrinogen, and enzymes), lipids, carbohydrates, hormones, vitamins, and salts. If a blood specimen is allowed to clot, the fibrinogen is consumed and the resultant fluid portion is called *serum*.

Erythropoiesis

All blood cells are thought to originate from an uncommitted pluripotential stem cell, designated the *colony-forming unit–spleen*. This in turn gives rise to (1) the *lymphoid stem cell* and (2) the *myeloid*, or *hematopoietic, stem cell* (or *colony-forming unit–culture*). The hematopoietic stem cell is thought to be the common precursor of RBCs, granulocytes, monocytes, and platelets. Stem cells are not morphologically recognizable, but their existence has been shown by various culture techniques.

RBCs are formed in the bone marrow in a series of steps. The colony-forming unit–culture gives rise to a *burst-forming unit–erythroid*, which, in response to erythropoietin (see below), becomes a *colony-forming unit–erythroid*. This entity differentiates through morphologically identifiable stages, during which the nucleus condenses and the cell gradually shrinks: pronormoblast, basophilic normoblast, polychromatophilic normoblast, and orthochromic normoblast. This phase takes approximately 3 days. The nucleus is then extruded, forming the reticulocyte, which is slightly larger than the normal mature

RBC. The reticulocyte remains in the bone marrow 2–3 more days and is then released into the peripheral blood. The mature erythrocyte is round, biconcave, and about 7 μm in diameter. Circulating RBCs have a lifespan of about 120 days.

Erythropoiesis is initiated by *erythropoietin,* a hormone that is found in the plasma and is produced mainly in the kidney. (Some researchers think that erythropoietin is also produced by the liver.) Any reduction in oxygen tension in the kidney (eg, from hypoxemia, low hemoglobin level, arterial insufficiency) stimulates production of erythropoietin, which causes stem cells to differentiate into pronormoblasts, leading to increased production of RBCs. In addition, immature reticulocytes are prematurely released into the peripheral blood. A number of tumors are associated with inappropriate production of erythropoietin, leading to erythrocytosis. These include benign and malignant kidney tumors, cerebellar hemangioblastoma, pheochromocytoma, and adrenal adenoma.

The production of RBCs and hemoglobin requires many substances. Iron is needed for proliferation and maturation of erythrocytes. Folic acid and vitamin B_{12} are necessary for DNA replication and cell division. Also required are manganese; cobalt; copper; vitamins C, E, B_{12}, thiamine, riboflavin, and pantothenic acid; and the hormones erythropoietin, thyroxine, and androgens.

Anemia

The *anemias* are a diverse group of disorders that have in common a reduction in the amount of circulating hemoglobin or erythrocytes, resulting in a decrease in the amount of oxygen reaching the tissues of the body. Normal hemoglobin levels are different for men (14–18 g/dL) and women (12–16 g/dL). Likewise, normal hematocrit values differ (men, 40%–54%; women, 37%–47%).

Diagnosis and Clinical Evaluation

The anemias may be classified by etiology, pathophysiologic mechanism, or morphology; none of these methods is ideal as a diagnostic approach. From a clinical standpoint, morphologic classification may be the most useful because it differentiates the various causes according to RBC size, information that is usually available from a complete blood count at the time of presentation. Thus, the mean corpuscular volume (MCV) is used to create three general categories of anemia: *microcytic* (MCV <83), *normocytic* (MCV 84–95), and *macrocytic* (MCV >95). The amount of hemoglobin (chromicity) has been used in the past as a second criterion, but in general microcytic anemias are hypochromic whereas normocytic and macrocytic anemias are normochromic.

The evaluation of the anemic patient is then guided by the morphology of the individual's erythrocytes. The causes of *microcytic anemia* include iron deficiency, thalassemia, and sideroblastic anemia. *Normocytic anemia* may be caused by defective formation of RBCs or the presence of tumor cells in the bone marrow in such conditions as aplastic anemia, myeloproliferative diseases, metastatic cancer, renal and inflammatory diseases, and chronic infection. Normocytic anemia may also be caused by abnormal hemoglobin or increased destruction of RBCs, as in sickle cell anemia, acquired hemolytic anemias, hemolytic disease of the newborn, and hypersplenism. *Macrocytic anemia* may result from deficiency of vitamin B_{12} or folic acid in cases of pernicious anemia, sprue, poor diet, alcoholism, and pregnancy, and after gastrectomy. Macrocytic anemia is also caused by accelerated erythropoiesis associated with hemolysis, acute blood loss, marrow replacement, or liver disease.

Clinical Consequences

Mild anemia is often asymptomatic. As the disease worsens, however, physiological adaptation to the blood's diminished oxygen-carrying capacity becomes clinically apparent. Blood flow is redistributed, shifting from skin and kidney to more oxygen-dependent tissues such as the brain, heart, and muscles. This produces the pallor and cool skin typical of anemic patients. With exercise or increasingly severe anemia, cardiac output is increased to provide more oxygen to the body. Exercise intolerance or fatigue at rest reflects the inability of the blood to provide adequate oxygen to major organs. Susceptible persons can experience high-output cardiac failure. Infarction of major organs can result, especially in patients with preexisting vascular insufficiency.

Anemia of Chronic Disease

Usually presenting as a mild normocytic or microcytic anemia, *anemia of chronic disease* is the most common form of anemia in hospitalized patients. It develops in association with malignancy, chronic infections (infectious endocarditis, tuberculosis, osteomyelitis), and chronic inflammation, such as in connective tissue and inflammatory bowel diseases. A hemoglobin level of less than 9 g/dL and a hematocrit value of less than 27% are unusual in this condition and should prompt an investigation into other possible causes, such as occult blood loss or iron deficiency. Anemia of chronic disease results from a combination of shortened RBC survival, impaired iron metabolism, and failure of the bone marrow to adequately increase RBC production. Iron deficiency anemia can now be distinguished from anemia of chronic disease by serum transferrin receptor assays.

Anemia in Elderly Patients

Studies have shown that the incidence of anemia increases each decade over age 60, especially in men. It has been suggested that the hematologic standards used for older men be adjusted for age. Evaluation of mild anemia (hemoglobin 12–14 g/dL) in this population fails to find a cause in most cases. These cases have sometimes been called *physiologic anemia* and attributed to the aging process. Below 12 g/dL, however, treatable causes—especially iron deficiency and hypothyroidism—are often discovered. Regardless of the hemoglobin level, however, all cases of iron deficiency anemia in this age group must be worked up.

Sickle Cell Disease

Affecting 0.2%–0.4% of the black population in the United States, sickle cell disease is a chronic anemia caused by an abnormal beta chain in the hemoglobin molecule. The resulting abnormal hemoglobin S, constituting 90%–100% of the hemoglobin in homozygous persons, causes intravascular hemolysis (sickling) that presents as painful episodes of vascular occlusion. Joint, bone, and abdominal pain are common, as are pulmonary and cerebral infarction. Heterozygotes have up to 50% hemoglobin S and are generally asymptomatic; they are said to have *sickle cell trait.*

Treatment of Anemia

Treatment is directed at the underlying cause whenever possible. Iron deficiency can be corrected with oral iron supplementation, provided there is adequate absorption and no source of chronic blood loss, such as gastrointestinal bleeding.

A recombinant form of the protein erythropoietin is available and approved for use in anemic patients with end-stage renal failure who are undergoing or awaiting hemodialysis, in whom such treatment is extremely effective. Erythropoietin is also being studied for use in anemia of chronic disorders and myelodysplastic diseases and in boosting hemoglobin levels prior to autologous blood donation. Erythropoietin appears to be effective in each of these situations, although higher doses are necessary than in renal failure.

Ocular manifestations of anemia include distended, tortuous retinal veins, hemorrhages, and cotton-wool spots. Retrobulbar neuritis may occur as part of the demyelinating disorder seen in pernicious anemia (vitamin B_{12} deficiency).

The eye is frequently affected by sickle cell disease. Hyphemas often cause marked elevation of intraocular pressure due to trabecular obstruction by RBCs that sickle in the hypoxic environment of the anterior chamber. Fundus abnormalities include choroidal vascular occlusion, angioid streaks, and venous tortuosity. Arteriolar occlusions, usually in the equatorial region, lead to hemorrhage *(salmon patches)* and neovascular tufts *(sea fans)*. See BCSC Section 12, *Retina and Vitreous,* for illustrations and further discussion of the ocular manifestations of sickle cell disease.

The use of general anesthesia can precipitate a sickling crisis in patients with sickle cell disease. Although the exact mechanism is not known, hypotension, hypovolemia, and hypoxemia are all thought to add to the likelihood of a crisis. The patient must therefore be meticulously monitored. *Hydroxyurea* has been proven effective in reducing the frequency and intensity of sickle cell crises and improving hematologic parameters.

Disorders of Hemostasis

A basic understanding of the hemostatic process and the manifestations associated with specific abnormalities helps the ophthalmologist with both medical and surgical management. (See Fig 7-1 for a diagram of blood-clotting pathways.) For the purpose of laboratory test interpretation, the coagulation cascade can be divided into intrinsic and extrinsic pathways. However, it is now understood that this is an oversimplification. For example, factor IX (an intrinsic factor) can be activated by factor VII (an extrinsic factor).

Hemostasis is initiated by damage to a blood vessel wall. This event triggers constriction of the vessel, followed by accumulation and adherence of platelets at the site of injury. Coagulation factors in the blood are activated, leading to formation of a fibrin clot. Slow fibrinolysis ensues, dissolving the clot while the damage is repaired. Circulating inhibitors are also present, modulating the process by inactivating coagulation factors to

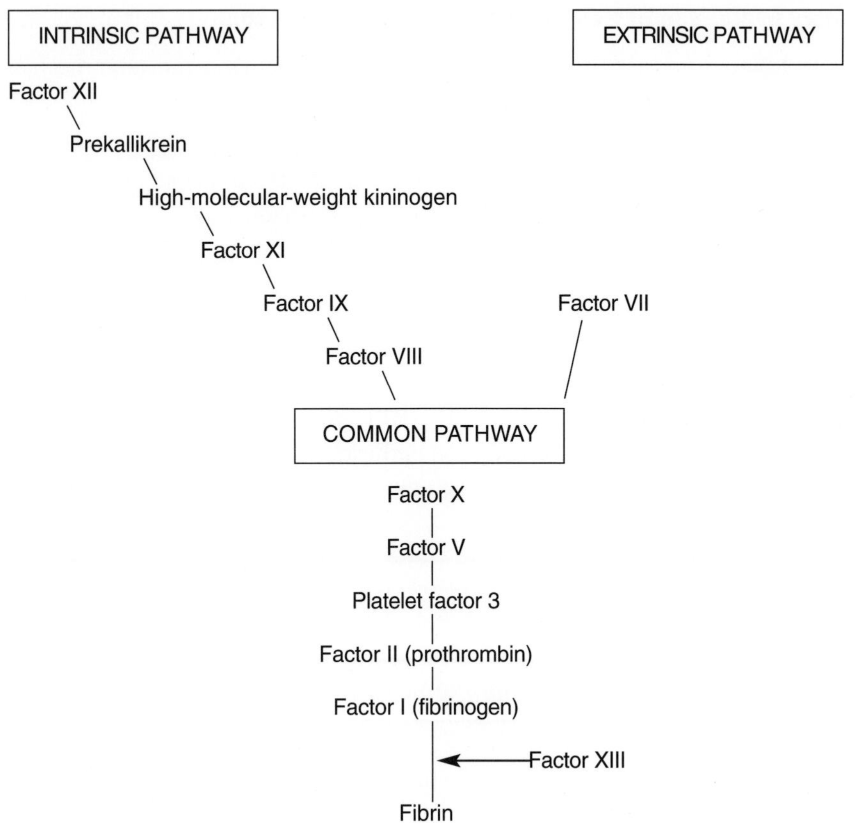

Figure 7-1 Blood-clotting pathways.

prevent widespread clotting. Normal endothelium plays a critical role in naturally anti-coagulating blood by preventing fibrin accumulation. The following physiologic anti-thrombotic systems can produce this effect:

- Antithrombin III
- Protein C and protein S
- Tissue factor pathway inhibitor
- The fibrinolytic system

Antithrombin III acts to inactivate thrombin. Activated protein C, with its cofactor protein S, functions as a natural anticoagulant by destroying factors Va and VIIa. Thrombin itself activates protein C. Although inherited deficiencies of antithrombin III, protein C, or protein S are associated with a lifelong thrombotic tendency, tissue factor pathway inhibitor deficiency has not yet been related to the hypercoagulable state (see later discussion of thrombotic disorders).

Laboratory Evaluation of Hemostasis and Blood Coagulation

Various techniques are used to assess the status of a patient's hemostatic mechanisms. Following are some of the most common tests:

- *Platelet count.* Minor bleeding may occur at platelet counts below 50,000/μL. Abnormal bleeding at higher platelet counts suggests abnormal platelet function. Below 20,000/μL, spontaneous bleeding may be serious.
- *Bleeding time.* A small dermal wound is created, and the duration of bleeding is recorded. This is a screening test of the vascular and platelet components of hemostasis. Because disorders of blood vessels are rare, the results essentially reflect platelet number and function. Bleeding time is prolonged when platelet counts drop below 50,000-100,000/μL.
- *Partial thromboplastin time (PTT).* The PTT requires all of the coagulation factors involved in the intrinsic and common pathways. The PTT is most commonly used to measure the effect of heparin therapy. Platelet abnormalities do not affect the result of this test.
- *Prothrombin time (PT).* The PT measures the integrity of the extrinsic and common pathways. It requires a 30% concentration of the vitamin K–dependent factors II, VII, and X (though not factor IX, a part of the intrinsic pathway) and therefore is prolonged in conditions affecting these factors (see below). The PT is most commonly used to monitor anticoagulant therapy. The action of heparin may slightly prolong PT.

In recent years, efforts have been made to tailor anticoagulation therapy to the problem being treated. For example, treatment or prevention of deep venous thrombosis is thought to require less oral anticoagulation therapy than endocardial mural thrombi or cardiac replacement valves. However, because of intra- and interlaboratory variation in test results, it has been difficult to standardize therapeutic dosages. To solve this problem, the international normalized ratio (INR) has been developed. The INR modifies the standard PT ratio (patient PT/control PT) to reflect the particular thromboplastin reagent used by a laboratory. The resulting reported INR value is an expression of the ratio of the patient's PT to the laboratory's mean normal PT. Thus, for prevention or treatment of deep vein thrombosis, the recommended INR value (comparable to subsequent values measured over time or across different laboratories) is 2.0–3.0; for tissue replacement valves, 2.0–3.0; for mechanical replacement valves, 2.5–3.5.

Clinical Manifestations of Hemostatic Abnormalities

Hemorrhage resulting from hemostatic derangement must be differentiated from hemorrhage caused by localized processes. The presence of generalized or recurrent bleeding suggests abnormal hemostasis. *Petechiae* (small capillary hemorrhages of the skin and mucous membranes) and *purpura* (ecchymoses) are typical of platelet disorders and vasculitis. Subcutaneous hematomas and hemarthroses characterize coagulation abnormalities. Bleeding due to trauma may be massive and life threatening in coagulation disorders, whereas bleeding is more likely to be slow and prolonged when platelet function is impaired.

Vascular Disorders

A number of inherited and acquired disorders of blood vessels and their supporting connective tissues result in pathological bleeding. *Hereditary hemorrhagic telangiectasia* (Osler-Weber-Rendu disease) is an autosomal dominant condition characterized by localized dilation of capillaries and venules of the skin and mucous membranes. The lesions increase over a period of decades, often leading to profuse bleeding.

Several inherited connective tissue disorders are associated with hemorrhage. *Ehlers-Danlos syndrome* is characterized by hyperplastic fragile skin and hyperextensible joints; it is dominantly inherited. In *osteogenesis imperfecta*, also a dominant trait, bone fractures and otosclerosis (leading to deafness) are common. In both of these conditions, easy bruising and hematomas are common. *Pseudoxanthoma elasticum*, a recessive disorder, is much rarer but is often complicated by gastrointestinal hemorrhage. *Marfan syndrome* is sometimes associated with mild bleeding as well as with aortic dissection.

Scurvy, the result of severe ascorbic acid deficiency, is associated with marked vascular fragility and hemorrhagic manifestations resulting from abnormal synthesis of collagen. In addition to the classic findings of perifollicular petechiae and gingival bleeding, intradermal, intramuscular, and subperiosteal hemorrhages are common. *Amyloidosis* is another acquired disorder in which petechiae and purpura are common.

All of the inherited vascular disorders have associated ocular findings. Conjunctival telangiectasias occur in hereditary hemorrhagic telangiectasia. Blue sclerae are typical of osteogenesis imperfecta. Ocular manifestations of Ehlers-Danlos syndrome include microcornea, myopia, and angioid streaks; retinal detachment and ectopia lentis have also been reported. Angioid streaks also occur in patients with pseudoxanthoma elasticum. Almost all patients with Marfan syndrome have some degree of ectopia lentis; severe myopia and retinal detachment are common.

Platelet Disorders

By far the most common cause of abnormal bleeding, platelet disorders may result from an insufficient number of platelets, inadequate function, or both. Mild derangement of platelet function may be asymptomatic or may cause minor bruising, menorrhagia, and bleeding after surgery. More severe dysfunction leads to petechiae, purpura, gastrointestinal bleeding, and other types of serious bleeding.

Thrombocytopenia

The number of platelets may be reduced by decreased production, increased destruction, or abnormal distribution. Production may be suppressed by many factors, including radiation, chemotherapy, alcohol use, malignant invasion of the bone marrow, aplastic anemia, and vitamin B_{12} or folic acid deficiency.

Accelerated destruction may occur through immunologic or nonimmunologic causes. *Idiopathic thrombocytopenic purpura (ITP)* is the result of platelet injury by antiplatelet antibodies. The acute form of ITP usually occurs in children and young adults, often following a viral illness, and commonly undergoes spontaneous remission. Chronic ITP is more common in adults and is characterized by mild manifestations; spontaneous remission is uncommon. Treatment consists of corticosteroid therapy or splenectomy.

Danazol is also effective in treating ITP, and when combined therapy is necessary, danazol allows the use of lower doses of corticosteroids. A neonatal form occurs in babies born to women with ITP; this form results from transplacental passage of antiplatelet antibodies. Recovery follows physiologic clearance of the antibodies from the child's circulation.

Many drugs have been implicated as causes of immunologic platelet destruction; readers are referred to the source textbooks for details. Another important cause is *post-transfusion isoantibody production,* which occurs predictably after transfusions containing platelets, unless human leukocyte antigen typing is undertaken, and leads to decreasing efficacy of later platelet transfusions.

Nonimmune causes of thrombocytopenia include *thrombotic thrombocytopenic purpura* and the syndromes of intravascular coagulation and fibrinolysis (discussed below). In addition to the symptoms of thrombocytopenia, thrombotic thrombocytopenic purpura is characterized by thrombotic occlusions of the microcirculation and hemolytic anemia. Fever, neurologic symptoms, anemia, and renal dysfunction occur with abrupt onset, with death occurring in days to weeks in the majority of untreated cases. Early treatment with exchange plasmapheresis has improved the survival rate to over 80%. Additional treatment includes antiplatelet drugs, corticosteroids, and splenectomy.

Abnormal distribution of platelets is most commonly caused by splenic sequestration. The usual clinical setting is hepatic cirrhosis, and the level of thrombocytopenia is mild. Patients with severely depressed platelet counts probably also have accelerated platelet destruction in the spleen.

Platelet dysfunction

Patients in this category usually come to the physician's attention because of easy bruising, epistaxis, menorrhagia, or excessive bleeding after surgery and dental work. Unlike patients with marked thrombocytopenia, patients with platelet dysfunction rarely have petechiae.

Hereditary disorders of platelet function are rare. Much more important clinically are the acquired forms, of which drug ingestion is the most common cause. As with drugs causing antiplatelet antibodies, the list of causative agents is very long. A single aspirin tablet taken orally irreversibly inhibits platelet aggregation for the lifespan of the circulating platelets present, causing a modest prolongation of the bleeding time for at least 48–72 hours following ingestion. This reaction has remarkably little effect in normal persons, although intraoperative blood loss may be slightly increased. However, in patients with hemophilia, severe thrombocytopenia, or uremia and in those on warfarin or heparin therapy, bleeding may be significant.

Nonsteroidal anti-inflammatory drugs cause reversible inhibition of platelet function in the presence of the drug; the effect disappears as the drug is cleared from the blood. Other commonly used drugs that may affect platelet function include ethanol, tricyclic antidepressants, and antihistamines.

In addition to uremia, clinical conditions associated with abnormal platelet function include liver disease, multiple myeloma, systemic lupus erythematosus, chronic lymphocytic leukemia, and Hermansky-Pudlak syndrome (an autosomal recessive form of oculocutaneous albinism).

Disorders of Blood Coagulation

Hereditary coagulation disorders

Inherited abnormalities involve all of the coagulation factors except factors III and IV. The most common and most severe is factor VIII deficiency, called *hemophilia A*, or *classic hemophilia*. Typical manifestations of this X-linked disease include severe and protracted bleeding, after even minor trauma, and spontaneous bleeding into joints (hemarthroses), the central nervous system, and the abdominal cavity.

Treatment involves infusion of coagulation factor VIII. Transfusion of pooled human factor VIII in the past had always carried a significant risk of transmission of hepatitis B virus; in the 1980s, transmission of the human immunodeficiency virus became a major problem as well. Those risks have now been mostly eliminated with the availability of recombinant factor VIII. Up to 10% of patients with hemophilia A develop antibodies, presumably due to sensitization following administration of factor VIII. These anticoagulants can also develop in normal elderly patients, in nonhemophiliac patients after drug reactions, and in those with collagen vascular diseases. Clinical manifestations range from mild bleeding to full-blown hemophilia. The PTT is prolonged, and the PT is normal. Treatment involves various regimens of coagulation factor replacement and immunosuppression to try to eliminate the inhibitor.

Von Willebrand disease, another relatively common hereditary disorder, is caused by deficiency or abnormality of a portion of the factor VIII molecule called von Willebrand's factor. This deficiency causes platelet adhesion abnormalities, leading to bleeding symptoms that are mild in most cases and may escape detection until adult years.

Acquired Coagulation Disorders

Vitamin K deficiency

Vitamin K is required for the production of factors II (prothrombin), VII, IX, and X in the liver. Normal diets contain large amounts of vitamin K, which is also synthesized by gut flora. Causes of vitamin K deficiency include biliary obstruction and various malabsorption syndromes (including sprue, cystic fibrosis, and celiac disease), in which intestinal absorption of vitamin K is reduced. Suppression of endogenous gastrointestinal flora, seen commonly in hospitalized patients on prolonged broad-spectrum antibiotic therapy, decreases intestinal production of vitamin K. However, clinical deficiency occurs only if dietary intake is also diminished. Nutritional deficiency is unusual but may occur with prolonged parenteral nutrition. Laboratory evaluation reveals prolongation of both PT and PTT. Most forms of vitamin K deficiency respond to subcutaneous or intramuscular administration of 20 mg of vitamin K_1, with normalization of coagulation defects within 24 hours. Vitamin K_1 should not be given intravenously because of the risk of sudden death from an anaphylactoid reaction.

One special form of vitamin K deficiency is *hemorrhagic disease of the newborn*, which is the result of a normal mild deficiency of vitamin K–dependent factors during the first 5 days of life and the absence of the vitamin in maternal milk. This condition is now rare in developed countries because of the routine administration of vitamin K to newborns.

Liver disease

Hemostatic abnormalities of all types may be associated with disease of the liver, the site of production of all the coagulation factors except factor VIII. As liver dysfunction develops, levels of the vitamin K–dependent factors decrease first, followed by factors V, XI, and XII; both PT and PTT are prolonged. Thrombocytopenia, primarily the result of hypersplenism, and a prolonged bleeding time due to platelet dysfunction are common. In addition, intravascular coagulation and fibrinolysis (see below) are common, further complicating the clinical picture.

Mild hemorrhagic symptoms are common in patients with significant liver disease. Severe bleeding is usually gastrointestinal in origin, arising from peptic ulcers, gastritis, and esophageal varices. Treatment is difficult at best and consists of blood and coagulation factor replacement. Local measures, such as vasopressin infusion or balloon tamponade of bleeding varices, can sometimes control potentially catastrophic bleeding.

Disseminated intravascular coagulation (DIC)

DIC is a complex syndrome involving widespread activation of the coagulation and fibrinolytic systems within the general circulation. Utilization and consumption of coagulation factors and platelets produce bleeding; formation of fibrin and fibrin degradation products (fibrin split products) leads to occlusion of the microcirculation, various forms of organ failure, and occasionally thrombosis of larger vessels. Laboratory findings may vary but usually include thrombocytopenia, hypofibrinogenemia, and elevated levels of fibrin split products. PT and PTT are usually, though not invariably, prolonged.

Clinically, two forms of DIC are recognized. *Acute DIC* is characterized by the abrupt onset of severe, generalized bleeding. The most common causes are obstetrical complications (most notably abruptio placentae and amniotic fluid embolism), septicemia, shock, massive trauma, and major surgical procedures. Treatment, other than specific measures aimed at the underlying disease, is controversial. Among the modalities used are heparinization and replacement of blood, platelets, and fibrinogen.

Chronic DIC is associated with disseminated neoplasms, some acute leukemias, and autoimmune diseases. Laboratory values range from normal to moderately abnormal; levels of coagulation factors may even be elevated. Bleeding and thrombosis (especially leg-vein thrombosis and pulmonary embolism) may occur, but in most patients the syndrome remains undiagnosed unless renal failure results from intravascular coagulation in the kidney. In these patients, the disease has been demonstrated via biopsy to detect fibrin in renal tissue. On occasion, chronic DIC may convert to the acute form.

Thrombotic disorders (thrombophilia)

The "hypercoagulable states" encompass a group of inherited or acquired disorders that increase the risk of thrombosis. The primary hypercoagulable states are caused by abnormalities of specific coagulation proteins involving inherited mutations in one of the antithrombotic factors. The trigger for a thrombotic event is often the development of one of the acquired secondary hypercoagulable states superimposed on an inherited state of hypercoagulability. The secondary hypercoagulable states cause a thrombotic tendency by complex and often multifactorial mechanisms.

Primary Hypercoagulable States

Antithrombin III deficiency

Antithrombin III deficiency leads to increased fibrin accumulation and a lifelong propensity to thrombosis.

Protein C deficiency

Protein C deficiency leads to unregulated fibrin generation because of impaired inactivation of factors VIIIa and Va, two essential cofactors in the coagulation cascade.

Protein S deficiency

Protein S is the principal cofactor of activated protein C, and therefore its deficiency mimics that of protein C.

Activated protein C resistance

Inherited activated protein C resistance causing thrombophilia was originally detected by the finding that the activated PTT of the plasma of affected persons could not be appropriately prolonged by the addition of exogenous activated protein C in vitro. The great majority of these subjects are now recognized to harbor a single specific point mutation in the factor V gene, termed *factor V Leiden*. This mutation is remarkably frequent (3%–7%) in healthy white populations but appears to be far less prevalent or even absent in certain black and Asian populations.

Prothrombin gene mutation

The prothrombin gene mutation has been associated with elevated plasma levels of prothrombin; it is second only to factor V Leiden as a genetic risk factor for venous thrombosis.

Hyperhomocystinemia

Hyperhomocystinemia is due to elevated blood levels of homocysteine and leads to severe neurologic developmental abnormalities in the homozygous state. Adults with heterozygous deficiency state may have only thrombotic tendencies. Acquired causes of hyperhomocystinemia in adults commonly involve nutritional deficiencies of pyridoxine, vitamin B_{12}, and folate, all cofactors in homocysteine metabolism. High blood concentrations of homocysteine constitute an independent risk factor for both venous and arterial thrombosis; in contrast, all of the other primary hypercoagulable states are associated only with venous thromboembolic complications, usually involving the lower extremities. The initial treatment of acute venous thrombosis in these patients is not different from treatment in those without genetic defects.

Secondary Hypercoagulable States

Malignancy may stimulate thrombosis directly by elaborating procoagulant substances that initiate chronic DIC. This appears to be most prominent in patients with pancreatic cancer, adenocarcinoma of the gastrointestinal tract or lung, and ovarian cancer. *Myeloproliferative disorders* (polycythemia vera, essential thrombocythemia, chronic myelogenous leukemia, and myelofibrosis) are major causes of thrombosis and paradoxical bleeding, as is the related stem cell disorder *paroxysmal nocturnal hemoglobinuria.* The *phospholipid antibody syndrome* is characterized by both venous and arterial thrombosis, including recurrent spontaneous abortions, deep venous thrombosis, and cerebrovascular arterial thrombotic events. Ophthalmic complications include retinal vein and artery occlusion, retinal vasculitis, choroidal infarction, and anterior ischemic optic neuropathy. Tests for patients with this syndrome include anticardiolipin antibodies, lupus anticoagulants, and biological false-position VDRL. The hypercoagulability associated with *pregnancy* involves a progressive state of DIC throughout the course of pregnancy, activated in the uteroplacental circulation. *Oral contraceptives* induce similar changes. The *postoperative state* and *trauma* are significant causes of venous thrombosis. Detailed discussion of treatment of these various and complex disorders is beyond the scope of this text.

Therapeutic anticoagulation

Many clinical situations require intentional disruption of the hemostatic process. The effect of aspirin on platelet function has already been discussed.

Heparin is a mucopolysaccharide that binds antithrombin III, inhibiting the formation of thrombin. It is given intravenously or subcutaneously, and therapy is assessed by measuring the PTT. Aspirin should not be given to patients on heparin because the resultant platelet dysfunction may provoke bleeding.

The orally administered warfarin derivatives, of which warfarin sodium (Coumadin) is the most widely used, inhibit the production of normal vitamin K–dependent coagulation factors (II, VII, IX, and X). Therapeutic effect is assessed by measuring the patient's INR. One critical issue is the long list of commonly used drugs that interact with warfarin. These interactions may cause an unintended increase or decrease in the INR, depending on the drug.

Heparin and the warfarin derivatives are used to prevent the formation of new thrombi and the propagation of existing thrombi, but neither affects the original clot. Thrombolytic agents such as *streptokinase, urokinase,* and *tissue plasminogen activator* are used to dissolve existing thrombi, most notably in the very early stages of myocardial infarction resulting from coronary artery thrombosis. These agents are also currently being used for early treatment of thrombotic stroke; this form of treatment increases the risk of converting a thrombotic stroke into a hemorrhagic stroke.

Asherson RA, Merry P, Acheson JF, et al. Antiphospholipid antibodies: a risk factor for occlusive ocular vascular disease in systemic lupus erythematosus and the "primary" antiphospholipid syndrome. *Ann Rheumatol Dis.* 1989;48:358–361.

Provan D, O'Shaughnessy DF. Recent advances in haematology. *BMJ.* 1999;318:991–994.

Schafer A. Approach to the patient with bleeding and thrombosis. In: Goldman L, Bennett JC, eds. *Cecil Textbook of Medicine.* Vol 1. 21st ed. Philadelphia: WB Saunders; 2000:991–995.

Schafer A. Thrombotic disorders: hypercoagulable states. In: Goldman L, Bennett JC, eds. *Cecil Textbook of Medicine.* Vol 1. 21st ed. Philadelphia: WB Saunders; 2000:1016–1021.

CHAPTER 8

Rheumatic Disorders

Recent Developments

- Cyclooxygenase 2 (COX-2)–selective nonsteroidal anti-inflammatory drugs (NSAIDs) are introduced to minimize gastrointestinal damage.
- Leflunomide (Arava) is a new disease-modifying antirheumatic drug (DMARD) approved for the treatment of rheumatoid arthritis. Leflunomide inhibits pyrimidine synthesis, thereby targeting rapidly dividing cell populations.
- Two new agents for cytokine-based therapy of rheumatoid arthritis are etanercept (Enbrel) and infliximab (Remicade). Both agents are inhibitors of tumor necrosis factor α (TNF-α).

Introduction

The rheumatic disorders are a heterogeneous collection of diseases that include rheumatoid arthritis, the seronegative spondyloarthropathies, juvenile rheumatoid arthritis, systemic lupus erythematosus, scleroderma, polymyositis and dermatomyositis, Sjögren syndrome, relapsing polychondritis, Behçet syndrome, and the vasculitides, including polyarteritis nodosa, allergic granulomatosis, Wegener granulomatosis, giant cell arteritis, and Takayasu arteritis. Ocular involvement is common in the rheumatic diseases but varies among the different disorders.

Rheumatoid Arthritis

Rheumatoid arthritis (RA) is the most common rheumatic disorder, affecting approximately 1% of adults. RA is classically an additive, symmetrical, deforming, peripheral polyarthritis characterized by synovial membrane inflammation. All joints may be involved, but this disorder affects primarily the small joints of the hands and feet. Like all inflammatory arthritides, RA is associated with the *gel phenomenon,* a stiffness at rest that improves with use; patients often complain of morning stiffness. Approximately 80% of patients with RA are positive for a rheumatoid factor, which is an autoantibody directed against immunoglobulin G. Seropositive RA aggregates in families. Human leukocyte antigen DR4 (HLA-DR4) is found in 70% of Caucasian seropositive patients.

Extra-articular disease in RA may affect a wide variety of nonarticular tissues. Rheumatoid nodules, located subcutaneously on extensor surfaces, occur in approximately 25% of patients with RA. The lungs may be affected with rheumatoid pleural effusions, pleural nodules, pulmonary nodules, and occasionally interstitial fibrosis. Cardiac disease includes pericarditis and rheumatoid nodules involving the conducting system, heart valves, or both. Mild anemia of chronic disease is the rule. *Felty syndrome* is a triad of RA, splenomegaly, and leukopenia. Patients with Felty syndrome often have hyperpigmentation, chronic leg ulcers, and recurrent infections. Rheumatoid vasculitis affects fewer than 1% of patients with RA. It generally presents either as peripheral polyneuropathy or as refractory skin ulcers. Patients may develop digital gangrene or occasionally visceral ischemia. The most common neuropathy is median nerve compression caused by synovitis of the wrist.

Ophthalmologic Considerations

Ocular manifestations of RA include Sjögren syndrome, scleritis, episcleritis, and marginal corneal ulcers. Baseline ophthalmic evaluation of patients with RA is suggested to monitor for retinal toxicity from hydroxychloroquine therapy. Most reported retinal complications of this drug have occurred in patients who have taken a cumulative dosage of more than 800 g. The ocular manifestations of RA are discussed in BCSC Section 6, *Pediatric Ophthalmology and Strabismus;* and Section 9, *Intraocular Inflammation and Uveitis.* Retinal complications from hydroxychloroquine are discussed in Section 12, *Retina and Vitreous.*

Therapy

Treatment of RA is approached in a stepwise additive fashion, with the initial therapy being an NSAID. All of the different NSAIDs (eg, aspirin, indomethacin, naproxen, sulindac) appear to be about equally effective, although the response of the individual patient may vary from one drug to another. COX-2–selective NSAIDs are newer agents introduced to minimize gastrointestinal damage (see later discussion of NSAIDs).

The second phase of treatment is to add a *remittive agent,* also known as a *slow-acting antirheumatic drug (SAARD).* Although these second-line agents are sometimes called *DMARDs,* true disease modification is difficult to document. Many think that these agents may improve the natural disease course. These agents are classified by toxicity as follows:

- *Least toxic:* hydroxychloroquine, oral gold, and sulfasalazine
- *More toxic:* methotrexate, parenteral gold, azathioprine, cyclosporine, and penicillamine
- *Most toxic:* chlorambucil, cyclophosphamide

These drugs often take several months to have an effect but can induce a remission of the active arthritis and are thought to retard joint destruction. *Methotrexate* is often used very early in the disease course; many rheumatologists prefer this SAARD agent because it is more effective and better tolerated than some of the other agents listed. Because of their toxicity, the most potent immunosuppressive drugs are reserved only for severe and unresponsive cases. Low-dose *prednisone* (5–10 mg orally per day) is sometimes added to the treatment regimen to increase the patient's mobility and functional capacity. Therefore, if an NSAID alone is inadequate, most rheumatologists add a SAARD, with or without low-dose corticosteroids, very early in the disease course. Leflunomide is a new DMARD approved for the treatment of RA. It inhibits pyrimidine synthesis, targeting rapidly dividing cell populations. Two new agents approved for cytokine-based therapy of RA are etanercept, a TNF-α receptor blocker, and infliximab, an anti–TNF-α monoclonal antibody.

Joint surgery for pain and impaired function is useful at virtually all stages of RA.

Seronegative Spondyloarthropathies

The seronegative spondyloarthropathies include ankylosing spondylitis, reactive arthritis (formerly known as *Reiter syndrome*), arthritis with inflammatory bowel disease (enteropathic arthritis), juvenile spondyloarthropathy, acne-associated arthritis, Whipple disease, and psoriatic arthritis. "Seronegative" refers to the uniform absence of serum immunoglobulin M antibodies to immunoglobulin G (rheumatoid factor). These spondyloarthropathies are linked by their statistical association with the antigen type HLA-B27 and by their overlapping features, but they are distinguished by their somewhat different clinical patterns.

Ocular Findings

The most common ophthalmic manifestation of these diseases is nongranulomatous acute anterior uveitis. Indeed, acute anterior uveitis shares with the seronegative spondyloarthropathies a statistical association with HLA-B27: approximately 50% of patients with nongranulomatous acute anterior uveitis are positive for HLA-B27. See BCSC Section 9, *Intraocular Inflammation and Uveitis*, for illustrations and further discussion of these conditions.

Ankylosing Spondylitis

Ankylosing spondylitis is characterized by involvement of the axial skeleton and bony fusion (ankylosis). Inflammation occurs particularly at the enthesis, the point where ligaments and tendons attach to bone. The cause is unknown, but the strong association with HLA-B27 suggests a genetic predisposition. Although more than 90% of Caucasian patients with ankylosing spondylitis possess HLA-B27, only 6%–8% of the general population is positive for HLA-B27. The prevalence of ankylosing spondylitis is approximately 0.1%–0.2% of the population. Men are affected three times more commonly than women; moreover, the radiographic features seem to evolve more slowly in women.

The classic features of ankylosing spondylitis are chronic low back pain, fusion of the axial skeleton (spinal ankylosis), and sacroiliitis. The demonstration of sacroiliitis on x-ray examination of the sacroiliac joints is the sine qua non for the diagnosis of spondylitis. The end stage of this process is a completely fused and immobilized spine, also known as a *bamboo* or *poker spine*. In addition to the spinal arthritis that is the hallmark of the disease, patients may develop arthritis of the shoulders and hips, limited chest expansion, and restrictive lung disease. Other extra-articular features include apical pulmonary fibrosis, ascending aortitis, aortic valvular incompetence, and heart block. The primary ocular manifestation of ankylosing spondylitis is recurrent, acute, nongranulomatous iridocyclitis, which occurs in approximately 25% of these patients.

Reactive Arthritis (Reiter Syndrome)

Reactive arthritis, formerly known as Reiter syndrome, was originally defined by the classic triad of arthritis, nongonococcal urethritis, and conjunctivitis. It is now recognized that most patients present with arthritis alone. Like ankylosing spondylitis, reactive arthritis has a clear genetic predisposition in that 63%–95% of patients are positive for HLA-B27. It has become clear that reactive arthritis develops in a genetically susceptible host following an infection by bacteria such as *Chlamydia trachomatis* in the genitourinary tract or by *Salmonella, Shigella, Yersinia,* or *Campylobacter* organisms in the gastrointestinal tract. Fragments of *Yersinia, Salmonella,* and *Chlamydia* organisms have been identified in the synovial tissues of patients with reactive arthritis, but intact organisms have not been cultured. The male/female ratio is at least 5:1.

The arthritis of reactive arthritis typically appears within 1–3 weeks of the inciting urethritis or diarrhea. It is an asymmetrical, episodic oligoarthritis affecting primarily the lower extremities, in particular the large joints such as the knees or ankles. Other particular features include periostitis, particularly heel pain, interphalangeal arthritis of the toes and fingers producing "sausage digits," and sacroiliitis. Mucocutaneous lesions include urethritis in men and cervicitis in women, circinate balanitis, painless oral ulcers, nail lesions, and keratoderma blennorrhagicum. Patients may also have systemic symptoms including fever and weight loss. The disease tends to follow an episodic and relapsing course. Systemic treatment includes NSAIDs and sulfasalazine in addition to appropriate antibiotic therapy. Patients should undergo HIV testing prior to consideration of immunosuppressive therapy.

Ophthalmologic considerations

Conjunctivitis is one of the hallmarks of the disease and is part of the original triad described by Reiter. The more serious ocular manifestation is uveitis, which, as in ankylosing spondylitis, is an acute, nongranulomatous, recurrent iridocyclitis that occurs in 15%–25% of patients with reactive arthritis.

Enteropathic Arthritis

Enteropathic arthritis is associated with ulcerative colitis and Crohn disease. *Ulcerative colitis* is an inflammatory disorder of the gastrointestinal mucosa with diffuse involvement of the colon. *Crohn disease* is a focal granulomatous disease involving all areas of the bowel and affecting both the large and the small intestine. Crohn disease is also known as *regional enteritis, granulomatous ileocolitis,* and *granulomatous colitis.* Symptoms of inflammatory bowel disease include diarrhea, bloody diarrhea, and cramping abdominal pain.

Extraintestinal manifestations of inflammatory bowel disease include dermatitis, mucous membrane disease, ocular inflammation, and arthritis. Skin disorders occur in approximately 15% of patients with inflammatory bowel disease and include erythema nodosum (in Crohn disease) and pyoderma gangrenosum (in ulcerative colitis). Enteropathic arthritis occurs in up to 22% of patients and has two distinct variants. *Peripheral arthritis* is predominantly a nondeforming oligoarthritis of the lower extremity. The activity of enteropathic arthritis parallels the activity of the bowel disease. The second type is *ankylosing spondylitis,* which is present in at least 7%–12% of patients with enteropathic arthritis. The activity of the spondylitis is unrelated to the activity of the bowel disease. Multiple series have shown that 50% of patients with spondylitis and enteropathic arthritis are positive for HLA-B27, which predisposes them to spondylitis and iridocyclitis. Ocular inflammation—including iridocyclitis, scleritis, and less commonly retinal vasculitis—occurs in approximately 3%–11% of patients with enteropathic arthritis.

Psoriatic Arthritis

Psoriatic arthritis, an inflammatory arthropathy, occurs in about 6% of patients with psoriasis and may occur before the skin lesions have appeared. The pattern of joint involvement varies, but the radiographic feature of whittling of the distal phalanges ("pencil-in-cup" appearance) is distinctive. NSAIDs are the mainstay of treatment for this form of arthritis, which runs a fairly benign course.

Juvenile Spondyloarthropathy

Juvenile spondyloarthropathy has replaced the term *juvenile rheumatoid arthritis* because only a small portion of affected children have the same disease as adults with RA.

Subsets of juvenile spondyloarthropathy have been identified. First, older children (over age 10) may develop a seropositive (rheumatoid factor–positive), rheumatoid-like polyarthritis. Among this subgroup, girls are more commonly affected than boys. The arthritis is an additive, symmetrical, deforming polyarticular arthritis identical to adult RA; tends to be persistent; and results in severe morbidity. Ocular disease is uncommon in this subgroup.

Second is a systemic variant known as *Still disease.* The male/female ratio is approximately 1:1, and this disease affects young children, generally under age 5. The systemic manifestations sometimes occur before the onset of the arthritis, which generally presents as a polyarthritis. The systemic features predominate and include fever, a salmon-colored evanescent maculopapular rash, lymphadenopathy, hepatitis, spleno-megaly, serositis, an elevated erythrocyte sedimentation rate (ESR), and leukocytosis. Ocular disease is generally not associated with this variant.

Third is a constellation of early-childhood oligoarthritis associated with antinuclear antibodies and a high risk of chronic iridocyclitis and blindness. Periodic eye examinations are important to detect occult ocular inflammation. (See BCSC Section 6, *Pediatric Ophthalmology and Strabismus;* and Section 9, *Intraocular Inflammation and Uveitis.*)

Fourth is an early-childhood polyarthritis that is seronegative for rheumatoid factor and antinuclear antibodies.

Systemic Lupus Erythematosus

Systemic lupus erythematosus (SLE) is generally regarded as the prototypical autoimmune disease. The cause of SLE is unknown, but familial aggregation of autoimmune diseases and association with the HLA types DR2 and DR3 suggest a genetic predisposition. Pathogenetically, SLE is characterized by B-cell hyperreactivity, polyclonal B-cell activation, hypergammaglobulinemia, and a plethora of autoantibodies. These autoantibodies include antinuclear antibodies, antibodies to DNA (both single-stranded DNA [anti-ssDNA] and double-stranded or native DNA [anti-dsDNA or anti-nDNA]), and antibodies to cytoplasmic components. SLE classically has been considered an immune complex disease in which immune complexes incite an inflammatory response and lead to tissue damage.

SLE affects women five times as often as men, and the disease may affect almost any organ system. Cutaneous disease, which occurs in approximately 70%–80% of patients, is most often manifested by the characteristic butterfly rash across the nose and cheeks, also known as a *malar flush*. Other cutaneous manifestations include discoid lesions, vasculitic skin lesions such as cutaneous ulcers or splinter hemorrhages, purpuric skin lesions, and alopecia. Less common skin lesions include a maculopapular eruption, lupus profundus, bullous skin lesions, and urticarial skin lesions. Mucosal lesions, characteristically painless oral ulcers, occur in 30%–40% of patients. Photosensitivity occurs in many patients with SLE.

About 80%–85% of patients with SLE experience articular disease at some point, either polyarthralgias or a nondeforming, migratory polyarthritis. Cutaneous nodules, myalgias, and myositis are far less common. Systemic features, including fatigue, fever, and weight loss, occur in over 80% of patients with lupus. Renal disease is present in approximately 50%–75% of patients with SLE. Clinically, it presents as either proteinuria with nephrotic characteristics or glomerulonephritis with an active urinary sediment. Lupus nephritis is a major cause of the morbidity and mortality of SLE.

Raynaud phenomenon occurs in 30%–50% of patients. Cardiac disease includes pericarditis, occasionally myocarditis, and Libman-Sacks endocarditis. Pleuropulmonary lesions include pleuritic chest pain and, less commonly, pneumonitis. Hepatosplenomegaly and adenopathy occur in over 50% of patients with SLE.

Central nervous system (CNS) involvement occurs in more than 35% of patients with SLE, and manifestations are typically transient. Peripheral neuropathy and cranial nerve palsies are less common. The most common manifestations of CNS lupus are headache, seizures, an organic brain syndrome, and psychosis. Transverse myelitis is an uncommon manifestation in patients with SLE but often occurs in association with optic neuritis.

SLE frequently affects the hematologic system. Patients often have an anemia of chronic disease but may also develop an autoimmune hemolytic anemia. Leukopenia, in particular lymphopenia, is a characteristic feature. Thrombocytopenia occurs in approximately one third of patients.

Because of the diffuse manifestations of SLE, diagnostic criteria have been established.

These include:

- Malar rash
- Discoid lupus
- Photosensitivity
- Oral ulcers
- Arthritis
- Serositis (pleuritis, pericarditis)
- Renal disorder (proteinuria, nephritis)
- Neurologic disorder (seizures, psychosis)
- Hematologic disorder (hemolytic anemia, leukopenia, lymphopenia, thrombocytopenia)
- Immunologic disorder (positive results with LE cell test, anti-DNA test, anti-Sm test; false-positive test result for syphilis)
- Antinuclear antibody

Four or more of these criteria are needed for a diagnosis of SLE. It should be emphasized that these criteria are used in clinical investigation and not for patient management.

Ophthalmologic Considerations

The major ocular manifestations of SLE are:

- Involvement of eyelid skin with cutaneous disease, most often discoid lesions
- Secondary Sjögren syndrome
- Retinal vascular lesions
- Neuro-ophthalmic lesions

Retinal vascular manifestations are the most common form of ophthalmic involvement in patients with SLE. They consist of cotton-wool spots with or without intraretinal hemorrhages. The prevalence varies from 3% of outpatients to 28%–29% of hospitalized patients. Neuro-ophthalmic involvement in SLE includes cranial nerve palsies, lupus optic neuropathy, and central retrochiasmal disorders of vision. The cerebral disorders of vision include hallucinations, visual field defects, and cortical blindness.

Treatment is controversial but may include bed rest during episodes of disease activity, avoiding physiologic stresses on the body, and avoiding sun exposure. Helpful medications include NSAIDs, antimalarials, glucocorticoids, and cytotoxic drugs.

Scleroderma

Scleroderma, also known as *progressive systemic sclerosis,* is a rheumatic disease of unknown cause characterized by fibrous and degenerative changes in the viscera, skin, or both. Scleroderma is much more common in women and rare in childhood. There is no known cure. The disorder may be localized (confined to the skin, subcutaneous tissue, and muscle) or systemic (which may be diffuse or limited). Localized scleroderma is not a severe illness and may allow a normal lifespan. The limited form of systemic scleroderma, known as *CREST* (calcinosis, Raynaud phenomenon, esophageal involvement, *s*clerodactyly, and *te*langiectasias), involves internal organs less frequently and therefore carries a better prognosis than the diffuse form. In addition to the thickening and fibrous replacement of the dermis, the disease is characterized by vascular insufficiency and vasospasm. The hallmark of scleroderma is the skin change, which consists of thickening, tightening, and induration, with subsequent loss of mobility and contracture. The disease most characteristically begins peripherally and involves the fingers and hands, with a subsequent centripetal spread up the arms to involve the face and body. Telangiectasia and calcinosis are common. More than 95% of scleroderma patients experience Raynaud phenomenon, and some develop digital ulcers.

Organ involvement is common and includes esophageal dysmotility with gastro-esophageal reflux in over 90% of patients. The small and large intestines may be involved with decreased motility, malabsorption, and diverticulosis. Cardiopulmonary disease is manifested primarily by pulmonary fibrosis, which results in restrictive lung disease with a decreased diffusing capacity. The consequences of the interstitial fibrosis include pulmonary hypertension and right-sided heart failure. Conduction abnormalities and arrhythmias result from cardiac fibrosis. Musculoskeletal features include polyarthralgias, tendon friction rubs, and occasionally myositis.

Renal disease is a major cause of mortality and is often associated with the onset of malignant hypertension and a rapid progression to renal failure. This process is sometimes known as *scleroderma renal crisis* or *scleroderma kidney.* This complication was uniformly fatal until the late 1970s; however, aggressive antihypertensive therapy sometimes reverses the scleroderma renal crisis. Angiotensin-converting enzyme inhibitors are effective in treating the hypertension associated with scleroderma renal disease and in delaying the progression to renal failure.

Overlap syndromes occur between scleroderma and other diseases. The best-known overlap syndrome is *mixed connective tissue disease,* which has features of SLE, systemic sclerosis, and myositis. This syndrome is characterized by antibodies to ribonuclear protein, and it has been suggested that some of its clinical features respond to steroids.

Ophthalmologic Considerations

Ocular manifestations of scleroderma include eyelid involvement resulting in tightness and blepharophimosis (but only rarely corneal exposure); conjunctival vascular abnormalities, including telangiectasia and vascular sludging; and keratoconjunctivitis sicca. Occasionally, a patient develops retinopathy of malignant hypertension, with cotton-wool spots, intraretinal hemorrhages, and optic disc edema, as a result of scleroderma renal crisis.

Polymyositis and Dermatomyositis

Polymyositis and dermatomyositis are inflammatory diseases of skeletal muscle characterized by pain and weakness in the involved muscular groups. Typically, weakness begins insidiously and involves the proximal muscle groups, particularly those of the shoulders and hips. *Dermatomyositis* is distinguished from *polymyositis* by the presence of cutaneous lesions. These skin lesions are an erythematous to violaceous rash variably affecting the eyelids (heliotrope rash), cheeks, nose, chest, and extensor surfaces. The knuckles of the fingers may develop plaques known as *Gottron papules.* The diagnosis of myositis is based on the characteristic clinical features and abnormal laboratory findings. Laboratory abnormalities include elevated serum levels of skeletal muscle enzymes, abnormal electromyography results, and muscle damage and inflammation as revealed by muscle biopsy.

Polymyositis and dermatomyositis have been classified into seven groups:

- Primary idiopathic polymyositis
- Primary idiopathic dermatomyositis
- Dermatomyositis (or polymyositis) associated with malignancy
- Childhood dermatomyositis (or polymyositis)
- Polymyositis or dermatomyositis associated with collagen vascular disease (overlap group)
- Miscellaneous: eosinophilic myositis, localized nodular myositis, and others

Dermatomyositis with malignancy occurs most often in patients over age 50 and rarely in young patients. Vasculitis is common in patients with childhood dermatomyositis. Inflammatory myositis with a defined connective tissue disease is usually associated with SLE or scleroderma.

Ophthalmologic Considerations

Other than the heliotrope rash of dermatomyositis, ocular involvement is relatively uncommon in inflammatory myositis. Occasionally, ophthalmoplegia is due to involvement of the extraocular muscles by the myositis.

Sjögren Syndrome

Sjögren syndrome was originally described as a triad of dry eyes, dry mouth, and RA. Subsequently, it became apparent that Sjögren syndrome could coexist with a variety of other connective tissue diseases, including SLE and scleroderma (secondary Sjögren syndrome) or without a definable connective tissue disease (primary Sjögren syndrome).

The cause of the dry eyes and dry mouth in patients with Sjögren syndrome is a mononuclear inflammatory infiltrate into the lacrimal and salivary glands, resulting in glandular destruction and dysfunction. Several studies have demonstrated the usefulness of minor salivary gland biopsy in documenting the presence of such an inflammatory infiltrate. Patients with Sjögren syndrome often have autoantibodies to the Ro and La antigens; these antigens are also known as SSA (Sjögren syndrome A) and SSB (Sjögren syndrome B), respectively. Preliminary criteria for the diagnosis of Sjögren syndrome have been published, including parameters referring to oral and ocular symptoms, ocular signs, salivary gland involvement, histopathologic features, and the presence of autoantibodies anti-Ro/SSA and anti-La/SSB. The presence of four of six items confers high sensitivity and specificity (Table 8-1). There appears to be a subset of patients with primary Sjögren syndrome who have vasculitis, hyperglobulinemia, CNS lesions, and an increased risk of malignancy, particularly lymphoma. Treatment is aimed at symptomatic

---

Table 8-1 Preliminary Criteria for the Classification of Sjögren Syndrome

1. Ocular symptoms
   A positive response to at least 1 of the following 3 questions:
      (a) Have you had daily, persistent, troublesome dry eyes for more than 3 months?
      (b) Do you have recurrent sandy or gravelly feeling in the eyes?
      (c) Do you use tear substitutes more than 3 times a day?
2. Oral symptoms
   A positive response to at least 1 of the following 3 questions:
      (a) Have you had a daily feeling of dry mouth for more than 3 months?
      (b) Have you had recurrent or persistently swollen salivary glands as an adult?
      (c) Do you frequently drink liquids to aid in swallowing dry foods?
3. Ocular signs
   Objective evidence of ocular involvement determined on the basis of a positive result on at least 1 of the following 2 tests:
      (a) Schirmer-1 test ($\leq$5 mm in 5 minutes)
      (b) Rose bengal score ($\geq$4, according to the van Bijsterveld scoring system)
4. Salivary gland involvement
   Objective evidence of salivary gland involvement, determined on the basis of a positive result on at least 1 of the following 3 tests:
      (a) Salivary scintigraphy
      (b) Parotid sialography
      (c) Unstimulated salivary flow ($\leq$1.5 mL in 15 minutes)
5. Histopathologic findings
   Focus score$\geq$1 on minor salivary gland biopsy
   (focus defined as an agglomeration of at least 50 mononuclear cells, focus score defined as the number of foci/4mm^2 of glandular tissue)
6. Autoantibodies
   Presence of at least 1 of the following autoantibodies in the serum: Antibodies to Ro (SSA) or La (SSB) antigens or antinuclear antibodies or rheumatoid factor

A patient is considered as having probable Sjögren syndrome if 3 of 6 criteria are present, and as definite if 4 of 6 criteria are present.

---

relief and substitution of the missing secretions. (See also BCSC Section 8, *External Disease and Cornea.*)

Relapsing Polychondritis

Relapsing polychondritis is an episodic disorder characterized by recurrent, widespread, potentially destructive inflammation of cartilage, the cardiovascular system, and the organs of special sense. The most common clinical features are auricular inflammation, arthropathy, and nasal cartilage inflammation. Auricular chondritis and nasal chondritis are the features that most often suggest the diagnosis. Laryngotracheobronchial disease may lead to a fatal complication from laryngeal collapse. Involvement of the internal ear, cardiovascular system, and skin are less common. Cardiovascular lesions include aortic insufficiency (due to progressive dilation of the aortic root) and vasculitis. Skin lesions are most often due to cutaneous vasculitis. Over 30% of patients have an associated autoimmune disease such as systemic vasculitis, SLE, or RA; Sjögren syndrome; and even Hodgkin disease or diabetes mellitus.

The pathogenesis of relapsing polychondritis appears to be due to autoantibodies to collagen types II, IX, and XI. This condition appears to be mediated by CD4+ lymphocytes. In some reported cases, the autoantibody titer has correlated with the clinical course and severity of the disease. Ocular manifestations occur in about 50% of patients with relapsing polychondritis. The most common ocular conditions are conjunctivitis, scleritis, uveitis, and retinal vasculitis.

Vasculitis

The spectrum of vasculitis is outlined in Table 8-2. The *polyarteritis group of systemic necrotizing vasculitis* is characterized by necrotizing vasculitis of the medium and small-sized muscular arteries. *Hypersensitivity vasculitis,* also known as *allergic vasculitis* or *leukocytoclastic vasculitis,* is characterized by involvement of the postcapillary venules with infiltration of polymorphonuclear leukocytes and leukocytoclasis. *Wegener granulomatosis* is characterized by granuloma formation and vasculitis. *Temporal,* or *giant cell, arteritis* is characterized by involvement of large- and medium-sized arteries with chronic inflammation, giant cells, and internal elastic lamina damage.

Systemic Necrotizing Vasculitis

Polyarteritis nodosa

The polyarteritis group of systemic necrotizing vasculitis is subdivided into classic polyarteritis nodosa (PAN) and allergic granulomatosis (Churg-Strauss angiitis). Both types are characterized by necrotizing vasculitis of the medium-sized and small muscular arteries. The lesions are segmental, and lesions in different stages of development are present simultaneously. Medium-sized arteries often develop aneurysms, which can be detected by angiography. In classic PAN, eosinophilia and granulomas are absent and there is no history of allergy. Renal involvement is common, related to either vasculitis or glomerulonephritis. Hypertension develops as a consequence of the renal disease, and

---

Table 8-2 Outline of the Vasculitides

Systemic necrotizing vasculitis
  Classic polyarteritis nodosa
  Allergic granulomatosis (Churg-Strauss angiitis)
  Overlap syndrome
Hypersensitivity vasculitis
  Serum sickness
  Henoch-Schonlein purpura
  Vasculitis with connective tissue disease
  Vasculitis with malignancy
Wegener granulomatosis
Lymphomatoid granulomatosis
Giant cell (temporal) arteritis
Takayasu arteritis

---

gastrointestinal disease with infarction of the viscera can occur. Neurologic disease can present as a mononeuritis multiplex or as CNS lesions.

The mean age of onset of PAN is 40–50 years, and men are affected more often than women. Survival in patients with untreated PAN is poor. However, most patients are now treated with a combination of corticosteroids and an immunosuppressive drug such as cyclophosphamide, and this therapy appears to improve disease control and long-term outcome.

Ocular manifestations occur in approximately 10%–20% of patients with PAN and include hypertensive retinopathy in patients with renal disease, ischemic retinopathy from the vasculitis, CNS lesions resulting in visual loss (eg, homonymous hemianopia), cranial nerve palsies, scleritis, and marginal corneal ulceration. *Cogan syndrome*, manifested by interstitial keratitis, hearing loss, tinnitus, and vertigo, is associated with PAN in up to 50% of cases (see also BCSC Section 8, *External Disease and Cornea*).

Allergic granulomatosis (Churg-Strauss angiitis)

An allergic diathesis, particularly asthma, is present in allergic granulomatosis. Lung disease is the sine qua non for diagnosis. Eosinophilia is generally present, and pathological examination often shows granulomas with eosinophilic tissue infiltration. In addition to the arteriole fibrinoid necrosis of classic PAN, the small vessels, capillaries, and venules are often involved. The vasculitis-related ocular complications of classic PAN also occur in allergic granulomatosis. Additionally, conjunctival granulomas have been reported in patients with allergic granulomatosis.

Wegener Granulomatosis

Wegener granulomatosis was originally described as the classic triad of necrotizing granulomatous vasculitis of the upper respiratory tract, necrotizing granulomatous vasculitis of the lower respiratory tract, and focal segmental glomerulonephritis. The clinical features of Wegener granulomatosis include granulomatous inflammation of the paranasal sinuses in 90% of cases, nasopharyngeal disease in 63%, cutaneous vasculitis in 45%, and vasculitis affecting the nervous system in 25%. Ocular disease occurs in up to 60% of patients with Wegener granulomatosis and includes scleritis with or without peripheral keratitis, orbital pseudotumor, and vasculitis-mediated retinal vascular or neuro-ophthalmic lesions. Serum antibodies that react with cytoplasmic components of neutrophils are present in most patients. Approximately 80% of patients with Wegener granulomatosis are serum positive for a cytoplasmic pattern of anti-neutrophil cytoplasmic antibodies (ANCA). (See also BCSC Section 9, *Intraocular Inflammation and Uveitis*.)

Prior to the use of immunosuppressive drugs, Wegener granulomatosis was a uniformly fatal disease, with a mean untreated survival of 5 months. With corticosteroid treatment, the mean survival increased to 12.5 months; long-term survival occurred only in patients with limited disease. However, the use of cytotoxic drugs has dramatically improved the outcome for patients with Wegener granulomatosis.

Treatment generally consists of cyclophosphamide 1–2 mg/kg/day, and prednisone initially at 1 mg/kg/day, subsequently tapered to an every-other-day schedule and then discontinued. Cyclophosphamide is continued for 1 year after a complete remission has been achieved; the drug is then tapered off. The best results with this treatment regimen have been reported by the National Institutes of Health, where remission was achieved in 93% of patients. Although some patients experience relapse when the cyclophosphamide is discontinued, a second remission can be achieved with reinduction therapy. Complications of this treatment include leukopenia, hemorrhagic cystitis, gonadal dysfunction, alopecia, and neoplasia.

Giant Cell (Temporal) Arteritis

Giant cell arteritis (GCA) has been described in all races, although whites are most often affected. It is a disease of the elderly, rarely occurring in patients under age 50. It is particularly common in northern climates such as Scandinavia, Great Britain, and the northern United States. Autopsy studies in Scandinavia have estimated the prevalence of GCA at 1.1% of the population.

The clinical features of GCA include headache, polymyalgia rheumatica, jaw claudication, constitutional symptoms such as fever and malaise, and ophthalmic symptoms. The signs of GCA include tenderness over the temporal artery, a pulseless temporal artery, scalp tenderness, fever, and loss of vision. Polymyalgia rheumatica is a symptom complex of proximal muscle pain and weakness that may occur by itself without overt GCA.

The most common laboratory abnormality in GCA is with the ESR: the ESR is elevated in more than 90% of patients. A recent study suggested that a marked acute-phase reactant response, defined by an elevated ESR and an elevated serum C-reactive protein, appears to have strong predictive value in identifying patients with GCA. Care must be taken in interpreting the ESR because the method used must be known. For example, the Westergren method yields markedly elevated ESRs. In patients with GCA tested by the Westergren method, the median ESR is 96 mm/hour, with a range of 50–132 mm/hour. Studies stating that the normal ESR in elderly patients can be as high as 40 mm/hour have used the Westergren method. The Wintrobe method uses a closed-end tube and yields lower ESR rates. The mean ESR in patients with GCA tested by the Wintrobe method is 51 mm/hour, with a range of 38–59 mm/hour.

The definitive test for GCA is the temporal artery biopsy. Approximately 18%–45% of patients with polymyalgia rheumatica have GCA as determined by temporal artery biopsy. The characteristic features with temporal artery biopsy are occlusion of the vessel lumen with either thrombus or subintimal edema and cellular proliferation. There are fragmentations of the internal elastic lamina and a patchy degeneration of smooth muscle cells. Granulomatous inflammation of the vessel wall affects the media, adventitia, and subintima. The inflammatory material is composed of lymphocytes, plasma cells, histiocytes, epithelioid cells, and giant cells. Temporal artery biopsies occasionally reveal negative results on one side and positive results on the other. Two studies have suggested that the prevalence of false-negative unilateral biopsies is 4%–5%. False-negative results are due to the presence of areas without histologic involvement in the temporal artery biopsy.

GCA is treated with systemic corticosteroids. Because untreated GCA can cause blindness, treatment should be initiated as soon as the diagnosis is suspected. The initial prednisone dosage is approximately 1 mg/kg/day (60–80 mg daily). Generally, the symptoms respond promptly within several days. Alternate-day steroids are ineffective in the initial treatment of GCA.

Some studies have suggested that GCA is a self-limited disease that will run its course in 1–2 years. These studies recommend steroid therapy for 1–2 years. Treatment is generally instituted at the initial high dose and slowly tapered using the ESR and clinical symptoms to monitor disease. Occasionally, longer-lasting disease requires longer-term treatment.

Ophthalmologic considerations

The most frequent ocular manifestation of GCA is ischemic optic neuropathy. Other ocular manifestations include amaurosis fugax; ischemic retinopathy; occasionally, diplopia, ophthalmoplegia, or both due to ischemia in the extraocular muscles; the ocular ischemic syndrome; choroidal ischemia; and cortical blindness. (Ocular involvement by GCA is discussed in BCSC Section 5, *Neuro-Ophthalmology.*)

Takayasu Arteritis

Takayasu arteritis affects large arteries, particularly branches of the aorta. It occurs primarily in children and young women. The disease is rare in the West but common in the Far East, particularly Japan. Other names for Takayasu arteritis include *aortic arch arteritis, aortitis syndrome,* and *pulseless disease.*

The disease may involve the entire aorta or be localized to any segment of the aorta or its primary branches. The inflammatory process is characterized by a panarteritis with a granulomatous inflammation. The involved vessels may ultimately become narrowed or obliterated, resulting in ischemia to the supplied tissues. Areas of weakened vascular wall may develop dissections or aneurysms.

Systemic features such as fatigue, weight loss, or low-grade fever are common. Evidence of vascular insufficiency due to large-artery narrowing or reduction leads to the characteristic pulseless phase. The disease is most often diagnosed via arteriography. Treatment is generally with systemic corticosteroids, which may successfully suppress the disease. Cyclophosphamide or methotrexate is added in resistant cases. Surgical reconstruction of damaged vessels may be necessary.

Ophthalmologic considerations

The most characteristic ocular findings are retinal arteriovenous anastomoses, best demonstrated by fluorescein angiography. Earlier, milder changes are small-vessel dilation and microaneurysm formation; more severe ischemia may result in peripheral retinal nonperfusion, neovascularization, and vitreous hemorrhage.

Behçet Syndrome

Behçet syndrome was initially described as a triad of oral ulcers, genital ulcers, and uveitis with hypopyon. It is now recognized as a multisystem illness. The disease is most common in the Middle East and Far East, particularly Japan. Oral ulcers are the most common clinical feature, affecting 98%–99% of patients. Genital ulcers occur in 80%–87%; skin disease occurs in 69%–90% and includes erythema nodosum, superficial thrombophlebitis, and pyoderma. Some 44%–59% of patients have asymmetrical, nondeforming, large-joint polyarthritis that frequently responds to steroids.

Vascular disease, which occurs in 10%–35% of patients, can present as migratory superficial thrombophlebitis, major vessel thrombosis, arterial aneurysms, or even peripheral gangrene. CNS disease, found in 10%–30% of patients, has been classically divided into three types: brain stem syndrome, meningoencephalitis, and confusional states. Most often patients present with combinations of the three. The major cause of mortality in Behçet syndrome is CNS involvement.

Treatment

The clinical impression of most authors is that corticosteroids can delay disease progression but do not alter the ultimate outcome. Since the early 1970s, immunosuppressive drugs have been used in the treatment of Behçet syndrome. *Chlorambucil* (0.1–0.2 mg/kg/day) has been the most frequently used drug. Other studies have used cyclophosphamide (1–2 mg/kg/day). In many cases, immunosuppressive drugs have arrested the disease process, and studies have suggested that long-term remission can be induced with 1–2 years of treatment. The indications for immunosuppressive drugs have been either ocular or neurologic Behçet syndrome. Cyclosporine has also been reported to be highly effective in the treatment of Behçet syndrome, but it has the side effect of nephrotoxicity.

Ophthalmologic Considerations

The most common ocular manifestations are iridocyclitis, with or without hypopyon, and retinal vasculitis. The natural history of retinal vasculitis in Behçet syndrome is poor. The majority of untreated patients lose all or part of their vision within 5 years. See also BCSC Section 9, *Intraocular Inflammation and Uveitis.*

Medical Therapy for Rheumatic Disorders

Medications are used for analgesia, an anti-inflammatory effect, and immunosuppression.

Endogenous Corticosteroids

The adrenal cortex synthesizes three types of corticosteroids: glucocorticoids, mineralocorticoids, and androgens. Only the glucocorticoids have anti-inflammatory activity. Although the mechanism of the anti-inflammatory effect is complex, it appears to involve the inhibition of prostaglandin synthesis by preventing the release of the prostaglandin precursor, arachidonic acid, from membrane phospholipids.

In addition to their anti-inflammatory activity, glucocorticoids have a variety of other effects. Gluconeogenesis is promoted, with concomitant reduction in protein and negative nitrogen balance. Fat oxidation, synthesis, storage, and mobilization are also affected. Glucocorticoids exert a broad range of effects on circulating leukocytes. They produce lymphocytopenia, which lasts for about 24 hours. Circulating neutrophils increase because mature neutrophils are released from bone marrow and movement from blood to other tissues decreases. Other circulating leukocytes decrease after glucocorticoid administration. Associated mineralocorticoid activity increases sodium retention and potassium excretion.

Exogenous Corticosteroids

The molecular structure of the steroid nucleus can be modified to dissociate glucocorticoid from mineralocorticoid activity. Although synthetic glucocorticoids have been produced with various levels of biological potency, the goal of dissociating beneficial anti-inflammatory effects from the harmful side effects of glucocorticoid activity has not been achieved. In some instances, administering the total 48 hour dose of corticosteroids during the early morning every other day can reduce undesirable metabolic effects. Alternate-day therapy is preferred for maintenance whenever feasible and is reported to be particularly effective in asthma, SLE, uveitis, and nephrotic syndrome. However, alternate-day therapy may not be adequate in severe conditions such as renal transplantation or certain hematologic and malignant disorders. Furthermore, this regimen is not effective with steroids that have prolonged effects, such as those with substitution at the 16 position of the steroid nucleus (triamcinolone, paramethasone, betamethasone, and dexamethasone).

The ophthalmologist must be aware of both ocular and systemic toxicity in patients who are receiving systemic steroids. Ocular side effects of systemic steroids include posterior subcapsular cataracts, glaucoma, mydriasis, ptosis, papilledema associated with pseudotumor cerebri, reactivation or aggravation of ocular infection, and delay of wound healing. Systemic complications may include peptic ulceration, osteoporosis, compression fracture, negative nitrogen balance, aseptic necrosis of the femoral head, muscle and skin atrophy, hyperglycemia, hypertension, edema, weight gain, hyperosmolar nonketotic coma, hypokalemia, mental changes, pseudotumor cerebri, changes in body fat distribution resulting in cushingoid habitus, and growth retardation in children.

Another frequently overlooked complication of systemic steroid therapy is the effect of rapid withdrawal from the drugs. Several patterns of response to steroid withdrawal have been described. They include hypothalamic-pituitary-adrenal (HPA) axis suppression with or without symptoms, exacerbation of the disease being treated, and physical or psychological dependence with otherwise normal function. The rate of steroid withdrawal should be determined by the degree of HPA suppression (related to dose and duration of therapy) and the response of the underlying disease.

A variety of schedules have been suggested. Glucocorticoids given in large doses for 1–3 days probably suppress HPA function only temporarily, so they can be withdrawn suddenly or gradually over 1 week. After 1 or more months of treatment, a dosage-reduction protocol is usually followed. Otherwise, sudden withdrawal of steroid therapy may produce adrenal insufficiency, with the symptoms of fatigue, weakness, arthralgias, anorexia, nausea, orthostatic hypotension, fainting, dyspnea, and hypoglycemia. In severe cases, adrenal suppression may be fatal. After steroid therapy has been discontinued, adrenal function may not return to normal for 1 year or more; thus, supplementary steroids may be needed if the patient has a serious illness or undergoes surgery during this recovery period.

Some patients become psychologically dependent on glucocorticoids, particularly those who have been given repeated courses of therapy for recurring problems such as asthma or certain dermatologic conditions. Because initiation of glucocorticoid therapy causes euphoria and rapid relief, it may be difficult to convince the patient to accept repeated withdrawals of medication and the attendant discomforts.

Because of the likelihood of withdrawal symptoms, even physiologic doses of long-term steroids (20 mg of hydrocortisone or 5 mg of prednisone a day) should be gradually tapered off. Moreover, patients presently on long-term corticosteroid therapy or who have undergone significant corticosteroid therapy within the previous 9 months should wear an identification bracelet that describes the need for supplemental steroids during acute stress or illness and prior to any major surgical procedure.

Nonsteroidal Anti-Inflammatory Drugs

A wide variety of nonsteroidal anti-inflammatory agents have been developed in recent years to treat RA and other rheumatic diseases. Approximately 17 million Americans take NSAIDs daily; 50% of NSAID prescriptions are written for people over age 60 for management of osteoarthritis. The names of and starting dosages for some of these agents are listed in Table 8-3. Aspirin and indomethacin are also included for comparison. All of these agents inhibit prostaglandin synthesis, although they may have other actions that add to their therapeutic efficacy. These drugs are all analgesic, antipyretic, and anti-inflammatory. Their relative efficacy remains largely untested, and individual patients vary in their responsiveness to these drugs.

Complications from NSAID use result in about 100,000 hospitalizations and 10,000 to 20,000 deaths per year. The most common side effects of oral nonsteroidal anti-inflammatory agents are gastrointestinal symptoms, including nausea, vomiting, diarrhea, anorexia, and abdominal pain. Gastrointestinal bleeding and ulceration may occur. In 1999, selective COX-2 inhibitors were introduced. The benefit of the selectivity is to

Table 8-3 Nonsteroidal Anti-inflammatory Drugs

Drug	Starting Dose
Aspirin*	3.6 g daily in divided doses
Indomethacin (Indocin)	25 mg tid
Diclofenac (Voltaren)	50 mg bid
Etodolac (Lodine)	300 mg bid or tid
Flurbiprofen (Ansaid)	50 mg PO bid
Ibuprofen (Motrin)*	400 mg qid
Ketoprofen (Orudis)*	75 mg tid
Ketorolac (Toradol)	10 mg PO q4–6h (max 40 mg)
Nabumetone (Relafen)	1000 mg once a day
Naproxen (Naprosyn)*	250 mg bid
Oxaprozin (Daypro)	1200 mg once a day
Piroxicam (Feldene)	20 mg qid
Sulindac (Clinoril)	150 mg bid
COX-2 inhibitors	
Rofecoxib (Vioxx)	12.5 mg once a day
Celecoxib (Celebrex)	200 mg once a day
Valdecoxib (Bextra)	10 mg once a day

* Available over the counter.

minimize gastrointestinal damage and possibly renal toxicity. (Due to an increased risk of cardiovascular disease, the COX-2 inhibitor rofecoxib (Vioxx) was recently pulled off the market.) Oral NSAID agents can interfere with platelet function and clotting as well as cause marrow suppression, hepatic toxicity, depressed renal function, and CNS symptoms, including headache, dizziness, and confusion. Asthmatic attacks and other hypersensitivity reactions may occur in susceptible patients.

The exact role of nonsteroidal agents in treating ocular inflammation remains uncertain. Systemic *indomethacin*, for example, appears to be effective in treating scleritis. Many of the drugs have also been tried for postsurgical analgesia and as anti-inflammatory agents in patients with uveitis or cystoid macular edema. In general, these drugs are not as effective as corticosteroids. Several topical nonsteroidal anti-inflammatory agents have been approved for ocular use. *Flurbiprofen* (Ocufen) is used primarily to control intraoperative miosis during anterior segment surgery. *Diclofenac* (Voltaren) has been approved for the treatment of postoperative inflammation following cataract surgery. *Ketorolac tromethamine* (Acular) is approved for treating the symptoms of allergic conjunctivitis but has also been studied for the relief of pain following corneal injuries or erosions. Both ketorolac and diclofenac are used to relieve postoperative pain following excimer laser photorefractive keratectomy.

Beginning in the summer of 1999, corneal events possibly associated with the use of topical NSAIDs began to be reported. The problems ranged from punctate keratopathy to corneal melts. As of December 2001, epidemiologic studies were in progress to investigate the possible relationship. Theories regarding pathways that could explain the observed events include induced apoptosis and induction of matrix metalloproteinases, a family of collagenolytic enzymes. Indomethacin has been noted to cause corneal deposits and perhaps retinal toxicity, although this remains unproven. Ibuprofen has been reported to cause optic neuritis.

O'Brien RP, Li QJ, Sauerburger F, et al. The role of matrix metalloproteinases in ulcerative keratolysis associated with perioperative diclofenac use. *Ophthalmology.* 2001;108:656–659.

Price FW. New pieces for the puzzle: nonsteroidal anti-inflammatory drugs and corneal ulcers [editorial]. *J Cataract Refract Surg.* 2000;26.

Methotrexate

Used as an anti-inflammatory agent at oral doses beginning at 7.5 mg weekly, methotrexate has become a second-line drug for RA. Major side effects include hepatic fibrosis, marrow toxicity, and sterility.

Hydroxychloroquine

Hydroxychloroquine is a relatively safe medication (with a small risk of retinopathy; regular eye examinations are recommended) used as a second-line agent for RA.

Sulfasalazine

Sulfasalazine is used in RA with moderate side effects, usually gastrointestinal upset.

Gold Salts

Gold salts are used much less frequently now because of modest efficacy and a high side-effect profile involving hematologic, renal, and dermatologic reactions.

Anticytokine Therapy

Anticytokine therapy involves inhibiting the activity of tumor necrosis factor alpha (TNF-α) by receptor blockade (etanercept [Enbrel]) or with an anti–TNF-α monoclonal antibody (infliximab [Remicade]) or adalimumab [Humira]).

Immunosuppressive Agents

Alkylating agents such as cyclophosphamide (hematologic and gastrointestinal toxicity) and antimetabolites such as azathioprine are used in resistant cases.

Cyclosporine (hypertension and renal toxicity) is also used in difficult cases.

Leflunomide (Arava) inhibits pyrimidine synthesis, targeting rapidly dividing cell populations (liver toxicity, possible birth defects).

Dionne R. Relative efficacy of selective COX-2 inhibitors compared with over-the-counter ibuprofen. *Int J Clin Pract.* Suppl 2003;(135):18–22.

Elward K. Rheumatoid arthritis. In: Griffith HW, ed. *Griffiths 5 Minute Clinical Consult.* Baltimore: Lippincott Williams & Wilkins; 1999:88–89.

Flach A. Topically applied nonsteroidal anti-inflammatory drugs and corneal problems: an interim review and comment. *Ophthalmology.* 2000;107:1224–1266.

Hayreh SS, Podhajsky PA, Raman R, et al. Giant cell arteritis: validity and reliability of various diagnostic criteria. *Am J Ophthalmol.* 1997;123:285–296.

Kary S, Burmester GR. Anakinra: the first interleukin-1 inhibitor in the treatment of rheumatoid arthritis. *Int J Clin Pract.* 2003;47:231–234.

Manthorpe R, Asmussen K, Oxholm P. Primary Sjögren's syndrome: diagnostic criteria, clinical features, and disease activity. *J Rheumatol.* 1997;24(suppl 50):8–11.

Miceli-Richard C, Dougados M. Leflunomide for the treatment of rheumatoid arthritis. *Expert Opin Pharmacother.* 2003;4:987–997.

Schumacher HR, ed. *Primer on the Rheumatic Diseases.* 12th ed. Atlanta: Arthritis Foundation; 2001.

Spiegel BM, Targownik L, Dulai GS. The cost-effectiveness of cyclooxygenase-2 selective inhibitors in the management of chronic arthritis. *Ann Intern Med.* 2003;138:795–806.

Strand V. Recent advances in the treatment of rheumatoid arthritis. *Clin Cornerstone.* 1999; 2:38–47.

CHAPTER 9

Endocrine Disorders

Recent Developments

- Newer oral agents for management of type 2 diabetes mellitus include

    Glimepiride (Amaryl). A sulfonylurea; stimulates pancreatic insulin secretion

    Metformin (Glucophage). A biguanide; decreases hepatic glucose production, decreases intestinal glucose absorption, and improves insulin sensitivity (increases peripheral uptake and utilization)

    Rosiglitazone (Avandia) and *pioglitazone (Actos).* Thiazolidinediones; increase insulin sensitivity

- In 2002, the prevalence of diabetes was estimated at 8.7% among adults over the age of 20 in the United States. Obesity, which has risen 57% since 1991, is the leading cause, according to the Centers for Disease Control and Prevention.
- Cigarette smoking may be an independent and modifiable determinant of type 2 diabetes.
- Current cigarette smoking in patients with Graves disease is associated with an increased incidence of ophthalmopathy that parallels the number of cigarettes smoked per day.
- Cigarette smoking is a risk factor for thyroid disease.

Diabetes Mellitus

The definition and diagnosis of diabetes mellitus have changed considerably in recent years. Diabetes mellitus is now defined as a group of metabolic diseases characterized by hyperglycemia resulting from defects in insulin secretion, insulin action, or both. The American Diabetes Association Expert Panel recommends a diagnosis of diabetes when one of the following three criteria is met (and confirmed with retesting by any of the three methods on a subsequent day) in nonpregnant adults:

- A random plasma glucose level of 200 mg/dL or greater, plus classic signs and symptoms of diabetes mellitus, including polydipsia, polyuria, and unexplained weight loss
- A fasting plasma glucose level of 126 mg/dL or greater on at least two occasions
- A fasting plasma glucose level of less than 126 mg/dL but a 75 g 2 hour oral glucose tolerance test plasma glucose level of 200 mg/dL or greater

Classification

Diabetes is subdivided into several major groups, as outlined in Table 9-1.

Type 1 diabetes

Type 1 diabetes was previously called *insulin-dependent diabetes mellitus* or *juvenile-onset diabetes*. This form of diabetes is due to a deficiency of endogenous insulin secretion secondary to destruction of insulin-producing beta cells in the pancreas.

Most type 1 diabetes is due to immune-mediated destruction characterized by the presence of various autoantibodies. The rate of destruction varies but is usually rapid in children and slow in adults. One or more autoantibodies are present in 90% of patients at initial presentation of fasting hyperglycemia. There are strong human leukocyte antigen (HLA) associations and multiple genetic predispositions related to type 1 diabetes. These patients are also prone to other autoimmune disorders such as Graves disease, Hashimoto thyroiditis, Addison disease, vitiligo, and pernicious anemia.

In some persons, no autoantibodies are present; in such patients the disease is called *type 1 idiopathic*. Most of these patients are of African or Asian ancestry and have a strong inheritance pattern for diabetes, but the HLA association is absent.

Type 2 diabetes

Type 2 diabetes was formerly known as *non–insulin-dependent diabetes mellitus*. This group accounts for 90% of Americans with diabetes and has a strong genetic predisposition. Type 2 patients are usually, but not always, older than age 40 at presentation. Obesity is a frequent finding and, in the United States, is present in 80%–90% of these patients. Increased visceral fat, leading to an increased waist-to-hip ratio, is an even more significant risk factor than obesity. This form of diabetes is frequently undiagnosed for years because the hyperglycemia develops slowly and symptoms are not severe enough to warrant attention. Although symptoms may be minimal, these patients are at increased risk for microvascular and macrovascular complications. Such patients are not prone to ketoacidosis and rarely require insulin.

Autoimmune destruction of beta cells does not occur in this type of diabetes. Beta cell function is impaired, but in response to fasting hyperglycemia, basal insulin secretion is normal or increased initially. Patients with type 2 disease do not produce sufficient insulin to overcome increased demand caused, at least in part, by insulin resistance. Insulin resistance can lead to a defect in insulin secretion; similarly, impaired beta cell function can lead to a disturbance in insulin action. This explains why both impaired insulin secretion and insulin resistance occur in patients with type 2 diabetes once the disease is fully established. Obesity by itself leads to insulin resistance and predisposes to or exacerbates the state.

In a significant number of these patients, the elevated plasma glucose level can revert to normal with caloric restriction and weight loss. Patients with type 2 disease are therefore initially treated with dietary counseling to promote weight loss and optimal health. If needed, oral agents (or less commonly insulin) are used.

Other specific types of diabetes

The following paragraphs describe other forms of diabetes that are outlined in Table 9-1.

Genetic defects of the beta cell Several types of diabetes are due to monogenetic defects in beta cell function that frequently present as hyperglycemia before age 25 (MODY = *m*aturity *o*nset *d*iabetes of the *y*oung). In these patients, insulin secretion is impaired, with minimal or no defect in insulin action. Inheritance is autosomal dominant.

Point mutations in mitochondrial DNA have been found to be associated with impaired hearing and diabetes.

Autosomal dominant genetic defects resulting in inability to convert proinsulin to insulin have been identified in a few families. Other families have been identified that produce a mutant insulin with impaired receptor binding.

Genetic defects in insulin action Insulin receptor mutations are associated with disease severity, ranging from hyperinsulinemia and modest hyperglycemia to severe diabetes. Physical findings may include acanthosis nigricans, and women may experience virilization and enlarged cystic ovaries.

Diseases of the exocrine pancreas Diseases of the exocrine pancreas used to be considered part of secondary diabetes. Damage to the pancreas itself may result in diabetes.

Endocrinopathies Endocrinopathies were formerly part of secondary diabetes. Multiple hormones (growth hormone, cortisol, glucagon, epinephrine) act as antagonists to insulin's action. Excesses of these hormones in disease states may initiate diabetes that typically resolves when the hormonal excess is corrected.

Diabetes induced by drugs or other chemicals Certain chemicals may impair insulin secretion, directly damage beta cells, or impair insulin activity.

Infections Certain viruses are associated with beta cell destruction.

Uncommon forms of immune-mediated diabetes Anti–insulin receptor antibodies may cause hyperglycemia by blocking insulin activity or hypoglycemia by acting like an insulin agonist.

Other genetic syndromes sometimes associated with diabetes See Table 9-1.

Gestational diabetes mellitus

Gestational diabetes mellitus complicates about 4% of all pregnancies in the United States and is defined as any degree of glucose intolerance with onset or first recognition during pregnancy. In 30%–50% of affected women, type 2 diabetes develops within 10 years of initial diagnosis (Table 9-2).

Table 9-1 Etiologic Classification of Diabetes Mellitus

I. Type 1 diabetes* (β-cell destruction, usually leading to absolute insulin deficiency)
    A. Immune mediated
    B. Idiopathic
II. Type 2 diabetes* (may range from predominantly insulin resistance with relative insulin deficiency to a predominantly secretory defect with insulin resistance)
III. Other specific types
    A. Genetic defects of β-cell function
        1. Chromosome 12, HNF-1α (MODY3)
        2. Chromosome 7, glucokinase (MODY2)
        3. Chromosome 20, HNF-4α (MODY1)
        4. Mitochondrial DNA
        5. Others
    B. Genetic defects in insulin action
        1. Type A insulin resistance
        2. Leprechaunism
        3. Rabson-Mendenhall syndrome
        4. Lipoatrophic diabetes
        5. Others
    C. Diseases of the exocrine pancreas
        1. Pancreatitis
        2. Trauma/pancreatopathy
        3. Neoplasia
        4. Cystic fibrosis
        5. Hemochromatosis
        6. Fibrocalculous pancreatopathy
        7. Others
    D. Endocrinopathies
        1. Acromegaly
        2. Cushing's syndrome
        3. Glucagonoma
        4. Pheochromocytoma
        5. Hyperthyroidism
        6. Somatostatinoma
        7. Aldosteronoma
        8. Others
    E. Drug- or chemical-induced
        1. Vacor
        2. Pentamidine
        3. Nicotinic acid
        4. Glucocorticoids
        5. Thyroid hormone
        6. Diazoxide
        7. β-Adrenergic agonists
        8. Thiazides
        9. Dilantin
       10. α-Interferon
       11. Others
    F. Infections
        1. Congenital rubella
        2. Cytomegalovirus
        3. Others
    G. Uncommon forms of immune-mediated diabetes
        1. "Stiff-man" syndrome
        2. Anti-insulin receptor antibodies
        3. Others

Continued

H. Other genetic syndromes sometimes associated with diabetes
   1. Down syndrome
   2. Klinefelter syndrome
   3. Turner syndrome
   4. Wolfram syndrome
   5. Friedreich ataxia
   6. Huntington chorea
   7. Laurence-Moon-Biedl syndrome
   8. Myotonic dystrophy
   9. Porphyria
   10. Prader-Willi syndrome
   11. Others
IV. Gestational diabetes mellitus (GDM)

---

* Patients with any form of diabetes may require insulin treatment at some stage of the disease. Such use of insulin does not, of itself, classify the patient's condition.

(Modified from American Diabetes Association. Clinical practice recommendations 2001. *Diabetes Care.* 2001;24[Suppl].)

Table 9-2 Diagnosis of Gestational Diabetes Mellitus With a 100 G or 75 G Glucose Load

	mg/dL	mmol/L
100 g glucose load		
Fasting	95	5.3
1 h	180	10.0
2 h	155	8.6
3 h	140	7.8
75 g glucose load		
Fasting	95	5.3
1 h	180	10.0
2 h	155	8.6

Two or more of the venous plasma concentrations must be met or exceeded for a positive diagnosis. The test should be performed in the morning after an overnight fast of between 8 and 14 h and after at least 3 days of unrestricted diet ($\geq$150 g carbohydrate per day) and unlimited physical activity. The subject should remain seated and should not smoke throughout the test.

(Modified from American Diabetes Association. Clinical practice recommendations 2001. *Diabetes Care.* 2001;24[Suppl].)

Impaired glucose tolerance and impaired fasting glucose (IFG)

Impaired glucose tolerance is defined as a 75 g oral glucose tolerance test yielding a fasting plasma glucose level of less than 126 mg/dL; 0.5, 1.0, or 1.5 hour plasma glucose levels of 200 mg/dL or greater; and 2 hour plasma glucose levels of 140–200 mg/dL. A new category, impaired fasting glucose, requires a fasting plasma glucose level of between 110 mg/dL and 126 mg/dL. These values were based on large epidemiologic studies. Although these patients are not at risk for retinopathy or nephropathy, they have an elevated risk of macrovascular disease (eg, coronary artery disease) compared with persons who have normal glucose tolerance. Also, 30%–50% of patients with impaired glucose tolerance develop type 2 diabetes within 10 years of diagnosis.

Report of the Expert Committee on the Diagnosis and Classification of Diabetes Mellitus. *Diabetes Care.* 2001;24(suppl 1): at http://journal.diabetes.org/FullText/Supplements/ DiabetesCare/Supplement101/S5.htm

Pathophysiology

In normal persons, the mean fasting venous plasma glucose level measured by enzymatic methods (glucose oxidase or hexokinase) is 60–109 mg/dL. A level greater than 126 mg/ dL is abnormal and consistent with the diagnosis of diabetes mellitus. Measurements of venous or capillary whole blood yield values approximately 10%–15% lower.

A number of homeostatic mechanisms act to maintain the plasma glucose level. The plasma glucose level is reduced by only one hormone, insulin. In contrast, there are six hormones that increase plasma glucose: somatotropin, adrenocorticotropin, cortisol, epinephrine, glucagon, and thyroxine. Each of these hormones combines with a specific receptor on the surfaces of responsive cells. The hormones are secreted as needed to maintain normal serum glucose levels. The interaction on the cellular surface initiates a chain of postreceptor enzymatic and biochemical events. In the fed state, anabolism is initiated by increased secretion of insulin and growth hormone. This leads to conversion of glucose to glycogen for storage in the liver and muscles, synthesis of protein from amino acids, and the combining of fatty acid and glucose in adipose tissue to form triglycerides.

In the fasting state, catabolism results from the increased secretion of contrainsulin hormones. In this set of interactions, glycogen is reduced to glucose in the liver and muscles; proteins are broken down into amino acids in muscles and other tissues and transported to the liver for conversion to glucose or ketoacids; and triglycerides are degraded into fatty acids and glycerol in adipose tissue for transport to the liver for conversion to ketoacids and glucose (or for transport to muscle for use as an energy source).

The normal lean adult secretes approximately 33 units of insulin per day. In the obese overfed adult, insulin secretion can increase almost fourfold to approximately 120 units per day. In this state, the plasma glucose may rise only slightly, but pancreatic beta cell mass increases. When serum insulin levels are elevated, the number of insulin receptors on the surface of insulin-responsive cells actually decreases and formerly insulinsensitive tissues become resistant to the glucose-lowering effects of both endogenous and exogenous insulin, even in great amounts. This condition may progress to fasting hyperglycemia and type 2 diabetes. Compared with persons at ideal body weight, the risk of hyperglycemia is two times as great in persons who are 20% above ideal body weight; four times as great at 40% above; eight times as great at 60% above; 16 times as great at 80% above; and 32 times as great at 100% above. Ninety percent of Americans who are at risk for fasting hyperglycemia can avoid it by maintaining ideal body weight or by losing excess weight.

Therapeutically induced weight loss can reverse the metabolic consequences of obesity. Insulin requirements are increased during the growth spurts of pregnancy and puberty and in the presence of excessive amounts of exogenously administered or endogenously produced anti-insulin hormones. Thus, hyperthyroidism, Cushing syndrome, acromegaly, pheochromocytoma, pregnancy, and puberty can all induce enough metabolic stress to precipitate fasting hyperglycemia.

Insulin production falls if the pancreatic beta cell mass is reduced below a critical level, as in type 1 disease. In such cases, sometimes less than 3 units per day are produced. Fasting hyperglycemia and resultant persistent catabolism may lead to fatal diabetic ketoacidosis or hyperglycemic hyperosmotic coma if insulin therapy is not started. Cellular insulin receptors are increased in number, and tissues are sensitive to exogenous insulin.

Clinical Presentations

The classic findings of diabetes mellitus are polyuria, polydipsia, and polyphagia. When diabetes is initially detected, however, most patients—particularly those with type 2 disease—are asymptomatic. Other important Historical findings include complications of pregnancy or giving birth to large babies, reactive hypoglycemia, advanced vascular disease, impotence, leg cramps or pains, dry mouth, and burning feet.

Physical findings, particularly in type 2 diabetes, may include obesity, hypertension, arteriopathy, neuropathy, genitourinary abnormalities (especially recurrent *Candida* infections or bacterial bladder or kidney infections), periodontal disease, foot abnormalities, skin abnormalities, and unusual susceptibility to infections.

Diagnosis and Screening

Table 9-3 lists the criteria for diagnosing diabetes mellitus. Note that hemoglobin A_{1c} (HbA_{1c}) measurement is not currently recommended for diagnosing diabetes.

Criteria for diabetes testing in asymptomatic persons are given in Table 9-4.

Management

Diet and exercise

Adherence to nutrition and meal planning principles is a challenging but essential component of successful diabetes management. A registered dietitian should be part of the management team. Diet planning considerations should include lifestyle and nutrition goals as well as specific biochemical and other physiologic parameters for the individual. Insulin requirements are then matched to the patient's diet, not vice versa. Although the concept of a "one type fits all" diabetic diet is no longer recommended, meals should be consistent, regularly spaced, and low in cholesterol, with less than 10% of calories coming from saturated fat and 10%–20% of calories derived from protein, depending on renal function.

If type 2 diabetes is diagnosed and the patient is overweight, a diet (prudent low fat, low cholesterol) is begun and an exercise routine is initiated with the goal of approaching ideal weight. This goal is often not realized, but even a modest weight loss of 10 to 20 lbs may ameliorate or cause a remission of the diabetes. Extensive and continuing counseling on weight reduction may be necessary.

Isotonic exercises requiring rhythmic and repetitive large-muscle activity over a continuous period increase endurance and fitness. These cardiovascular training programs must promote the use of oxygen (aerobic exercise). A good exercise program aids with

---

Table 9-3 Criteria for the Diagnosis of Diabetes Mellitus

1. Symptoms of diabetes plus casual plasma glucose concentration≥200 mg/dL (11.1 mmol/L). Casual is defined as any time of day without regard to time since last meal. The classic symptoms of diabetes include polyuria, polydipsia, and unexplained weight loss.
2. Fasting plasma glucose ≥126 mg/dL (7.0 mmol/L). Fasting is defined as no caloric intake for at least 8 h.
3. 2 h plasma glucose ≥200 mg/dL (11.1 mmol/L) during an oral glucose tolerance test (OGTT). The test should be performed as described by WHO* using a glucose load containing the equivalent of 75 g anhydrous glucose dissolved in water.

In the absence of unequivocal hyperglycemia with acute metabolic decompensation, these criteria should be confirmed by repeat testing on a different day. The third measure (OGTT) is not recommended for routine clinical use.

* World Health Organization. *Diabetes Mellitus: Report of a WHO Study Group.* Geneva: WHO; 1985 (Tech. Rep. Ser., no. 727).

(Modified from American Diabetes Association. Clinical practice recommendations 2001. *Diabetes Care.* 2001;24[Suppl].)

Table 9-4 Criteria for Testing for Diabetes Mellitus in Asymptomatic Patients in Whom Diabetes Has Not Been Diagnosed

1. Testing for diabetes should be considered in all persons at age 45 years and older; if results are normal, testing should be repeated at 3-yr intervals.
2. Testing should be considered at younger ages or performed more frequently in persons who:
   - Are obese (≥120% desirable body weight or a BMI ≥27 kg/m^2)
   - Have a first-degree relative with diabetes
   - Are members of a high-risk ethnic population (eg, African American, Hispanic American, Native American, Asian American, Pacific Islander)
   - Have delivered a baby weighing >9 lb or have a diagnosis of gestational diabetes mellitus
   - Are hypertensive (≥140/90)
   - Have an HDL cholesterol level ≤35 mg/dL (0.90 mmol/L) and/or a triglyceride level ≥250 mg/dL (2.82 mmol/L)
   - Were shown to have impaired glucose tolerance or impaired fasting glucose

---

The oral glucose tolerance test or fasting plasma glucose test may be used to diagnose diabetes; however, in clinical settings, the fasting plasma glucose is greatly preferred because of ease of administration, convenience, acceptability to patients, and lower cost.

(Modified from American Diabetes Association. Clinical practice recommendations 2001. *Diabetes Care.* 2001;24[Suppl].)

---

the weight-loss program and improves fitness. Before an exercise program is prescribed for anyone over age 35, a determination must be made that the heart is normal and that there are no contraindications. Anyone who has been sedentary and out of condition should start slowly and work up to more demanding activities.

Insulin therapy

Approximately 1 million North Americans require insulin therapy. Such therapy is indicated in diabetic patients who are at or below ideal body weight with sustained hyperglycemia, ketoacidosis, a hyperosmotic state, or pregnancy. The use of insulin in type 2 diabetes actually decreases target-cell insulin receptors, increases food intake, and promotes weight gain. Therefore, patients who are above ideal body weight, who have not experienced ketoacidosis, and are not pregnant should not be treated with insulin initially.

The Diabetes Control and Complications Trial demonstrated that intensive therapy aimed at maintaining near-normal glucose levels had a large and beneficial effect on delaying the development and retarding the progression of long-term diabetic complications. These levels were obtained either by three or more daily self-administered insulin injections or via a battery-powered external or implantable insulin pump. One study showed that severe hypoglycemia may be less common with implantable pumps that deliver insulin intravenously or intraperitoneally than with subcutaneous regimens. Intensive therapy decreased the risk of development and progression of retinopathy, nephropathy, and neuropathy by 40%–76%. The beneficial effects increased over time but came with a threefold increased risk of hypoglycemia. Accordingly, intensive therapy is recommended for most patients with type 1 disease, but with careful self-monitoring of blood glucose levels to prevent hypoglycemic episodes.

Many types of insulin are available with variations in type (bovine, porcine, human), degree of purity (amount of proinsulin), rapidity of onset, duration of effect, and formulation (single formulation or combination). Bovine and porcine insulin differ slightly from each other and from human insulin. Despite the difference in amino acid sequence and tendency to induce antibody formation, their potency is similar to that of human insulin and they seldom cause immune-mediated problems. All insulins available in the United States are highly purified, containing less than 50 parts per million (ppm) of proinsulin. A more highly purified porcine insulin ($<$10 ppm proinsulin) is available for patients who develop immune-mediated complications (insulin resistance or local or systemic insulin allergy) from the less purified varieties. Rapid-acting insulins include regular, crystalline zinc, or lispro (Humalog). Intermediate-acting insulins are insulin zinc suspension (Lente) or isophane insulin suspension (NPH insulin). Long-acting insulins are extended insulin zinc preparations (Ultralente).

Complications of insulin therapy *Hypoglycemia* is the most significant complication of insulin therapy. Stimulation of adrenal medulla overactivity with hyperepinephrinemia may result in anxiety, palpitation, perspiration, pallor, tachycardia, hypertension, and dilated pupils. Neurologic dysfunction is manifested as headache, paresthesia, blurred vision, drowsiness, irritability, bizarre behavior, mental confusion, combativeness, and a variety of other symptoms. Short-term hypoglycemia can lead to accidental injury, criminal behavior, or death. Prolonged hypoglycemia can result in irreversible brain damage or death.

Hypoglycemia is usually caused by inadequate carbohydrate intake secondary to a missed or delayed meal, vigorous exercise, decreased hepatic gluconeogenesis, or an excessive dose of insulin. The condition needs to be promptly verified by testing for a venous plasma glucose level of lower than 50 mg/dL. Patients who are still able to swallow should be given candy, soft drinks, orange juice, food, or glucose. For those unable to swallow, 25 g of intravenous glucose or 1 mg of subcutaneous or intramuscular glucagon is administered. The patient needs to be observed until recovery is complete, and the plasma glucose test is repeated with additional food given.

The *Somogyi phenomenon* is the occurrence of post-hypoglycemic rebound hyperglycemia. In 1959, Somogyi postulated that stimulation of counter-regulatory hormone secretion by hypoglycemia could lead to subsequent hyperglycemia. Critics have argued that hyperglycemia is merely the consequence of waning insulin; however, it has been convincingly demonstrated that rebound hyperglycemia can occur in the absence of waning insulin. The incidence of the Somogyi phenomenon is not known, but it is probably not frequent. Hypoglycemia as mild as 50–60 mg/dL of plasma glucose (which may be asymptomatic) can activate counter-regulation. Current evidence indicates that catecholamines and growth hormone are the major factors involved.

The *dawn phenomenon* is simply an exaggeration of a normal physiologic process, which can result in substantial hyperglycemia. It is characterized by early morning hyperglycemia not preceded by hypoglycemia or waning of insulin. The dawn phenomenon is thought to be caused by a surge of growth hormone secretion shortly after the patient falls asleep, which leads to overproduction of glucose by the liver and diminished use of glucose by muscle tissue, without a compensatory increase in insulin secrction. Some patients with diabetes have excessive surges of growth hormone secretion, producing severe morning hyperglycemia. This phenomenon can occur with equal frequency in type 1 and type 2 diabetes, but its severity varies, making this condition difficult to treat. Management consists of increasing a patient's before-supper intermediate-acting insulin or delaying the insulin administration to before bedtime. Thus, additional insulin is provided for the period in which growth hormone–induced insulin resistance occurs.

Allergies and local reactions to insulin Lipoatrophy (loss of fat) or lipohypertrophy (accumulation of fat) may occur at sites of insulin injection. In the past, lipoatrophy was due to lipolytic impurities in insulin preparations. The use of purified human insulins has made this phenomenon rare. Lipohypertrophy can be eliminated via proper rotation of injection sites so that no single site is injected more often than once a month.

True insulin allergy is caused by IgE antibodies and is characterized by a hard erythematous indurated area at the injection site, which is usually pruritic. The allergic reaction develops 1–4 weeks after initiation of insulin therapy and usually clears as therapy continues. Generalized anaphylaxis, hives, and angioedema may also develop and must be treated with desensitization techniques.

Immunologic insulin resistance may occur in patients who require more than 200 units of insulin per day for plasma glucose control. These patients also have an insulin-neutralizing antibody titer (IgG and IgA) greater than 30 units per liter of serum. Many cases of apparent insulin resistance are caused by down-regulation of the number of receptors as a result of obesity. Congenital absence of these receptors and insulin receptor antibodies are rare causes of insulin resistance. In this situation, highly purified pork or human insulin is indicated. Human and pork insulins are equally efficacious. However, human insulin is less immunogenic than animal insulin in cases of insulin resistance. Patients with insulin resistance requiring over 200 units per day have been successfully treated with U-500 regular insulin.

Oral agents

The United Kingdom Prospective Diabetes Study reported the following findings with regard to oral agents:

- Hypoglycemic medications are used when diet and exercise have failed to induce a remission. Intensive control (insulin or sulfonylurea drugs or both, median HgA_{1c} 7.0%) compared with conventional treatment (diet therapy initially, augmented with pharmacological therapy in 80% of patients, median HbA_{1c} 7.9%) of type 2 diabetes significantly reduces progression of retinopathy and slows progression to renal failure.
- There is a trend toward less nonfatal myocardial infarction among the intensive treatment group.
- There was no excess mortality from insulin and sulfonylureas.
- No significant difference among hypoglycemic agents was found in the intensive treatment group.

The sulfonylureas (Table 9-5) have been widely used in the United States and Canada since 1967 for type 2 diabetes. Their major mechanism of action is stimulation of pancreatic insulin secretion, although some studies have suggested a peripheral augmentation of insulin action.

The major problem with sulfonylurea therapy is that approximately one third of patients who begin therapy do not become normoglycemic ("primary failures"). Furthermore, over a 5 year period, 85% of those who initially respond to the drug experience

Table 9-5 Sulfonylureas Currently Available in the United States

Generic Name	Daily Dose Range (mg)	Duration (h)	Comments
First generation			
Chlorpropamide	100–750	>36	Disulfiram-like effect; can lead to hyponatremia or prolonged hypoglycemia; administer once a day
Tolbutamide	500–3000	6–12	Metabolized in liver; safest sulfonylurea to use in patients with renal insufficiency
Acetohexamide	250–1500	12–18	Metabolized in liver to active metabolites
Tolazamide	100–1000	12–24	—
Second generation			
Glyburide	2.5–20	18–24	Administer once or twice a day unless patient develops hypoglycemia; has fewer side effects and drug interactions than first-generation drugs
Glipizide	5–40	12–18	Administer once or twice a day
Glimepiride	1–8	24	Administer once a day

(Modified from American Diabetes Association. Clinical practice recommendations 2001. *Diabetes Care.* 2001;24[Suppl].)

secondary failure to control blood sugar. Weight reduction is a far more effective method of normalizing blood sugar and is the method of choice. The sulfonylureas are also contraindicated in diabetics who are pregnant or in those who have had ketoacidosis.

The most significant adverse effect of the sulfonylureas is hypoglycemia, which although infrequent may be severe and prolonged. Extrapancreatic effects include blood dyscrasias, increased fibrinolytic activity, photosensitivity, corneal opacities, water retention, jaundice, liver enzyme inhibition, and increased secretion of stomach acid. Therapy also causes an altered EEG in epilepsy. The sulfonylureas are usually not effective in nonobese patients with type 2 disease and often are associated with weight gain.

Sulfonylureas compete for carrier protein–binding sites with many other drugs, including sulfonamides, salicylates, phenylbutazone, monoamine oxidase inhibitors, thiazides, and barbiturates. Because the pharmacologic effect of these drugs may be increased when they are displaced from their albumin-combining sites, combination drug therapy may have unforeseen toxic consequences. It is also difficult to maintain stable anticoagulation therapy in a patient taking sulfonylureas because these agents compete with anticoagulants for the same binding sites. In addition, the effects of alcohol are potentiated by sulfonylureas.

Second-generation sulfonylurea agents, *glipizide* (Glucotrol), *glyburide* (DiaBeta, Micronase), and *glimepiride* (Amaryl) differ from the first-generation agents in structure and potency. On a weight-for-weight basis, the newer sulfonylureas are approximately 50–100 times more potent than first-generation agents and are effective at nanomolar rather than micromolar blood levels. Although both glipizide and glyburide have very short half-lives (2–4 hours, about 5 hours for glimepiride), blood levels and duration of action are dissociated so that these drugs generally need to be given only once daily. Although these newer agents are more potent than the first-generation sulfonylureas in facilitating insulin release, this enhanced beta-cytotrophic effect is not associated with better control of hyperglycemia. Complications are less frequent with the second-generation agents because of their nonionic binding to albumin. Thus, patients may be less susceptible to drug interactions in that the second-generation sulfonylureas are not displaced by anionic drugs. The rates of primary and secondary failure with these new second-generation agents are virtually identical to those seen through the years with the first-generation drugs. If a patient has a primary or secondary failure of control with one sulfonylurea agent, a trial with another agent is indicated.

Nonsulfonylurea meglitinides *Repaglinide* (Prandin) and nateglinide (Starlix) are meglitinides whose mechanism of action and side effect profile are similar to the sulfonylureas. Because of their rapid onset of action, these agents are taken with meals two to four times daily. They can be used as single agents (eg, in patients with a sulfa allergy) or in combination therapy with other oral hypoglycemic agents.

Biguanides A major advance became available with the FDA's approval of *metformin* (Glucophage). Metformin therapy improves insulin sensitivity, as shown by a reduction in fasting plasma glucose and insulin. The drug's glucose-lowering effect in type 2 disease is attributed mainly to decreased hepatic glucose output and enhanced peripheral glucose uptake. Several other actions may contribute, such as increased intestinal use of glucose and decreased fatty acid oxidation. Metformin can be used as either first-line therapy or in combination with other hypoglycemic agents. When used appropriately, metformin appears to be a much safer agent, with an extremely low incidence of lactic acidosis. It is effective in nonobese as well as obese patients with type 2 diabetes and is not associated with weight gain or hypoglycemia. Metformin should not be prescribed to patients with elevated serum creatinine. The drug should also be discontinued before or during any studies involving iodinated contrast materials, withheld for 48 hours after the study, and restarted only after renal function has been reevaluated and found to be normal. Glucovance is a new combination drug that contains metformin and glyburide. It offers improved glycemic control and the convenience of two hypoglycemic agents in one pill.

α-Glucosidase inhibitors *Acarbose* (Precose) and *miglitol* (Glyset) are given with meals to delay digestion and absorption of complex carbohydrates, thereby limiting postprandial serum glucose levels. Although relatively safe, these agents often cause flatulence and are to be avoided in patients with intestinal disorders.

Thiazolidinediones This new class of orally active drugs, represented by *rosiglitazone* (Avandia) and *pioglitazone* (Actos), are thought to increase insulin sensitivity in muscle and adipose tissue and to inhibit hepatic gluconeogenesis, thereby increasing glycemic control while reducing circulating insulin levels. These agents activate the nuclear receptor peroxisome proliferator–activated receptor gamma, which controls adipocyte differentiation, lipid storage, and insulin sensitization as well as the nonmetabolic effects of control of host defense, cell proliferation, and tumorigenesis. The first available agent of this class, *troglitazone* (Rezulin), was withdrawn from the market in 2000 when the FDA noted that the rate of liver toxicity was less with rosiglitazone and pioglitazone. Thiazolidinediones may be used in concert with other oral agents or insulin.

Glucose Surveillance

Self–blood-glucose monitoring

Probably the most important advance in glycemic control is self–blood-glucose monitoring. It potentially permits the patient to achieve blood sugars in the normal physiologic range, thus allowing more ambitious treatment strategies. Home use of blood-glucose analyzers facilitates the normalization or near-normalization of metabolic control in diabetic patients requiring insulin. Blood-glucose analyzers are small electronic devices that measure the glucose in the blood. The patient obtains a drop of capillary blood by a finger stick and places it on a glucose oxidase–impregnated paper strip and inserts the strip into the reflectance meter for the determination. Blood-glucose analyzers for home use are safe and reasonably accurate when used as directed.

Self–blood-glucose monitoring is appropriate for any insulin-requiring diabetic who is well motivated and capable of adhering to a rigorous management program. It is also becoming the standard monitoring process for patients on oral agents who do not use insulin.

Glycosylated hemoglobin

Diabetes mellitus is characterized by constant fluctuation of blood sugar. Thus, periodic blood sugar measurement is inadequate for assessing long-term metabolic control; it indicates the blood sugar level only at the specific time the blood was drawn.

In recent decades, the measurement of *glycosylated hemoglobin levels* has significantly improved long-term glucose-control surveillance. All serum- and membrane-bound proteins are exposed to glucose, and these proteins undergo a nonenzymatic postsynthetic modification that results in the attachment of glucose to the protein (glycosylation). Higher concentrations of glucose and longer periods of exposure result in a higher concentration of glycosylated proteins. The time period reflected by the glycosylated protein concentration depends on the particular protein's turnover rate. Red blood cells and hemoglobin have a half-life of 60 days. Therefore, the glycosylated hemoglobin level reflects the mean blood glucose concentration over the preceding 2 months. Glycosylated hemoglobin has been called *fast hemoglobin* (HbA_1 or HbA_{1c}, depending on the assay). Chromatography can separate the glycosylated fractions designated HbA_{1a}, HbA_{1b}, and HbA_{1c}, with HbA_{1c} being the largest quantitatively. Assays for glycosylated hemoglobin are expressed as a percentage of total hemoglobin.

The glycosylated hemoglobin assay is useful because it is relatively unaffected by transient fluctuations in serum blood glucose and does not require patient cooperation. The HbA_{1c} assay is used to monitor the degree of chronic glucose control in both type 1 and type 2 disease. This assay is especially useful in uncooperative, unreliable patients. HbA_{1c} helps to differentiate transient glucose intolerance associated with stress from previously unrecognized diabetes and to clarify contradictory or confusing oral glucose tolerance test results. The American Diabetes Association recommends measuring levels at least twice a year. Nondiabetic values are less than 6, goal values in diabetics are less than 7; levels greater than 8 warrant further interventions (Fig 9-1).

Acute Complications of Diabetes

The acute complications of diabetes are *nonketotic hyperglycemic-hyperosmolar coma* and *diabetic ketoacidosis.* Either of these, if not recognized promptly and treated aggressively, can lead to death. Patients in severe ketoacidosis or in the nonketotic hyperosmolar state may experience a marked increase in the serum osmolality, primarily because of hyperglycemia. In addition, an adult with diabetic ketoacidosis might have lost as much as 12 L of water and up to 800 mEq of sodium and 80 mEq of potassium in the development of this imbalance. Patients typically present with a decreased pH, as manifested in a decreased CO_2 content.

In mild to moderate ketoacidosis, the imbalances may be corrected by administration of continuous intravenous insulin infusion, coupled with oral fluids containing potassium and sodium to replace water and electrolyte deficits. In anything but minimal ketoacidosis, an intravenous infusion of isotonic sodium chloride with potassium supplementation is begun and regular insulin administration is instituted. The subcutaneous route of insulin administration should be avoided initially in patients with marked dehydration, hypotension, or shock because of delayed absorption. Insulin treatment, beginning with an intravenous bolus of 5–10 units of regular insulin followed by intrave-

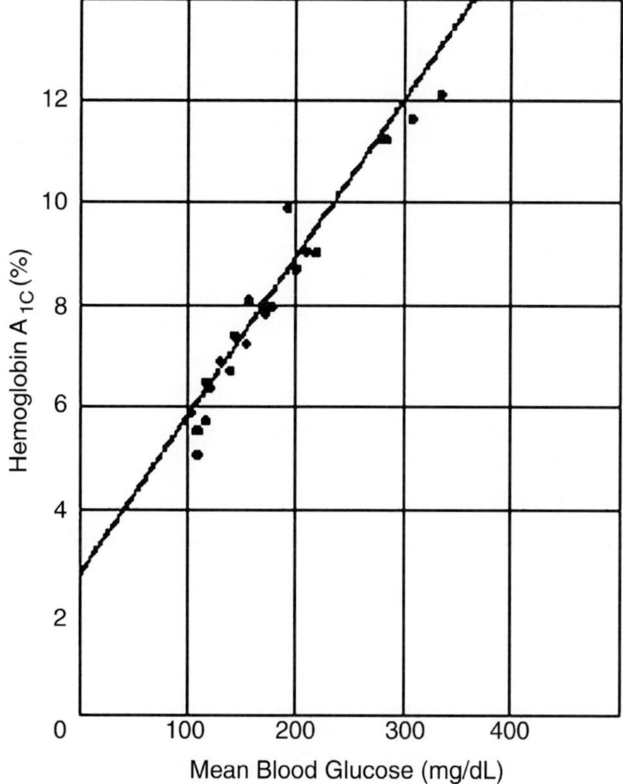

Figure 9-1 Twenty-one diabetic subjects monitored their blood glucose levels four to six times a day (pre- and postprandial) for 8 weeks. The arithmetic mean of all blood glucose values (200–300 measurements) for each subject was plotted against the subject's hemoglobin A$_{1c}$ (HbA$_{1c}$) level measured by high-performance liquid chromatography at the end of the 8 weeks. This graph depicts the relation between HbA$_{1c}$ and mean blood glucose levels; the correlation coefficient is high (r = 0.958).

nous infusion of 1–10 units of regular insulin per hour, is recommended, depending on the response. Blood pressure, urine flow, serum glucose, potassium, and sodium must be monitored hourly. When plasma glucose reaches 300 mg/dL, 5% dextrose should be added to the intravenous infusion to prevent hypoglycemia.

Long-Term Complications of Diabetes

The precise mechanism for the development of diabetic complications is elusive, but hyperglycemia plays some central role. Additional risk factors include hypertension, duration of disease, pregnancy, and possibly a genetic predisposition. The long-term complications of diabetes are usually secondary to vascular disease. Neuropathy, nephropathy, peripheral vascular disease, coronary atherosclerosis, secondary cerebral thrombosis, cardiac infarction, and retinopathy are all important causes of morbidity and mortality.

Nephropathy

Approximately 40% of patients who have had diabetes mellitus for 20 or more years have nephropathy (as demonstrated by a urinary protein level of more than 200 mg/day). Currently, 25%–33% of all patients with end-stage renal disease are diabetics. Renal failure eventually occurs in approximately 50% of patients who develop diabetes before age 20 and in 6% of those with onset after age 40. Almost invariably, nephropathy and retinopathy develop within a short time of each other.

Nephropathy is associated with the highest mortality, but tight control of blood glucose can delay and perhaps prevent the development of microalbuminuria (urine albumin levels of 30–300 mg/24 hours), the first sign of nephropathy. The progression is as follows: microalbuminuria (incipient nephropathy), macroalbuminuria (urine albumin >300 mg/24 hours), nephrotic syndrome, and finally end-stage renal disease. Controlling hypertension (particularly with angiotensin-converting enzyme inhibitors) and low-protein diets may decrease the rate of decline in glomerular filtration rate late in the course of nephropathy.

Neuropathy

Diabetic neuropathy is a common problem. Electrophysiologic diagnostic techniques indicate that 75%–80% of diabetic patients have neuropathological abnormalities at presentation. After 30 years of diabetes mellitus, 45%–50% of diabetic patients have signs of neuropathy and 15%–20% have symptoms of distal symmetrical polyneuropathy. Changes in nerve metabolism and function are thought to be mediated through increased polyol-pathway activity; reduced cellular *myo*inositol concentrations, with alterations in Na$^+$, K$^+$-ATPase activities; reduced membrane fluidity; and reduced oxygen uptake. Schwann cell synthesis of myelin is impaired, and axonal degeneration ensues. Thus, as with microvascular complications, the altered metabolic milieu leads to abnormal cell function.

In addition, microangiopathy of the endoneural capillaries leads to vascular abnormalities and microinfarcts of the nerves, with multifocal fiber loss. Symptoms in the feet and lower legs are most common. Foot pain, paresthesias, and loss of sensation occur frequently and probably result from both ischemic and metabolic abnormalities of nerves. Weakness may occur as part of mononeuritis or a mononeuritis multiplex and is usually associated with pain.

There is no specific treatment for diabetic neuropathy. Aldose reductase inhibitors (not yet commercially available) may improve nerve conduction slightly but do not produce major clinical improvement. The pain often responds to amitriptyline or carbamazepine. Phenytoin and phenothiazines are ineffective and should not be used.

Cerebrovascular and peripheral vascular disease

Cerebral thrombosis is approximately twice as prevalent in the diabetic as in the nondiabetic population. Peripheral vascular disease is 40 times as prevalent in the diabetic population, and 25% of those with diabetic peripheral vascular disease have peripheral neuropathy. The tibial and peroneal vessels are more frequently involved in diabetics than in nondiabetics, and the macrovascular lesions are more diffuse and extensive. Intermittent claudication of the calf, thigh, or buttock is a common complaint. More advanced disease may cause pain at rest. Initial findings may include absent peripheral pulses. In more advanced states, findings include tight shiny skin, hair loss, localized pallor or cyanosis, muscle atrophy, ulceration, gangrene, and diminished sensation. Delayed venous filling and delayed capillary flush may occur when the leg returns to a dependent position after several minutes of elevation.

Coronary artery disease

Coronary artery disease is the major cause of death in the United States. In diabetic patients, the risk is 2–10 times higher. Diabetic women are at an even higher risk than diabetic men, being more likely to sustain a myocardial infarction and to experience complications. Hypertension adds significantly to the risk of cardiovascular disease for diabetics. It is widely accepted that diabetic infarcts are frequently painless. The mortality rate in diabetic patients with an anterior myocardial infarction is twice that of nondiabetics. It is generally agreed that gross pathology of the coronary artery is similar among diabetics and nondiabetics. All controllable risk factors must be reduced. Metabolic management in the hospital must be directed toward avoiding both hypoglycemia and hyperglycemia. The physician may have to adjust myocardial infarction therapy because of coexisting diabetic complications.

Ophthalmologic Considerations

The most common acute ocular manifestation in diabetes is refractive change due to hyperglycemia. The most important *chronic* features of diabetes include retinopathy and accelerated cataract formation. Chronic diabetes causes additional problems, such as cranial mononeuropathies and an increased incidence of other retinal vasoocclusive phenomena. Chronic and acute vasoocclusive disease can lead to rubeosis and glaucoma. Diabetic retinopathy and associated conditions are discussed at length in BCSC Section 12, *Retina and Vitreous.*

> Flynn HW Jr, Smiddy WE, eds. *Diabetes and Ocular Disease: Past, Present, and Future Therapies.* Ophthalmology Monograph 14. San Francisco: American Academy of Ophthalmology; 2000.

Surgical Considerations in Diabetes

The stress of surgery exacerbates the metabolic abnormalities of diabetes mellitus; meticulous attention to plasma glucose control is necessary. The goals of treatment are to prevent hypoglycemia and ketoacidosis by keeping the plasma glucose levels between 150 and 250 mg/dL and to maintain fluid and electrolyte balance. The key to achieving these goals is frequent assessment of plasma glucose and plasma electrolytes. Additional regular insulin is given if plasma glucose exceeds 300 mg/dL, and the rate of glucose infusion is increased if the plasma glucose is less than 150 mg/dL. The choice of therapy is guided by the patient's usual treatment and the extent of surgery. All regimens require frequent plasma glucose measurement and appropriate modification of therapy. Rapid bedside methods of blood glucose determination facilitate management. Sliding-scale methods of insulin administration based on urine tests should be abandoned.

Patients treated with diet may not require specific therapy, but small doses of regular insulin should be given if the blood sugar exceeds 300 mg/dL. If temporary insulin therapy is needed, human insulin should be used to minimize the future risk of insulin allergy or resistance.

In patients treated with sulfonylureas, the drug should be omitted on the day of surgery. For minor operations, insulin is required only if the plasma glucose exceeds a certain level, perhaps 300 mg/dL. For major operations in which the patient will be on NPO status for some period, dextrose is administered intravenously with monitoring of plasma glucose. Insulin may be given subcutaneously or by IV push or infusion pump as determined in consultation with the anesthesiologist.

In *insulin-dependent patients* undergoing minor procedures, the morning insulin dose may be delayed until the procedure is completed and the patient is fed; this delayed dose is often reduced according to postoperative plasma glucose measurements. For major surgery, glucose is administered in the IV solution. Regular insulin is given subcutaneously or by IV push or infusion pump as indicated by blood glucose measurements and in consultation with the anesthesiologist.

Bell DS, Ovalle F. Long-term efficacy of triple oral therapy for type 2 diabetes mellitus. *Endocr Pract.* 2002;8:271–275.

Del Prato S, Heine RJ, Keilson L, et al. Treatment of patients over 64 years of age with type 2 diabetes: experience from nateglinide pooled database retrospective analysis. *Diabetes Care.* 2003;26:2075–2080.

De Witt DE, Hirsch IB. Outpatient insulin therapy in type 1 and type 2 diebetes mellitus: scientific review. *JAMA.* 2003;289:2254–2264.

Holmboe ES. Oral antihyperglycemic therapy for type 2 diabetes: clinical applications. *JAMA.* 2002;287:373–376.

Intensive blood-glucose control with sulphonylureas or insulin compared with conventional treatment and risk of complications in patients with type 2 diabetes (UKPDS 33). *Lancet.* 1998;352:837–853.

Inzucchi SE. Oral antihyperglycemic therapy for type 2 diabetes: scientific review. *JAMA.* 2002;287:360–372.

Rosak C. The pathophysiologic basis of efficacy and clinical experience with the new oral antidiabetic agents. *J Diabetes Complications.* 2002;16:123–132.

Thyroid Disease

Physiology

Functionally, the thyroid gland can be thought of as having two parts. *The parafollicular* (or C) cells secrete calcitonin and do not play a role in thyroid physiology. Thyroid *follicles* are made up of a single layer of epithelial cells surrounding colloid, which consists mostly of thyroglobulin, the storage form of the thyroid hormones T_4 and T_3.

T_4 (thyroxine), the main secretory product of the thyroid gland, contains four iodine atoms; deiodination of T_4, which occurs mainly in the liver and kidney, gives rise to T_3, the metabolically active form of thyroid hormone. Eighty percent of serum T_3 is derived through deiodination; the remainder is secreted by the thyroid. Only a small fraction of the hormones circulate free in the plasma (0.02% of total T_4 and 0.3% of total T_3); the remainder is bound to the proteins thyroxine-binding globulin (TBG), transthyretin, and albumin.

Thyroid function is regulated by the interrelationships of hypothalamic, pituitary, and thyroid activity. Thyrotropin-releasing hormone is secreted by the hypothalamus, causing the synthesis and release of thyrotropin (or thyroid-stimulating hormone, TSH) from the anterior pituitary. TSH, in turn, stimulates the thyroid, leading to release of T_4 and T_3. T_4 and T_3 inhibit the release of TSH and the TSH response to thyrotropin-releasing hormone at the level of the pituitary.

The main role of the thyroid hormones is regulation of tissue metabolism through effects on protein synthesis. Normal development of the central nervous system requires adequate amounts of thyroid hormone during the first 2 years of life. Hypothyroidism results in irreversible mental retardation (cretinism). Normal growth and bone maturation also depend on sufficient hormone levels.

Testing for Thyroid Disease

Detection of thyroid disease and evaluation of the efficacy of therapy require the use of various combinations of laboratory tests. Greater availability of direct measurement of free T_4 and the "sensitive" TSH test have greatly simplified the testing process.

Measurement of serum T_4

Total serum T_4 is composed of two parts: protein-bound and free hormone. Total T_4 levels can be affected by changes in serum TBG levels while euthyroidism is maintained and free T_4 levels remain normal. TBG and total T_4 are elevated in pregnancy and with use of oral contraceptives while free T_4 levels remain normal. Low TBG and total T_4 levels are associated with chronic illness, protein malnutrition, hepatic failure, and use of glucocorticoids.

For many years, laboratory determination of *total T_4* by radioimmunoassay was the most commonly used direct measurement of thyroid function. Free T_4 was then calculated indirectly via multiplication of total T_4 by the T_3 resin uptake (itself an indirect determination of the fraction of unbound thyroid hormone in the serum). Direct determination of free T_4 has become widely available, however, improving the accuracy of thyroid function testing.

Measurement of serum T_3

Serum T_3 levels may not accurately reflect thyroid gland function for two reasons: first, because T_3 is not the major secretory product of the thyroid; and second, because many factors influence T_3 levels, including nutrition, medications, and mechanisms regulating the enzymes that convert T_4 to T_3. Determination of T_3 levels is indicated in patients who may have T_3 thyrotoxicosis. This is an uncommon condition in which clinically hyperthyroid patients have normal T_4 and free T_4 but elevated T_3 levels.

Measurement of serum TSH

TSH secretion by the pituitary is tightly controlled by negative feedback mechanisms regulated by serum T_4 and T_3 levels. TSH levels begin to rise early in the course of hypothyroidism and fall early in hyperthyroidism, even before free T_4 levels are outside the normal range. Therefore, the serum TSH level is a sensitive indicator of thyroid dysfunction.

Until recently, available tests were not sensitive enough to differentiate between normal and reduced TSH levels; the thyroid-releasing hormone test was required to make the distinction. In recent years, immunoradiometric assays of TSH levels, which can detect TSH levels down to 0.05 mU/L, have made it possible to differentiate low normal values from low TSH levels. Through the addition of a fluorophor, an enzyme, or a chemiluminescent molecule, sensitivity is further enhanced down to 0.005 mU/L.

The TSH test is useful for (1) screening for thyroid disease, (2) monitoring replacement therapy in hypothyroid patients (TSH levels respond 6–8 weeks after changes in hormone replacement dosage), and (3) monitoring suppressive therapy for thyroid nodules or cancer.

In screening for thyroid disease, the combination of free T_4 and sensitive TSH assays has a sensitivity of 99.5% and a specificity of 98%.

Serum thyroid hormone binding protein tests

TBG concentrations can be measured directly by immunoassay. However, it is rarely necessary to determine the levels of circulating TBG and transthyretin in the clinical setting. The T_3 resin uptake test can be used to estimate thyroid hormone binding.

Radioactive iodine uptake (RAIU)

A 24-hour test of the thyroid's ability to concentrate a dose of radioactive iodine, RAIU is not always accurate enough to assess thyroid metabolic status. The RAIU test is mainly used in determining whether a patient's hyperthyroidism is due to Graves disease (elevated RAIU, >30%–40%), toxic nodular goiter (normal to elevated), and subacute thyroiditis (low to undetectable, <2%–4%).

Testing for antithyroid antibodies

Several antibodies related to thyroid disease can be detected in the blood. The most common is *thyroid microsomal antibody,* found in approximately 95% of patients with Hashimoto thyroiditis, 55% of those with Graves disease, and only 10% of adults with no apparent thyroid disease. Antibodies to thyroglobulin are also found in thyroid disease of various causes, including Hashimoto thyroiditis, Graves disease, and thyroid carcinoma. Patients with Graves disease may have antibodies against the TSH receptors, one of which results in stimulation of those receptors and another that inhibits binding of TSH to the receptor and does not stimulate thyroid function. High serum levels of thyroidstimulating immunoglobulin and the absence of antithyroperoxidase antibody are both risk factors for ophthalmopathy in Graves disease. Assays are being developed to detect antibodies against antigens present on extraocular muscles in Graves ophthalmopathy.

Thyroid scanning

Scanning with iodine-123 reflects concentration and binding, whereas using technetium-99m demonstrates iodide-concentrating capacity. Thyroid scanning is useful in distinguishing functioning (hot) from nonfunctioning (cold) thyroid nodules and in evaluating chest and neck masses for metastatic thyroid cancer.

Thyroid ultrasonography

Ultrasonography is used to establish the presence of cystic or solid thyroid nodules when palpation is inconclusive in suspicious cases. This modality detects nodules as small as 1 mm, although nodules this size are not of clinical significance. Thyroid ultrasonography is also useful in assessing the response of thyroid nodule size to suppressive therapy.

Biopsy or fine-needle aspiration biopsy

These techniques are used to obtain tissue samples for the evaluation of thyroid nodules. Fine-needle aspiration specimens require interpretation by an experienced cytopathologist. Needle aspiration is also used to drain fluid from cystic thyroid nodules.

Hyperthyroidism

Hypermetabolism caused by excessive quantities of circulating thyroid hormones results in the clinical syndrome of hyperthyroidism. This syndrome has many causes. Graves disease accounts for about 85% of cases of thyrotoxicosis. Toxic nodular goiter and thyroiditis account for most of the remaining cases.

Graves disease

Patients with Graves disease (also known as *diffuse toxic goiter*) exhibit various combinations of hypermetabolism, diffuse enlargement of the thyroid gland, ophthalmopathy, and pretibial myxedema. Although the exact cause is not known, Graves disease is thought to be an autoimmune disorder: 85%–90% of patients have circulating TSH receptor antibodies. Patients with ophthalmopathy usually have high titers of antibodies against the TSH receptors; antibodies to soluble human eye muscle antigens have also been found in these patients but not in patients with Graves disease without eye involvement.

Graves disease is common, with a 10:1 female preponderance. The incidence peaks in the third and fourth decades of life, and there is a strong familial component. Current smoking is associated with an increased incidence of ophthalmopathy that parallels the number of cigarettes smoked per day. The clinical syndrome is well known, consisting of nervousness, tremor, weight loss, palpitations, heat intolerance, emotional lability, muscle weakness, and gastrointestinal hypermotility. Clinical signs include tachycardia or atrial fibrillation, increased systolic and decreased diastolic blood pressure (widened pulse pressure), and thyroid enlargement. Pretibial myxedema—brawny, nonpitting swelling of the pretibial area, ankles, or feet—is present.

One notable situation for the ophthalmologist is *euthyroid* Graves disease. These patients present with ophthalmopathy but without coexisting hyperthyroidism. This clinical picture may appear in thyroid gland destruction by Hashimoto thyroiditis or in delayed-onset hyperthyroidism, in which other systemic manifestations appear months to years later. In some cases, however, patients have ophthalmic manifestations without ever demonstrating thyroid abnormalities.

Thyroid storm, a potentially fatal complication seen in some patients with hyperthyroidism, is a medical emergency. It presents with fever, abdominal pain, change in mental status, and tachycardia or other arrhythmias. Often brought on by stress or infection, thyroid storm once carried a mortality rate of 20%–40%; with current treatment, mortality is much lower. Treatment includes IV fluids, body cooling, antithyroid drugs (propylthiouracil, methimazole), sodium iodide (to inhibit release of preformed thyroid hormone), steroids, beta blockers, and treatment directed at any underlying precipitating factors.

Treatment of Graves disease is aimed at returning thyroid function to normal. A significant proportion of patients (30%–50%) experience remission in association with drug treatment directed at the thyroid. Later in the course of the disease, patients may experience relapse, hypothyroidism, or both.

The first step in treatment is to suppress thyroid secretion with one of the *thiourea derivatives propylthiouracil* and *methimazole (Tapazole)*. The drugs work by inhibiting the organification of iodine by the gland. Treatment is continued until clinical and laboratory indices show improvement. Side effects include rash (common), liver damage (rare), vasculitis (rare), and agranulocytosis (0.02%–0.05% of patients).

Long-term therapy of Graves disease involves several options. The aforementioned antithyroid drugs can be continued for 12–24 months in hopes of a remission. Partial surgical removal of the gland is frequently successful, although about half of such patients eventually become hypothyroid. The third and most common choice is radioactive iodine. Iodine-131 is highly effective, resulting in hypothyroidism in 80% of patients within 6–12 months; some of the remainder require a second treatment. Side effects are minimal, with no increased risk of thyroid carcinoma or leukemia. Steroids may be used to prevent progression of ophthalmopathy related to this treatment. Optimal management of thyroid orbitopathy remains in flux. Investigators have recently questioned the benefit of orbital radiotherapy for Graves ophthalmopathy. Prednisone and cyclosporine, alone or in combination, are also used for this problem. Surgical decompression is an option when involvement is more severe.

Toxic nodular goiter

In this condition, thyroid hormone–producing adenomas (either single or multiple) make enough hormone to cause hyperthyroidism. Hot nodules (those shown to be functioning on thyroid scan) are almost never carcinomatous and often result in hyperthyroidism. Toxic nodules may be treated with radioactive iodine or surgery.

Hypothyroidism

Hypothyroidism is a clinical syndrome resulting from a deficiency of thyroid hormone. *Myxedema* is the nonpitting edema caused by subcutaneous accumulation of mucopolysaccharides in severe cases of hypothyroidism; the term is sometimes used to describe the entire syndrome of severe hypothyroidism.

Primary hypothyroidism accounts for more than 95% of cases and may be acquired or congenital. Most primary cases are due to Hashimoto thyroiditis (discussed below under Thyroiditis), "idiopathic" myxedema (thought by many to be end-stage Hashimoto thyroiditis as well), and iatrogenic causes (after iodine-131 or surgical treatment of hyperthyroidism). *Secondary hypothyroidism,* caused by hypothalamic or pituitary dysfunction (usually after pituitary surgery), is much less common. As in hyperthyroidism, the female preponderance among adults with hypothyroidism is significant.

Clinically, the patient with hypothyroidism presents with signs and symptoms of hypometabolism and accumulation of mucopolysaccharide in the tissues of the body.

Many of the symptoms are nonspecific, and their relationship to thyroid dysfunction may not be recognized for quite some time: weakness, fatigue, lethargy, decreased memory, dry skin, deepening of the voice, weight gain (despite loss of appetite), cold intolerance, arthralgias, constipation, and muscle cramps.

Clinical signs include bradycardia, reduced pulse pressure, myxedema, loss of body and scalp hair, and menstrual disorders. In severe cases, personality changes ("myxedema madness") and death (following "myxedema coma") may occur.

Treatment of hypothyroidism is straightforward, requiring the normalization of circulating hormone levels with oral thyroid replacement medication. Levothyroxine is the most commonly used preparation. Serum T_4 and TSH levels are monitored at regular intervals to ensure that euthyroidism is maintained.

Thyroiditis

Thyroiditis may be classified as acute, subacute, or chronic. *Acute thyroiditis,* caused by bacterial infection, is extremely rare. *Subacute thyroiditis* occurs in two forms: granulomatous and lymphocytic. There are also two types of *chronic thyroiditis:* Hashimoto and Riedel.

Subacute granulomatous thyroiditis presents with a painful, enlarged gland associated with fever, chills, and malaise. Thyroid function tests may be helpful because they may reveal the unusual combination of an elevated T_4 level and a low RAIU. The patient may be hyperthyroid because of release of hormone from areas of thyroid destruction; pathological examination reveals granulomatous inflammation. The disease is self-limited and treatment is symptomatic, with either analgesics or, in severe cases, oral corticosteroids. After resolution, transient hypothyroidism, which becomes permanent in 5%–10% of patients, may occur. *Subacute lymphocytic thyroiditis* ("painless" thyroiditis), which commonly occurs 2–4 months post partum in mothers but may occur in isolation, presents with symptoms of hyperthyroidism and a normal or slightly enlarged but nontender gland. Pathological investigation shows lymphocytic infiltration resembling Hashimoto thyroiditis, suggesting an autoimmune cause. This disease is also self-limited, generally lasting less than 3 months. Hypothyroidism may ensue. Treatment is symptomatic.

Hashimoto thyroiditis is an autoimmune disease that appears to be closely related to Graves disease. Hashimoto thyroiditis has been found to be associated with specific HLA antigens (B46, DR3, DR4, DR5, DR9, and DR53) and is the most common cause of goitrous hypothyroidism in adults. Patients have antibodies to one or more thyroid antigens and an increased incidence of other autoimmune diseases such as Sjögren syndrome, systemic lupus erythematosus, idiopathic thrombocytopenic purpura, and pernicious anemia. Rarely, other endocrine organs—the adrenals, parathyroids, pancreatic islet cells, pituitary, and gonads—may be involved as well.

Patients with Hashimoto thyroiditis may present with hypothyroidism, an enlarged thyroid, or both. Pathological examination reveals lymphocytic infiltration. Treatment is aimed at normalizing hormone levels with thyroid replacement therapy. Patients with enlarged glands and airway obstruction that do not respond to TSH suppression may require surgery. The risk of primary thyroid lymphoma is slightly increased in patients with Hashimoto thyroiditis.

Riedel thyroiditis is a very rare disease consisting of a sclerosing fibrous infiltration of the thyroid gland associated with hypothyroidism, tracheal obstruction, retroperitoneal fibrosis, and sclerosing cholangitis. Surgery is required to relieve airway obstruction.

Postpartum thyroiditis occurs in about 5% of women after delivery, is usually painless and self-limited, and can cause hyper- or hypothyroidism (or first one problem and then the other). Postpartum thyroiditis often occurs in subsequent pregnancies and is often associated with antimicrosomal antibodies.

Thyroid Tumors

Virtually all tumors of the thyroid gland arise from glandular cells and are, therefore, adenomas or carcinomas. Functioning adenomas have been discussed previously (see the discussion of toxic nodular goiter under Hyperthyroidism).

On thyroid scan, 90%–95% of thyroid adenomas are nonfunctioning ("cold" nodules) and come to attention only if large enough to be physically apparent. Diagnostic testing involves a combination of approaches, including ultrasonography (cysts are benign and simply aspirated), fine-needle aspiration, and surgery, depending on the clinical situation. Treatment options for benign cold nodules are suppressive therapy, in which thyroid hormone replacement is used to suppress TSH secretion and its stimulatory effect on functioning nodules, and surgery.

Carcinomas of the thyroid are of four types: papillary, follicular, medullary, and anaplastic (undifferentiated). Non-Hodgkin lymphoma accounts for about 5% of thyroid malignancies. Treatment involves surgical excision or iodine-131 ablation.

Papillary carcinoma is the most common form of thyroid tumor. It is two to three times more common in women than in men. Tumors removed prior to extension outside the capsule of the gland appear to have no adverse effect on survival; the 20 year survival rate with extrathyroidal papillary carcinomas is about 40%.

Follicular carcinoma is also more common in women than in men. When noninvasive, such tumors are compatible with a normal lifespan. They tend to spread via blood vessel invasion to bone; metastases may appear years after apparent complete excision. The 10 year survival rate in patients with vascular invasion at the time of surgery is 30%.

Medullary carcinoma arises from the C cells and produces calcitonin. The lesion can occur as a solitary malignancy or as part of the multiple endocrine neoplasia syndrome type 2B, in which the carcinoma is associated with enlarged corneal nerves.

Anaplastic carcinoma, though rare, is the most malignant tumor of the thyroid gland and is found mainly in patients over the age of 60. With the giant cell form, the survival time is less than 6 months from time of diagnosis; with the small cell form, the 5 year survival rate is 20%–25%.

Fatourechi V. Subclinical thyroid disease. *Mayo Clin Proc.* 2001;76:413–416.

Ginsberg J. Diagnosis and management of Graves' disease. *CMAJ.* 2003;168:575–585.

Kennedy JW, Caro JF. Managing hyperthyroidism in the older patient. *Geriatrics.* 1996;51:22–32.

Kopp P. The TSH receptor and its role in thyroid disease. *Cell Mol Life Sci.* 2001;58:1301–1322.

Streetman DD, Khanderia U. Diagnosis and treatment of Graves disease. *Ann Pharmacother.* 2003;37:1100–1109.

CHAPTER 10

Geriatrics

The expanding percentage of elderly persons in the United States presents a growing challenge to primary care physicians and medical subspecialists. With increasing life expectancies (a record high of 75.5 years in 1991) and the aging of the post–World War II baby boomers, the population over the age of 65 has grown from 4% at the turn of the century to 12.6% in 1994. By some projections, in the year 2030, 20% of people will be over age 65 years, and by the year 2010 the number of seniors over the age 85 years will have doubled to 5.6 million persons. In addition, this subpopulation accounts for a disproportionately large share (one third) of the U.S. health care dollar.

Ophthalmology is one specialty that will be significantly affected by this demographic shift. Although ophthalmologists already care for elderly patients, there will be an increasing need for geriatric expertise in all the medical subspecialties, including ophthalmology. In addition, cataracts, age-related macular degeneration, ischemic optic neuropathy, giant cell arteritis, diabetic retinopathy, and glaucoma are all diseases that disproportionately affect older persons. These eye conditions are discussed elsewhere, but the ophthalmologist needs to consider the impact of visual loss on activities of daily living (ADL) and functional outcome.

Ophthalmologists may be expert in dealing with ophthalmic problems in the geriatric population, but they may lack experience in identifying and managing geriatric problems in general. In the past, most medical specialties (including ophthalmology) have followed the traditional medical paradigm of diagnosis of illness, treatment of disease, and measurement of objective outcomes (usually vision parameters such as visual acuity or visual field). The relatively new subspecialty of geriatrics emphasizes a different medical paradigm of functional assessment and a more holistic approach to patient care. For example, rather than measuring visual acuity as an independent and isolated outcome measure, a functional approach might incorporate improvement in ADL and independence.

Geriatricians have developed validated instruments for assessment of ADL. Practicing ophthalmologists probably would not use these instruments daily, but they must recognize the potential impact of visual loss on ADL as well as the importance of joining the geriatrician or primary care physician in complete evaluation and management. The new paradigm involves a multidisciplinary history and comprehensive physical examination incorporating measures of physical health (including visual function), psychosocial assessment (including mental health, social support), and functional assessment.

These goals were summarized by the National Institutes of Health Development Conference on Geriatric Assessment: "The multiple problems of older persons are uncovered, described, and explained, if possible, and the resources and strengths of the person are catalogued, the need for services assessed, and a coordinated care plan developed to focus interventions on the person's problems."

The ophthalmologist's role in this multidisciplinary evaluation is to communicate the visual limitations and visual needs of the older patient to the geriatrician and contribute to the integrated goals of the care plan. The role of the ophthalmologist is not to provide a comprehensive geriatric assessment but to screen and identify particular geriatric conditions (eg, depression, dementia).

The psychosocial assessment recognizes the age-related role changes and identifies and coordinates available services. The goals are to increase the level of functioning but maintain patient self-determination. The ophthalmologist should recognize the need for psychosocial assessment when there is a change in the patient's cognitive, affective, or functional abilities (eg, loss of visual function, new signs or symptoms of depression or dementia, inability to drive).

Appropriate referral and coordination of care with the geriatrician or primary care physician should accomplish the following:

- Identify the strengths and weaknesses of patients in their environment
- Assess cognitive, affective, functional, environmental, and economic issues
- Include any appropriate changes in social support and identify caregiver stress
- Explore possible placement issues and options

The ophthalmologist, although generally not the primary clinician involved in placement, should be aware of the placement options and refer appropriately.

Physiologic Aging and Pathological Findings of the Aging Eye

Aging changes of the eye occur naturally but with marked variability among individuals. The periorbital and eyelid skin and soft tissues atrophy with age. Dermatochalasis and levator dehiscence may produce secondary ptosis. Lid laxity may cause entropion, ectropion, and trichiasis. Lacrimal gland dysfunction, decreased tear production, meibomian gland disease, and goblet cell dysfunction may cause dry eye symptoms. As the patient ages, the conjunctiva undergoes atrophic changes and corneal sensitivity is reduced. The pupils become progressively miotic and less reactive to light. There is an increasing incidence of presbyopia, cataract, glaucoma, age-related macular degeneration, and diabetic retinopathy. Contrast sensitivity and visual field sensitivity are reduced. In addition, refractive error (of some type) is present in more than 90% of patients and remains a significant cause of visual disability in the nursing home patient.

The four leading causes of visual loss in the elderly are age-related macular degeneration, glaucoma, cataract, and diabetic retinopathy. Of the 33.9 million patients over age 65, approximately 100,000 persons will lose vision because of subretinal neovascular membrane formation due to age-related macular degeneration. Glaucoma increases with increasing age, and screening is recommended for patients over age 50. Cataract surgery is the most common surgical procedure in the elderly: more than 1.4 million procedures are performed annually.

Pharmacology

Medication use, number and frequency of medications, adverse reactions to medicines, and drug interactions increase with advancing age. Ophthalmologists need to be aware that ophthalmic medications may have adverse effects or interact with other medications in the elderly. Age-related pharmacokinetic changes include changes in drug absorption, distribution, metabolism, and elimination. A complete medication history is mandatory in all patients, including prescription medications, over-the-counter drugs, herbal agents, vitamins and supplements, and topical agents. Caution is needed when using new (less tested and proven in the elderly) agents.

The ophthalmologist should regularly review all of the patient's medications (including topical antibiotics, steroids, and antiglaucoma medications). Elderly patients (especially nursing home patients) often take multiple medications whose indications expired long ago. Review of the indications for current ophthalmic medications and discontinuation of unnecessary medications should reduce ophthalmology's contribution to polypharmacy. In addition, ophthalmologists should be familiar with all of the agents that they prescribe and their potential interactions with other medications the elderly patient is using. Finally, if medical therapy is needed, the ophthalmologist should recognize that compliance issues are often more complex in the elderly. Considerations include dosing frequency, difficulty in applying the medication or remembering complex dosing regimens (eg, dementia, arthritis, poor vision), the number of agents, and expense.

Outpatient Visits

Ophthalmology is largely an outpatient specialty. Access to the ophthalmologist's office can be a major structural barrier to eye care for the elderly. The ideal outpatient office should be designed to accommodate geriatric patients with various disabilities. Modifications to the geriatric-friendly office environment include:

- A safe, well-lit office that is close to drop-off areas and parking
- Automatic or assisted doors (doorways with pull levers or handles)
- Large-print, legible, and well-placed signs
- Wheelchair-accessible entranceways and waiting rooms
- Obstacle-free and well-lit, high-contrast walkways, hallways, and waiting areas (free of rugs, electrical cords, hazards for falls)
- Accessible bathrooms with elevated toilet seat, grab bars, and wheelchair-accessible sink

Elder Abuse

The ophthalmologist may be the first or only physician to see an elderly patient suffering from maltreatment. The signs of elder abuse (a form of domestic violence) may be subtle, and early recognition is key. The national prevalence of elder maltreatment is 4%–10%

and may affect 1.5 to 2 million older adults per year. The actual numbers are probably significantly higher because of underreporting of cases. External stress (eg, marital, financial, legal), dependent relationships (eg, abuser may be dependent on the elderly patient for finances or housing), existing psychopathology (eg, mental illness, substance abuse), social isolation, and misinformation (eg, about normal aging or about the patient's medical or nutritional needs) are the major risk factors for elder maltreatment. This maltreatment may take the form of abuse or neglect.

Physical neglect includes withholding of food or water, medical care, medication, or hygiene. Neglect may be intentional or unintentional. Neglect may be fostered by financial constraints or other lack of resources (eg, transportation, supervision). Elder maltreatment also includes physical and mental abuse, financial abuse or exploitation, and deprivation of basic rights (eg, decision making for care, privacy). The ophthalmologist should suspect elder maltreatment ("red flags") in the following circumstances:

- Repeated visits to the emergency room or office
- Conflicting or noncredible history from caregiver or patient
- Unexplained delay in seeking treatment
- Unexplained, inconsistent, vague, or poorly explained injuries
- History of being "accident-prone"
- Expressions of ambivalence, anger, hostility, or fear by the patient toward the caregiver
- Poor compliance with follow-up or care instructions
- Evidence of physical abuse (eg, skin bruises, lacerations, wounds in various stages of healing, unusually shaped bruises, burns, welts, patches of hair loss, or unexplained subconjunctival, retinal, or vitreous hemorrhage)

Sometimes it is necessary to obtain the history with the caregiver absent. Directed questions for the patient include "Has anyone at home tried to harm you?" "Has anyone tried to make you do things that you don't wish to do?" "Has anyone taken anything from you without your consent?"

Any suspected case of elder neglect or abuse should prompt a complete written report. Documentation of any suspicious injuries is mandatory, including type, size, location, color, and stage of healing. Mandatory reporting of elder abuse varies from state to state, and many localities have abuse hot lines for reporting maltreatment. The physician should be aware of local services for adult protection, community social service, and law enforcement agencies.

Surgical Considerations

The ophthalmologist should be aware of how pre- and perioperative evaluation and management differ for the elderly patient. As discussed previously, loss of visual acuity alone may not be an appropriate sole indication for surgical intervention (eg, cataract surgery). Functional assessment includes determining how visual loss affects ADL (eg, reading, driving, glare). Documentation of these functional impairments is important to preoperative assessment. In addition, issues of informed consent are important in patients with mild dementia or who have legal guardians or caregivers.

The ophthalmic surgeon should know some general principles regarding the preoperative assessment of elderly patients. Delirium and confusion affect up to 25% of elderly patients in the postoperative period. There are numerous causes for confusion in this setting, but many are preventable. Minimization of preoperative sedation or psychotropic medications, appropriate patient and family orientation by nursing or ancillary staff, and careful supervision and reassurance in the postoperative period can decrease postoperative confusion. Often, a confused elderly patient simply needs a familiar face or reassurance to regain calm. The use of restraints should be minimized. Confusion in patients with visual loss or who require visual rehabilitation may be exacerbated. In addition, patients with decreased vision following intraocular surgery may experience decreased mobility or be at increased risk for falls. Bed rest and immobilization can lead to disuse, pressure ulcers, and other problems. Active rehabilitation should be encouraged as soon as possible ("Bed is bad").

Although rare in outpatient ophthalmic surgery, surgical or anesthesia complications may produce life-threatening problems. The surgeon must pay careful attention to any preexisting directives (eg, do not resuscitate orders or living wills) prior to any surgical intervention (including laser treatments and periocular injections or anesthesia). By discussing possible treatment decisions early on—preferably before any serious illness arises or, if a serious illness is present, early in its course—the surgeon can avoid emergency decisions.

Some potential issues for discussion include limiting treatment, feeding tubes, antibiotics, and changes in living situation. It is best to candidly and openly discuss these important issues with the patient and the family (especially in cases of dementia) in the preoperative period; this allows them to consider these matters in the context of their belief systems and without the disorientation and confusion created by an emergency. The content, context, time, and date of such discussions should be well documented in the medical record and communicated to the patient, the family, and the primary care physician or geriatrician.

When difficult decisions do need to be made, the physician should not merely set forth a menu of possible choices but should provide information on probable outcomes (such as survival with CPR, which patients and family members tend to overestimate). Treatments that are futile need not be offered, but the question of what constitutes medical futility is complex.

Psychology of Aging

The psychology of aging is influenced by a wide range of factors, including physical changes, adaptive mechanisms, and psychopathology. Each elderly patient has a unique psychological profile and social life history. Deleterious changes are not universal; in fact, in the absence of disease, growth of character and the ability to learn continue throughout life.

As we age, the issue of loss becomes more prevalent. Losses—of status, physical abilities, loved ones, and income—become more frequent. A fear of loss of social and individual power, and with it an attendant loss of independence, is common. In addition, the reality of death has increasing influence on a person's psychological status.

Normal Aging Changes

Age-related changes in sensation and perception can have great influence, isolating an individual from the surrounding environment and requiring complex psychological reactions. There may be diminution of hearing and vision (see Ophthalmologic Considerations, below), slowing of intellectual and physical response time, and increasing difficulty with memory.

Many physical and intellectual abilities, however, are retained throughout life, and their loss should not be assumed to be part of the normal aging process. These include the senses of taste and smell, intelligence, the ability to learn, and sexuality. Any change in physical, intellectual, or emotional capabilities may reflect underlying organic or psychological disease.

Psychopathology

Functional disorders

Depression is common in the elderly; a clear precipitant (eg, physical ailments, bereavement) can often be identified. Suicide rates in older men are high; for reasons that are unclear, older women commit suicide much less commonly. The signs and symptoms of depression are similar to those seen in younger age groups, although elderly persons may place greater emphasis on physical complaints.

Depression is the most common disorder of mood in the elderly. The prevalence of clinical depression, including dysthymia and bipolar disease, is up to 3.1%. Depressive symptoms that do not meet the criteria for depression per se *(subsyndromal depression)* may occur in up to 15% of elderly patients. Major depressive disorder is characterized by episodes of at least 2 weeks of depressed mood or loss of interest with four or more of the following symptoms:

- Loss of appetite
- Weight loss
- Sleep disturbance, agitation, or retardation
- Loss of energy
- Feelings of worthlessness or guilt
- Difficulties in concentration and decision making
- Recurrent thoughts of suicide or death

Elderly depressed patients are *more likely* than younger patients to express somatic or hypochondriacal complaints, minimize depression symptoms (masked depression), and have psychotic delusional disease but *less likely* to report symptoms of guilt. The most frequent presentations of subclinical depression include new medical complaints, fatigue, poor concentration, exacerbation of existing symptoms and medical problems, preoccupation with health, and diminished interest in pleasurable activities.

The ophthalmologist's role is to recognize and refer the patient with depression. In particular, loss of function such as moderate or severe visual loss can precipitate depression. Frequent visits to the ophthalmology office, preoccupation with medical problems, recent death of a spouse, fatigue, poor concentration, and unexplained visual loss may be red flags for depression. Early recognition may be crucial because elderly patients are at highest risk for suicide (for men over age 65, the risk is five times higher than in the general population). In addition, most elderly patients who commit suicide have communicated suicidal ideation to family or friends. There is no evidence that questions about suicide increase the likelihood of suicide attempts.

Paranoia is usually the result of social isolation or reduced cognitive and sensory capabilities rather than the severe personality disorganization seen in younger patients. For example, a hearing-impaired person may have difficulty understanding what is being said and may imagine hostile motivations on the part of others. Although it may begin in adolescence, *hypochondriasis* more often begins in middle to late adulthood and is relatively common in the older population.

Organic disorders/dementia

Dementia is a collection of multiple, chronic, and acquired neurocognitive deficits (eg, memory, calculation, orientation, language, construction, purposeful activity, executive planning, or complex behavior control). Acute confusion (ie, delirium), focal deficits (eg, aphasia), and congenital defects (eg, mental retardation) should be excluded. The most common causes of dementia are Alzheimer disease, vascular (multi-infarct) disease, depression (pseudodementia), and frontal lobe disease. (Alzheimer disease is discussed at length in Chapter 12.) Although less than 15% of dementias are due to reversible causes, these should be ruled out (eg, vitamin B_{12} or folate deficiency, alcohol abuse, normal-pressure hydrocephalus, drug toxicity, thyroid disease, syphilis, seizure, central nervous system infection, tumor).

Some elderly depressed patients may have pseudodementia. These patients manifest prominent symptoms resembling dementia, with several important differences. Impairment of memory and orientation in pseudodementia has a sudden onset and rapid progression. There is often a prior history of depression, and depressive symptoms are present. Most important, the intellectual deficits are relieved by successful treatment of the depression.

Treatment

Functional disorders in the elderly are as amenable to treatment as they are in younger patients. Psychotherapy and pharmacologic therapy are effective and should be offered to all patients. Acute mental disorders due to a general medical condition (organic brain syndromes) may also be treatable and thus should be thoroughly worked up.

Ophthalmologic Considerations

Diminishing visual capabilities of any cause can contribute to behavioral disorders in the elderly. Depression, paranoia, and organic brain syndromes may be exacerbated. Optimizing visual function through optical correction, medical therapy of vision-impairing disorders, surgical correction of cataract, and low-vision aids can reduce symptoms of behavioral disorders and greatly improve the quality of life.

Osteoporosis

Osteoporosis is a condition of varied etiology involving a decrease in the mass of bone per unit volume (reduced bone density), leading to increased bone fragility and risk of fracture. It is the most common bone disorder confronting the clinician.

Osteoporosis is a significant, worldwide public health problem whose prevalence seems to be increasing. The disease is rare among black women and females of southern European ancestry. About 25% of white women over age 60 have documented spinal compression fractures in association with osteoporosis. As many as 50% of women develop vertebral fractures by age 75. After age 45, the incidence of distal forearm fractures increases markedly. By age 60, there are 10 times as many forearm fractures in women as in men of comparable age. The risk of hip fractures increases with age and, among women, reaches 20% by age 90; 80% of hip fractures are associated with preexisting osteoporosis. Approximately 17% of women with hip fractures die within 3 months of the fracture. In the United States, it is estimated that osteoporosis causes 1.5 million fractures each year at a cost of $14 billion.

Bone Physiology

Bone is a two-component system, with an organic and an inorganic phase. The organic phase *(osteoid)* consists of a matrix of collagen, glycoproteins and phosphoproteins, mucopolysaccharides, and lipids. The inorganic phase *(hydroxyapatite)* consists of an insoluble calcium-phosphate mineral. There are three types of bone cells: *osteoclasts,* which resorb bone; *osteoblasts,* which form bone; and *osteocytes,* which maintain bone structure and function. The outer portion of bone *(cortical bone)* composes 80% of total bone volume and consists of less than 5% soft tissue. The inner portion of bone *(trabecular bone)* is more porous and includes 75% soft tissue.

Bone is metabolically active and continually remodels throughout life along lines of mechanical stress. During late adolescence, bone mineral content increases rapidly. Bone mass peaks in the third decade of life. With age, the balance between bone resorption and bone formation is altered and bone mass decreases. By age 60, skeletal mass may be as little as 50% of that at age 30.

Risk Factors

Many risk factors are associated with osteoporosis, some of which are modifiable (Table 10-1). Peak bone mass (the maximum bone density reached by an individual, normally in young adulthood) appears to be the strongest correlate to lifetime fracture risk. Racial and sexual differences in peak bone mass at skeletal maturity may explain the high relative risk in white women compared with black women and white men (intermediate peak density and risk) and black men (highest peak bone density and lowest risk).

Sex hormones play a significant role: rates of osteoporosis are high in women after menopause or oophorectomy, in girls with gonadal dysgenesis, and in female long-

Table 10-1 Risk Factors for Osteoporotic Fracture

Nonmodifiable	Personal history of fracture as an adult
	History of fracture in first-degree relative
	Caucasian
	Advanced age
	Female
	Dementia
	Poor health/frailty
Potentially modifiable	Current cigarette smoking
	Low body weight (<127 lb)
	Estrogen deficiency:
	Early menopause (age<45) or bilateral oophorectomy
	Prolonged premenopausal amenorrhea (>1 yr)
	Low calcium intake
	Alcoholism
	Impaired eyesight despite adequate correction
	Recurrent falls
	Inadequate physical activity
	Vitamin D deficiency
	Poor health, frailty

distance runners with functional hypogonadism. Age-related factors include decreased formation of new bone, impaired calcium absorption (with secondary hyperparathyroidism and increased bone loss), and nutritional vitamin D deficiency. Other associated factors include insufficient dietary calcium intake, sedentary lifestyle, nulliparity, alcohol abuse, and cigarette smoking.

In addition, glucocorticoid excess, thyrotoxicosis of Graves disease, acromegaly, diabetes mellitus, and a variety of other systemic diseases and drugs are all associated with bone loss.

Clinical Features

The typical clinical picture in osteoporosis includes back pain, spinal deformity, loss of height, and fractures of the vertebrae, hips, and (less commonly) other bones. Multiple vertebral fractures over a period of years can lead to severe kyphosis, with a loss of height of 4–8 inches, and cervical lordosis ("dowager's hump").

Diagnostic Evaluation

Radiographic evaluation

Patients at risk with a history of back pain are evaluated for radiographic evidence of vertebral fracture. Radiographic changes only become visible when at least 30% of bone mass has been lost. The changes may be subtle because osteoporosis involves a generalized reduction in bone mass. The amount of loss necessary for detection by conventional radiography depends on the bone involved. The spinal column exhibits the most characteristic radiographic features of osteoporosis, with accentuation of the vertebral end plates, anterior wedging in the thoracic spinal column, biconcave compression ("ballooning," or "codfish vertebrae") in the lumbar region, and disc herniation into the vertebral body. The long bones exhibit cortical thinning with irregularity of endosteal surfaces. Osteoporosis caused by glucocorticoid excess presents a somewhat different picture, with radiographic changes in the skull, ribs, and pelvic rami.

Several other techniques allow more accurate measurement of bone density than can be obtained through conventional radiography. All of these methods measure the degree of attenuation of a beam of photons from an x-ray tube by targeted bones and surrounding soft tissues. Measurements of the spine are used to predict vertebral fractures, of the femoral neck to predict hip fractures, and of the wrist or heel to predict peripheral fractures. Results are compared with mean bone mineral density (BMD) values in young adults, the normal for women being within 1 standard deviation (SD) of this reference mean (the *T score*). The risk of fractures increases with age and with each SD below the mean; below 2 SD, the risk rises exponentially. *Osteoporosis* is defined as values more than 2.5 SD below the mean, whereas *osteopenia* is a value 2.0 SD below the mean. The *Z score* represents a patient's BMD compared with the mean value for persons of the same age and sex. A Z score less than 2.0 SD below the mean suggests accelerated bone loss and warrants further evaluation of a secondary cause (Table 10-2).

Dual-photon x-ray absorptiometry is presently the technique of choice because it allows for shorter examination time (a few minutes with current machines), greater accuracy, improved resolution, and longer source life. The radiation dose of this test is less than 5 millirem.

Dual-energy quantitative computed tomography scans the lower thoracic and upper lumbar vertebral bodies in cross section at numerous levels, and the computed tomographic values obtained are compared with standards for soft tissue, fat, and mineral. Dual-energy quantitative computed tomography is highly accurate but is more expensive than dual-photon x-ray absorptiometry and may be less reproducible. The x-ray dose is less than 3 millirem.

Who Should Be Tested?

- All postmenopausal women under age 65 who have one or more risk factors for osteoporotic fractures (besides menopause)
- All women aged 65 and over
- Postmenopausal women who present with fractures
- Women who are considering therapy for osteoporosis (if BMD testing would facilitate the decision)
- Women who have been on hormone replacement therapy for prolonged periods

Clinical Evaluation

If densitometric studies confirm the diagnosis of osteoporosis, a medical evaluation should be undertaken to rule out secondary causes (see Table 10-2). Serum calcium and phosphorus levels are usually normal, although slight hyperphosphatemia may be present in postmenopausal women. The alkaline phosphatase level is usually normal but may be slightly elevated following a fracture. Sustained elevation of alkaline phosphatase in the absence of liver disease suggests osteomalacia or skeletal metastasis.

Table 10-2 Causes of Secondary Osteoporosis

Primary osteoporosis	**Bone marrow disorders**
Juvenile	Multiple myeloma
Idiopathic (young adults)	Systemic mastocytosis
Involutional	Disseminated carcinoma
Endocrine	Lymphoma and leukemia
Hypogonadism	Pernicious anemia
Ovarian agenesis	Hemophilia
Glucocorticoid excess	Thalassemia
Hyperthyroidism	**Connective tissue diseases**
Hyperparathyroidism	Osteogenesis imperfecta
Diabetes mellitus	Homocystinuria
Acromegaly	Ehlers-Danlos syndrome
Addison disease	Marfan syndrome
Gastrointestinal	Ankylosing spondylitis
Subtotal gastrectomy	Rheumatoid arthritis
Malabsorption syndromes	**Miscellaneous**
Chronic obstructive jaundice	Immobilization
Primary biliary cirrhosis	Chronic obstructive pulmonary disease
Severe malnutrition	Chronic alcoholism
Hemochromatosis	Sarcoidosis
Parental nutrition	Chronic heparin administration
	Chronic use of anticonvulsant drugs
	Lithium use
	Tamoxifen (premenopausal use)

Treatment

General considerations

All patients with osteoporosis should adhere to a diet that supplies adequate amounts of calcium, protein, and vitamins. Weight-bearing exercise (eg, walking, jogging, and weight lifting) is important in the maintenance of bone mass. Limitation of alcohol intake and cessation of smoking are also beneficial. Back pain is treated with analgesics and physical therapy.

Calcium and vitamin D

Ingestion of elemental calcium is important for the maintenance of bone mass. The incidence of hip fractures appears to be significantly less in female populations wherein dietary calcium and vitamin D intake is high. The recommended daily intake is at least 1200 mg/day (roughly the equivalent of four 8-ounce glasses of milk) and vitamin D (400–800 IU per day for persons at risk of deficiency), but the average calcium intake in women is only about 375 mg/day. During pregnancy and lactation, much more calcium may be needed. This calcium may be obtained from dietary as well as pharmacologic sources. Calcium and vitamin D supplementation is recommended in patients on long-term steroid therapy to treat an underlying disease. Calcium is available in a variety of preparations, including calcium carbonate, citrate, gluconate, lactate, and phosphate. Calcium carbonate and phosphate have the highest concentration of elemental calcium, about 40%; calcium citrate has 21%, lactate 13%, and gluconate 9%. Calcium therapy may cause constipation, nausea, flatulence, bloating, hypercalcuria, and renal stones. Hypercalcemia does not occur in patients with normal renal function. However, massive doses of vitamin D can lead to dangerous hypercalcemia.

Pharmacologic therapy

Five medications are approved by the U.S. Food and Drug Administration for prevention or treatment of osteoporosis (Table 10-3). They are estrogen, alendronate, risedronate, raloxifene, and calcitonin.

Estrogen Numerous clinical studies have established that estrogens help to prevent osteoporosis. Estrogens produce significant calcium retention, decrease the imbalance between bone formation and resorption, and tend to decrease the progression of osteoporosis by slowing bone turnover. A recent study showed an increase in BMD in women taking estrogen or combination estrogen-progestin treatment (see below) compared with those taking placebo.

Estrogen therapy may preserve height and reduce the rate of vertebral and hip fracture (by 70% and 25%, respectively, in some studies), prevent vertebral deformity, and stabilize bone loss in postmenopausal women, amenorrheic premenopausal women, and patients who have undergone oophorectomy. The effectiveness of estrogen therapy may be enhanced when combined with calcium supplementation or calcitonin therapy. The benefit of estrogen treatment appears to be maximized when therapy is started at the onset of menopause and continued for at least 7–10 years, although such therapy has also been shown to have some benefit in older women with established osteoporosis.

Unopposed estrogen treatment increases the risk of endometrial carcinoma, but concurrent progestin therapy reduces this risk to that of the general population. The recent Women's Health Initiative randomized trial demonstrated an increased risk of breast cancer, ovarian cancer, heart disease, hypertension, thromboembolic diseases, ischemic stroke, and dementia in women taking hormone replacement therapy (HRT). In view of these findings, patients should be advised of the significant risks of HRT before starting this treatment for osteoporosis.

Bisphosphonates Alendronate and risedronate are second-generation bisphosphonates, a class of drugs that bind strongly to hydroxyapatite crystals, are adsorbed onto new bone matrix, and prevent bone resorption by inhibiting osteoclast activity. Bisphosphonates shift the balance between bone formation and resorption toward formation. High doses, however, interfere with the process of bone mineralization. The main side effects of bisphosphonates are gastrointestinal. As with other treatments for osteoporosis, calcium and vitamin D intake must be adequate.

Raloxifene Raloxifene is an agent in a class of compounds called *selective estrogen receptor modulators*, which have estrogen-agonistic effects on bone, lipids, and blood clotting and estrogen-antagonistic effects on the breast and uterus. Raloxifene has been shown to increase BMD and reduce the risk of vertebral fractures by 30%–50%.

Calcitonin Calcitonin is a hormone that interferes with osteoclast function and inhibits bone resorption. Derived from salmon, it has been used in the treatment of osteoporosis

Table 10-3 FDA-Approved Drugs for Osteoporosis Prevention and Treatment

Name	Dose	Indications	Side Effects and Risks	Estimated Reduction for Fracture
Estrogen	Depends on formulation of estrogen (eg, conjugated equine estrogen, 0.625 mg daily)	Prevention	Vaginal bleeding, breast tenderness, gallbladder disease; risk of breast cancer, deep vein thrombosis, pulmonary embolism; increased risk of heart disease and stroke	Vertebral, 50%–80% Nonvertebral, 25%
Alendronate	5 mg/day 10 mg/day	Prevention Treatment	Gastrointenstinal disturbances (abdominal pain, nausea, dyspepsia), esophageal ulcer (rare)	Vertebral, 50% Nonvertebral, 50%
Risedronate	5 mg/day	Treatment	Same as alendronate	Vertebral, 40% Nonvertebral, 40%
Raloxifene	60 mg/day 60 mg/day	Prevention Treatment	Deep vein thrombosis or pulmonary embolism, hot flashes, leg cramps	Vertebral, 40% Nonvertebral*
Calcitonin	200 IU intranasal/day (alternating nostrils)	Treatment	Nasal irritation, rhinitis	Vertebral, 40% Nonvertebral*

* No studies thus far have demonstrated benefit for nonvertebral fracture rate.

(Adapted from McGarry KA, Kiel DP. Postmenonpausal: strategies for preventing bone loss, avoiding fracture. *Postgrad Med J.* 2000;108:79–88.)

for many years but could only be given by subcutaneous or intramuscular injection. Recently, however, calcitonin nasal spray *(Miacalcin)* has become available. It is well tolerated and has shown some effectiveness in increasing bone density and reducing fractures. Adequate concomitant intake of calcium and vitamin D is necessary.

Osteoporosis in Men

Osteoporosis is perceived primarily as a disease of postmenopausal females. It should be noted, however, that women have only twice the incidence of hip fracture as men. Cigarette smoking, alcohol consumption, steroid therapy, and hypogonadism are associated with an increased incidence of osteoporosis in men, who also seem to benefit from the above-cited protective measures (with the exception of estrogen therapy).

Falls

The incidence and severity of falls increases with increasing age. Fall-related expenses totaled $13.8 billion in 1995. Accidental death is the fifth-leading cause of death in the elderly, and two thirds of these deaths are due to falls. Three fourths of these fall-related deaths occur in the 13% of the population over 65 years old. In the community-living elderly patient population, 33% of patients will fall and 5% of these falls will result in a fracture or hospitalization. Falls were the single largest cause of restricted activity in the elderly (18%). The hospital mortality rate of relatively isolated hip fracture is 6%; with multiple medical problems, the mortality rate may be as high as 22%. The incidence rate is much higher among patients in nursing homes or hospitals (up to three times higher): up to 10%–25% of these patients experience a serious fall causing fracture or hospitalization. Each year, 1800 fatal falls occur in nursing homes in the United States.

In addition to serious injury or death, falls have a significant psychosocial impact on patients (eg, fear of falling, postfall anxiety, depression, social isolation, and loss of mobility, self-confidence, independence, and function). The three most common risk factors for falls are gait or balance disorder, dizziness, or environment-related. Visual disorders, however, account for up to 4% of falls. The ophthalmologist's role in fall prevention includes recognition and treatment of visual disorders (including refractive error), multifactorial and multidisciplinary risk reduction, and preventive targeting of risk factors (eg, postural hypotension, multiple medications, and impairments in transferring, strength, balance, and gait). If the ophthalmologist recognizes that a patient is at risk for falls (according to vision or other risk factors), appropriate referral can provide help in safety and preventive measures in the home (eg, increasing lighting, removing obstacles from the environment, eliminating slippery surfaces, removing loose rugs and electrical cords, and using high-contrast colors, hand rails, better-fitting and nonskid footwear, and assistive devices). (See Table 10-4.)

Systemic Diseases

Ophthalmologists should be aware of the increased incidence of systemic disease in the elderly. The prevalence of anemia due to vitamin B_{12} deficiency increases with age. In

Table 10-4 Interior Safety Checks

Living room	Are scatter rugs firmly anchored with rubber backing?
	Are electrical cords in good repair, especially on heating pad?
	Light, heat, and ventilation:
	Is there adequate night lighting?
	Are stairways continually illuminated?
	Is temperature within comfortable range (70°-75°F)?
	Is the heater vented properly?
	Is there cross ventilation?
	Is furniture sturdy enough to give support?
	Is there a minimum of clutter, allowing enough room for easy mobility as well as lower fire hazard?
	Are emergency telephone numbers posted in a handy place and easily read, such as doctor, fire department, ambulance, paramedics, nearest relative?
	If the person has limited vision, does phone have enlarged dial?
Kitchen	Stove, refrigerator, and sink
	Is the stove free of grease and flammable objects?
	Is baking soda available in case of fire?
	Are matches used or is there a pilot light?
	Is the refrigerator working properly?
	Is sink draining well?
	Is food being stored properly?
	Is trash taken out daily?
	Is there a sturdy stepping stool in evidence?
	Are there skid-proof mats on the floor?
	In the bathroom, are safety measures observed?
	Are there handrails beside the tub and toilet?
	Are there skid-proof mats in the bathtub and/or shower?
	Are electrical outlets a safe distance from the tub?
Outside the home	Walks and stairs
	Are there raised or uneven places on the sidewalks?
	Are stairs in good repair?
	Are the top and bottom stairs painted white or a bright contrasting color to improve visibility?
	Are handrails securely fastened?
	Are screens on doors and windows in good repair?
	Is there an alternate exit for the house?

(From Hypertext modules in geriatric medicine. Computer-based self-instruction modules. Baylor College of Medicine, 1998.)

patients with low to normal serum vitamin B_{12} levels, increased serum and urinary methylmalonic acid and homocysteine may assist with the diagnosis. In addition, 30% of patients with early vitamin B_{12} deficiency have anemia, but 59% may have reversible memory deficits. For the ophthalmologist, patients with vitamin B_{12} deficiency may present with painless, bilateral, progressive visual loss; a central or cecocentral scotoma on visual field testing; and optic atrophy (temporal pallor). Concomitant alcohol and tobacco use should be discontinued.

The incidence of hypertension, cardiovascular disease, cerebrovascular disease, and diabetes (which is 10% in adults over age 65 and up to 40% in patients over age 80) increases with age; these conditions may affect the eye (eg, homonymous hemianopsia, hypertensive or diabetic retinopathy, amaurosis fugax). Pulmonary diseases such as tuberculosis are more frequent in the elderly (who account for 25% of active cases; 60% of deaths related to pulmonary disease occur in patients older than 65 years). Tuberculosis may cause anterior or posterior uveitis or present with neuro-ophthalmic manifestations. Antituberculosis therapy (eg, ethambutol and isoniazid) may produce toxic optic neuropathy. Herpes zoster affects 10% of patients over age 80 (who have decreased cell-mediated immunity). Herpes zoster ophthalmicus may produce uveitis or central nervous system manifestations (including ophthalmoplegia) in addition to vesicular dermatomal skin eruption and postherpetic neuralgia (which occurs in 10%–15% of patients). The early use of antiviral agents (eg, acyclovir, famciclovir) may reduce the duration of pain with and development of postherpetic neuralgia. Hyperthyroidism and Graves ophthalmopathy may occur in the elderly (up to 15%–25% of patients are older than 65 years). Thyroid disease may be iatrogenically precipitated by iodine-containing contrast (eg, contrast-enhanced computed tomography). One subgroup of elderly patients with a particular form of hyperthyroidism—apathetic thyrotoxicosis—may present with depression and apathy.

Cauley JA, Robbins J, Chen Z, et al. Effects of estrogen plus progestin on risk of fracture and bone mineral density: the Women's Health Initiative randomized trial. *JAMA.* 2003; 290:1729–1738.

Chapuy MC, Arlot ME, Duboeuf F, et al. Vitamin D3 and calcium to prevent hip fractures in elderly women. *N Engl J Med.* 1992;327:1637–1642.

Colley CA, Lucas LM. Polypharmacy: the cure becomes the disease. *J Gen Intern Med.* 1993; 8:278–283.

Consensus Development Conference. Diagnosis, prophylaxis, and treatment of osteoporosis. *Am J Med.* 1993;94:646–650.

Costa AJ. Elder abuse. *Prim Care.* 1993;20:375–389.

Fitten LJ, Perryman KM, Wilkinson CJ, et al. Alzheimer and vascular dementias and driving. *JAMA.* 1995;273:1360–1365.

McGarry KA, Kiel DP. Postmenopausal osteoporosis: strategies for preventing bone loss, avoiding fracture. *Postgrad Med J.* 2000;108:79–88.

Mokshadundam S, Barzel US. Thyroid disease in the elderly. *J Am Geriatr Soc.* 1993;41:1361–1369.

Norman EJ, Morrison JA. Screening elderly populations for cobalamin (vitamin B12) deficiency using the urinary methylmalonic acid assay by gas chromatography mass spectrometry. *Am J Med.* 1993;94:589–594.

Orwoll ES, Klein RF. Osteoporosis in men. *Endocrinol Rev.* 1995;16:87–116.

Physician's Guide to Prevention and Treatment of Osteoporosis. Washington, DC: National Osteoporosis Foundation; 1998.

Retchim SM, ed. Medical considerations in the older driver. *Clin Geriatr Med.* 1993;9:279–481.

Rubenstein LZ, Josephson KR, Robbins AS. Falls in the nursing home. *Ann Intern Med.* 1994;121:442–451.

CHAPTER 11

Cancer

Recent Developments

- Biological therapies utilizing the immune system now play a major role in the treatment of cancer.
- Angiogenesis inhibitors may prove to be a significant form of cancer therapy in humans.
- Genetic profiling of tumors may contribute significantly to their potential treatment.

Incidence

Cancer is the second-leading cause of death in the United States. Each year, about 1,170,000 new cases are diagnosed and some 550,000 deaths occur. More than 3 million Americans have survived cancer, and in more than 2 million of these the diagnosis was established longer than 5 years ago. About 23% of all deaths in the United States are due to cancer.

Cancer is actually many different diseases; questions of etiology, cancer prevention, and cancer cure must address the specific types of tumors. Nonmelanotic skin cancers are the most common tumors, but these cancers rarely produce major clinical problems. After these types, the most common forms of cancer in adult Americans (in decreasing order of incidence) are lung, breast, prostate, and colorectal. About 80% of adult cancers arise from the epithelial tissues; leukemias and sarcomas are relatively rare.

Cancer is the leading cause of death by disease in children under age 15 in the United States. The number of children diagnosed with cancer each year has risen from 12 per 100,000 in the early 1970s to 14 per 100,000 today. At the same time, death rates have dropped and survival rates have risen. The 5-year survival rate for all childhood cancers is now 71%, compared with about 51% in 1973. Cancer is diagnosed in more than 8500 children each year: 30% with leukemia, 12% with Hodgkin and non-Hodgkin lymphoma, and the remainder with solid tumors.

Etiology

Cancer is a genetic disease. It is caused by multiple mutations in genes that control cell division. Some of these genes, called *oncogenes*, stimulate cell division; others, called *tumor-suppressor genes*, slow this process. In the normal state, both types of genes work together, enabling the body to replace dead cells and repair damaged ones. Mutations in these genes cause cells to proliferate out of control. Such mutations can be inherited or acquired through environmental insults. (Cancer causes, therefore, are explained on the basis of chemical, viral, or radiation-related causes that occur in a complex milieu, including host genetic composition and immunobiological status). Between 60% and 90% of cases are understood on the basis of environmental origin. Several examples of environmental causes are cigarette smoking (lung cancer), asbestos (lung cancer and mesothelioma), vinyl chloride (hepatic angiosarcoma), benzidine (leukemia), dietary nitrates (gastrointestinal carcinoma), and lye injury (esophageal carcinoma).

Carcinogenic Factors

Chemical

Since the 1950s, definite changes have occurred in the cancer mortality rates in the United States. For example, lung cancer death rates have increased markedly in both men and women. This increase parallels the rise in cigarette smoking, but the higher death rate lags about 20 years behind the increase in smoking. The increased incidence of and mortality from lung cancer are particularly striking in women, in whom the mortality rate is increasing about 6% per year. Even though breast cancer remains more prevalent, lung cancer kills more women than does breast cancer. Most cases of lung cancer can be attributed to cigarette smoking. One promising development in lung cancer is the drop in the number of new cases diagnosed each year in men. Lung cancer deaths among men dropped nearly 7% between 1991 and 1995. The mortality rates from breast, colon, and rectal cancer have remained essentially unchanged since about 1960.

Stomach cancer has become fairly rare in the United States, presumably because of a decrease in human exposure to exogenous agents such as dietary nitrates and an increase in dietary vitamins. In the United States and Western Europe, mortality from lung, colon, and breast cancer is high and mortality from stomach cancer is low. In Japan, stomach cancer predominates and colon and breast cancer are relatively rare. After several generations, descendants of Japanese persons who migrated to the United States show a decreased incidence of stomach cancer and acquire the high incidence of colon cancer characteristic of the United States. Similarly, Japanese in Japan who adopt a Western diet and lifestyle have an increased rate of colon cancer and a decreased rate of stomach cancer, whereas people of Japanese ancestry in the United States who marry Japanese spouses and do not adopt a Western diet continue to show high stomach cancer and low colon cancer rates. These examples support the argument for the predominant role of environmental factors as opposed to genetic or inborn factors in the etiology of most human cancers.

The incidence of specific cancers in different subsets of the American population varies considerably. For example, the black population has a higher incidence of cancer of the prostate, uterine cervix, lung, esophagus, and oropharynx than does the white population; however, the black population also has a lower incidence of cancer of the breast and corpus uteri than does the white population.

Epidemiologic data suggest that as much as 80% of human cancer may be due to exogenous chemical exposure. If these chemicals could be properly identified, a major proportion of human cancers could be prevented by reducing host exposure or by protecting the host. A number of industrial processes or occupational exposures and numerous chemicals or groups of chemicals have been implicated in various forms of human cancer. Specific causes of major cancers, such as large bowel and breast cancer, have not been identified with certainty. Important matters needing resolution are:

- The extent to which cancers are caused by naturally occurring substances versus man-made chemicals
- The role of chemical versus viral agents
- The role of general nutritional factors
- The role of multifactor interactions

Radiation

The carcinogenic effects of ionizing radiation were discovered at the turn of the century when radiation caused an epidermoid carcinoma on the hand of a radiologist.

The general population is exposed to both naturally occurring ionizing radiation and man-made ionizing radiation. Natural radiation comes from cosmic rays; thorium, radium, and other radionuclides in the earth's crust; and potassium-40, carbon-14, and other naturally occurring radioactive elements in the body. The average dose for a person living at sea level is 0.8 mSv (80 mrem) per year. The average dose may be double for persons living at higher elevations (eg, Denver) because of more intense cosmic rays. The dose may also be larger where the content of radioactive material in the soil and subterranean rock is greater.

Man-made sources deliver an average of 106 mrem per year to each person. These sources include medical diagnostic equipment, technologically altered natural sources (such as phosphate fertilizers and building materials containing small amounts of radioactivity), global fallout from atmospheric testing of atomic weapons, nuclear power, high-altitude jet flight, occupational exposure, and consumer products such as color television sets, smoke detectors, and luminescent clocks and instrument dials.

Radiation exposure has been associated with cancer of almost every organ, system, and tissue in human and animal models. The carcinogenic effects result from molecular lesions caused by random interactions of radiation with atoms and molecules. Most molecular lesions induced in this way are of little consequence to the affected cell. However, DNA is not repaired with 100% efficiency, and mutations and chromosomal aberrations accrue with increasing radiation dose. Although these changes in genes and chromosomes have been postulated to account for the carcinogenic effect of radiation, the precise molecular mechanisms are unknown. Parameters that influence response of the target tissue include the total radiation dose, the dose rate, the quality of the radiation source, the characteristics of certain internal emitters (such as radioiodine), and individual host factors such as age at the time of radiation exposure and sex.

Viral

The role of viruses in the etiology of cancer has been studied extensively, but evidence is still too weak to permit the unequivocal conclusion that viruses cause tumors in humans. The inoculation of animals with specific viruses may produce tumors, and certain naturally occurring tumors in animals may be transmitted horizontally from animal to animal by viruses (eg, Lucke renal adenocarcinoma in the leopard frog, Marek lymphomatous disease in chickens, leukemia in cats and cattle). In humans, some papillomavirus infections produce warts that can become cancerous, and particles resembling viruses associated with the transmission of leukemia in animals have been found in human cancer patients. In addition, several human cancers show a definite correlation with viral infection and the presence and retention of specific virus nucleic acid sequences and virus proteins in the tumor cells (Burkitt lymphoma, nasopharyngeal carcinoma, carcinoma of the cervix, and hepatocellular carcinoma).

All of the DNA virus groups except the parvovirus family have been associated with cancer. This is notable because all the DNA viruses associated with cancer contain double-stranded DNA, whereas the parvoviruses contain only single-stranded DNA.

There are nine RNA virus groups, but only one is associated with oncogenicity: the retrovirus group. The retroviruses differ from all other RNA viruses in that they require a DNA intermediate to replicate. Retroviruses contain and specify an enzyme called *reverse transcriptase.* In the presence of the four nucleoside triphosphates, reverse transcriptase can synthesize DNA complementary to the single-stranded RNA contained in the virion, producing an RNA–DNA hybrid. The RNA in this RNA–DNA hybrid is then degraded, and a double-stranded linear DNA molecule forms. This double-stranded DNA molecule moves into the cell nucleus and is integrated into the cellular DNA as a provirus.

The papillomavirus of the papovavirus group has been associated with squamous cell carcinoma and laryngeal papilloma in humans. The hepatitis B virus has been associated with primary hepatocellular carcinoma in humans.

The human herpesviruses that are associated with disease include Epstein-Barr virus, herpes simplex virus type 1, herpes simplex virus type 2, cytomegalovirus, and varicella-zoster virus. The Epstein-Barr virus, which causes infectious mononucleosis, has been associated with Burkitt lymphoma and nasopharyngeal carcinoma. The herpes simplex virus type 1, which causes gingivostomatitis, encephalitis, keratoconjunctivitis, neuralgia, and labialis, has been associated with carcinoma of the lip and oropharynx. The herpes simplex virus type 2, which causes genital herpes, disseminated neonatal herpes, encephalitis, and neuralgia, has been associated with cancer of the uterine cervix, vulva, kidney, and nasopharynx. The cytomegalovirus, which causes cytomegalovirus disease, transfusion mononucleosis, interstitial pneumonia, and congenital defects, has been associated with prostate cancer, Kaposi sarcoma, and carcinoma of the bladder and uterine cervix. The varicella-zoster virus, which causes chickenpox, shingles, and varicella pneumonia, has not yet been associated with specific human cancers.

Genetic and familial factors

Host susceptibility is an established but poorly defined concept in human carcinogenesis. A heritable component may be more important in some forms of cancer (colon cancer) and less important in others (esophageal cancer). Certain cancers show an ethnic predilection.

Cancers may aggregate in a nonrandom manner in certain families. These cancers may be of the same type or dissimilar. Such cancer-cluster families may have several children with soft tissue sarcoma and relatives with a variety of cancers, especially of the breast in young women. Multiple endocrine neoplasia (types I and II) is yet another example of familial cancers. The recognition of family cancer syndromes permits early detection that may be lifesaving.

Genetic abnormalities are a feature of many cancers. These may be single-gene disorders or inborn chromosomal abnormalities. Heritable retinoblastoma is due in part to a 13q14 deletion. Other forms of cancer may be caused by mutation of multiple alleles, some of which are pleiotropic (ie, they may induce more than one form of cancer). An example is osteosarcoma occurring in the lower femurs of children with bilateral retinoblastoma. Such persons may also be unusually susceptible to the carcinogenic effect of radiotherapy for the eye tumor and develop a second primary tumor after an indefinite latency.

Therapy

Radiation

Ionizing radiation interacts with host tissues and malignant tumors by an energy transfer and a chemical reaction, with the release of free radicals and the decomposition of water into hydrogen, hydroxyl, and perhydroxyl ionic forms. These ionic forms probably react with DNA and RNA in vital enzymes, producing biological injury.

The injuries noted to date include mitotic-linked death and chromosomal aberrations such as breakage, sticking, and cross-bridging. Consequent cell death occurs in both normal tissue and malignant lesions. In radiotherapy, biochemical recovery and biological repair occur in the normal host, maintaining the integrity of vital systems.

The poorly differentiated lymphoid cells, intestinal epithelium, and reproductive cells are more readily damaged and recover more quickly than do the highly differentiated normal cells. Lymphocytes are therefore damaged by 100 rads and central nervous system tissue by 5000 rads. Surface irradiation of approximately 1000 rads produces skin erythema. The most serious damage is the late development of postradiation malignant changes in as many as 21% of patients, manifesting as squamous cell carcinoma and basal cell carcinoma. Bone absorption can produce osteogenic sarcomas and fibrosarcomas.

Radiation teratology is an area of ongoing interest. The most radiosensitive stage occurs during the period of organogenesis, 6–12 weeks after conception. The most common site of radiation damage is the central nervous system, producing microcephaly and mental retardation.

Ocular manifestations of fetal irradiation in the first trimester include microphthalmos, congenital cataracts, and retinal dysplasia. A 5 rad dose may cause congenital anomalies in a fetus. Fetal exposure to approximately 30–80 rads doubles the incidence of congenital defects; 500 rads (the LD_{50} for humans) generally induces an abortion.

The traditional source of ionizing radiation is x-rays, which are produced by linear accelerators and betatrons. Gamma rays, produced spontaneously as certain elements (such as radium, uranium, and cobalt-60) decay, are another source of ionizing radiation. *Internal radiotherapy* is the use of radioactive implants directly in a tumor or body cavity. This form of radiotherapy delivers a concentrated dose of radiation to a small area and is frequently used for cancers of the tongue, uterus, and cervix.

Effects of irradiation on the eye and adnexa

The ocular effects of irradiation depend not only on total dose, fractionation, and treatment portal size but also on associated systemic diseases such as diabetes and hypertension. Concomitant chemotherapy has an additive effect.

The lens is the most radiosensitive structure in the eye, followed by the cornea, the retina, and the optic nerve. The orbit is completely included in the treatment portal in diseases such as large retinoblastomas and melanomas; the orbit is partially included in diseases such as small melanomas and retinoblastoma and tumors of adjacent structures, such as the maxillary antrum, nasopharynx, ethmoid sinus, and nasal cavity. Usual doses range from 2000 to 10,000 rads. The total dose is usually fractionated during the treatment.

Doses to the lens as low as 200 rads in one fraction may cause a cataract. However, cataracts caused by low doses may be asymptomatic and may not progress. Cataracts caused by higher doses (700–800 rads) may continue to progress, causing considerable visual loss.

The average latent period for the development of radiation-induced cataracts is 2–3 years. The clinical picture of radiation retinopathy resembles that of diabetic retinopathy. Radiation retinopathy is very rare below the fractionated dose of 5000 rads over 5–6 weeks. At higher fractionated doses (7000–8000 rads), most patients develop radiation retinopathy. The usual interval between radiation and the development of radiation-induced retinopathy is 2–3 years. Radiation retinopathy may develop earlier in patients who are diabetic or on chemotherapy. The earliest clinical manifestation of radiation retinopathy is usually cotton-wool spots. After several months, they fade away, leaving large areas of capillary nonperfusion. Telangiectatic vessels grow in the retina into the areas of capillary nonperfusion. Microaneurysms may also develop. These ischemic changes may cause rubeosis iridis, which in turn may lead to rubeotic glaucoma.

Histologically, the capillary endothelial cell is the first type of cell to be damaged, followed closely by the pericytes and then the endothelial cells of the larger vessels. The new intraretinal telangiectatic vessels have thick collagenous walls. There may be spotty occlusion of the choriocapillaris.

Doses to the optic nerve in the range of 6000–7000 rads cause some injury in a small number of patients. Damage to the distal end of the optic nerve is called *radiation optic neuropathy*. Clinically, these patients have disc pallor with splinter hemorrhages. If the injury occurs to the more proximal part of the optic nerve, it resembles retrobulbar optic neuropathy. Affected patients may complain of unilateral headaches and ocular pain; the disc may not reveal edema or hemorrhage. The effect of radiation on lacrimal tissue depends on the total dose. Permanent damage is not common below 5000 rads.

With doses of 6000–7000 rads, a dry eye syndrome sometimes develops. This syndrome usually develops within a year and occasionally progresses to corneal ulceration and severe pain.

Chemotherapy

The goal of cancer chemotherapy is to destroy cancer cells by taking advantage of their metabolic activity, which is increased compared with normal cells. Effective drugs should have minimal long-term impact on normal cells, especially those with a rapid rate of turnover such as bone marrow and mucous membrane. A model treatment plan should allow normal cells to regrow more rapidly than tumor cells, permitting retreatment at appropriate intervals. Cancer inhibition takes place at several levels:

- Macromolecular synthesis
- Cytoplasmic organization
- Cell membrane synthesis

Most drugs destroy cells by first-order kinetics—that is, they kill a constant percentage (or log) of cells with each treatment.

It has been estimated that approximately 10^9, or 1 g, of tumor cells are required to be detected. A lethal number of cells is 10^{12}, or 1 kg. If a drug's kill log is 2–3, then three to five treatments would still be required for cure after all clinical disease has disappeared. This is the basis for continuing treatment after an apparent complete remission. Chemotherapy sometimes fails because tumor populations are not homogeneous; some cells are less sensitive to drugs and, therefore, the log or percentage kill is lower.

The sensitivity of a tumor population largely depends on the growth characteristics of the tumor cells. Some of the factors involved are cell cycle time, growth fraction (the percentage of cells undergoing division), number of tumor cells present, and tumor cell natural death rate.

Chemotherapeutic agents can be divided into the following basic groups: alkylating agents, antimetabolites, hormones, and natural products (Table 11-1).

Alkylating agents

Alkylating agents form covalent bonds within the nuclei, which cause cross-linking and abnormal base-pairing, producing lethal errors in dividing cells. Examples are mechlorethamine (nitrogen mustard), cyclophosphamide (Cytoxan), chlorambucil (Leukeran), melphalan (Alkeran), and busulfan (Myleran). Toxicity causes cytopenia, nausea, alopecia, hemorrhage, and pulmonary fibrosis. Cyclophosphamide is a precursor to its active metabolites, phosphoramide mustard and acrolein. Cyclophosphamide is well absorbed orally (90% bioavailability). Its active products are excreted in the urine and cause two unusual adverse effects, hemorrhagic cystitis and inappropriate retention of water. *Nitrosoureas* are a form of alkylating agent that are lipid soluble and cross the blood–brain barrier; therefore, drugs of this type have some effect on central nervous system tumors. Cisplatin also binds and cross-links (interfering with DNA synthesis) and acts like an alkylating agent. Its unique toxicity is renal failure, which can be reduced with hydration.

Table 11-1 Antineoplastic Drugs

Drugs by Class	Mechanism of Action	Tumors Commonly Responsive	Toxicity and Remarks
Alkylating agents Mechlorethamine (nitrogen mustard) Chlorambucil (Leukeran) Cyclophosphamide (Cytoxan) Melphalan (Alkeran) Ifosfamide (Ifex)	Alkylation of DNA with restriction of strands' uncoiling and replication	Hodgkin, malignant lymphoma, small cell lung Ca, Ca of breast and testis, CLL	Alopecia with high IV dosage; nausea and vomiting; myelosuppression; hemorrhagic cystitis (especially with ifosfamide), which can be ameliorated with mesna; muto- and leukemogenic; aspermia; permanent sterility possible
Antimetabolites Folate antagonist Methotrexate (MTX)	Folate antagonist with binding to dehydrofolate reductase and interference with (pyrimidine) thymidylate synthesis	Choriocarcinoma (female), Ca of head and neck, ALL, Ca of ovary, malignant lymphoma, osteogenic sarcoma	Mucosal ulceration; bone-marrow suppression; toxicity increased with renal function impairment or ascitic fluid (with pooling of drug). Leucovorin rescue can reverse toxicity at 24 h (10–20 mg q 6 h $\times$ 10 doses).
Purine antagonist 6-Mercaptopurine (6-MP)	Blocks de novo purine synthesis	Acute leukemia	Myelosuppression, alopecia
Pyrimidine antagonist 5-Fluorouracil (5-FU)	Interferes with thymidylate synthase to reduce thymidine production	GI neoplasms, Ca of breast	Mucositis, alopecia, myelosuppression, diarrhea and vomiting, hyperpigmentation. When given after MTX, synergistic effect is significant.
Cytarabine (Ara-C)	DNA polymerase inhibition	Acute leukemia (especially nonlymphocytic), malignant lymphoma	Myelosuppression, nausea and vomiting, cerebellar and conjunctival toxicities at high dosage, skin rash

ALL = acute lymphocytic leukemia; Ca = cancer; CLL = chronic lymphocytic leukemia; CML = chronic myeloid leukemia; IFN = interferon; SIADH = syndrome of inappropriate antidiuretic hormone secretion.

Table 11-1 Antineoplastic Drugs (Continued)

Drugs by Class	Mechanism of Action	Tumors Commonly Responsive	Toxicity and Remarks
Plant Alkaloids			
Vincas			
Vinblastine (Velban)	Mitotic arrest by alteration of microtubular proteins	Lymphomas, leukemias, Ca of breast, Ewing sarcoma, Ca of testis	Alopecia, myelosuppression, peripheral neuropathy, ileus
Vincristine (Oncovin)	As above	As above	Peripheral neuropathy, SIADH. Dose commonly "capped" at total of 2 mg in adults.
Paclitaxel (Taxol)	Promotes assembly of microtubules	Ca of breast, lung, ovary, head, neck, and bladder	Myelosuppression, alopecia, myalgia, arthralgia, neuropathy
Podophyllotoxins			
Etoposide (VePesid, VP-16)	Inhibition of mitosis by unknown mechanisms	Lymphoma, Hodgkin, Ca of testis, Ca of lung (especially small cell), acute leukemia	Nausea, vomiting, myelosuppression, peripheral neuropathy. Etoposide cleared by liver (teniposide by kidney); increased toxicity in renal failure.
Antibiotics			
Doxorubicin (Adriamycin)	Intercalation between DNA strands inhibits uncoiling of DNA	Acute leukemia, Hodgkin, other lymphomas, Ca of breast, Ca of lung	Nausea and vomiting, myelosuppression, alopecia. Cardiac toxicity at cumulative dosage >500 mg/m^2. Higher dosage tolerated when given by continuous IV.
Bleomycin	Incision of DNA strands	Squamous cell Ca, lymphoma, Ca of testis, Ca of lung	Anaphylaxis, chills and fever, skin rash; pulmonary fibrosis at dosage >200 mg/m^2; requires renal excretion
Mitomycin	Inhibits DNA synthesis by acting as a bifunctional alkylator	Gastric adenocarcinoma; colon, breast, and lung Ca; transitional cell Ca of the bladder	Local extravasation causes tissue necrosis; myelosuppression, with leukopenia and thrombocytopenia 4-6 wk after treatment; alopecia; lethargy; fever; hemolytic-uremic syndrome

ALL = acute lymphocytic leukemia; Ca = cancer; CLL = chronic lymphocytic leukemia; CML = chronic myeloid leukemia; IFN = interferon; SIADH = syndrome of inappropriate antidiuretic hormone secretion.

Table 11-1 Antineoplastic Drugs (Continued)

Drugs by Class	Mechanism of Action	Tumors Commonly Responsive	Toxicity and Remarks
Nitrosoureas			
Carmustine (BiCNU)	Alkylation of DNA with restriction of strands' uncoiling and replication	Brain tumors, lymphoma	Myelosuppression, pulmonary toxicity (fibrosis), renal toxicity
Lomustine (CeeNU)	Carbamoylation of amino acids in proteins	As above	As above
Inorganic ions			
Cisplatin (Platinol)	Intercalation and intracalation between DNA strands inhibits uncoiling of DNA	Ca of lung (especially small cell), testis, breast, and stomach; lymphoma	Anemia, ototoxicity, peripheral neuropathy, myelosuppression, nausea, vomiting
Biologic response modifiers			
IFN (Intron-A, Roferon-A)	Antiproliferative effect	Hairy cell leukemia, CML, lymphomas, Kaposi sarcoma (AIDS), renal cell Ca, melanoma	Fatigue, fever, myalgias, arthralgias, myelosuppression, nephrotic syndrome (rarely)
Enzymes			
Asparaginase (Elspar)	Depletion of asparagine, on which leukemic cells depend	ALL	Acute anaphylaxis, hyperthermia, pancreatitis, hyperglycemia, hypofibrinogenemia
Hormones			
Tamoxifen (Nolvadex)	Places cells at rest: binding of estrogen receptor	Ca of breast	Hot flushes, hypercalcemia, deep vein thrombosis
Flutamide (Eulexin)	Binding of androgen receptor	Ca of prostate	Decreased libido, hot flushes, gynecomastia

ALL = acute lymphocytic leukemia; Ca = cancer; CLL = chronic lymphocytic leukemia; CML = chronic myeloid leukemia; IFN = interferon; SIADH = syndrome of inappropriate antidiuretic hormone secretion.

(Adapted from *The Merck Manual of Diagnosis and Therapy*. 17th ed. Rahway, NJ: Merck Research Laboratories; 1999:990–993.)

Antimetabolites

Antimetabolites interfere with metabolic pathways of dividing cells, especially with DNA synthesis. They are commonly structural analogues or precursor molecules of cofactors and, therefore, interfere with biosynthetic enzymes or become incorporated into abnormal or nonfunctional products lethal to the cells.

Antimetabolites include three basic groups. The *antifolates* (methotrexate) interfere with dihydrofolate reductase, an enzyme important in the reduction of folate and dihydrofolate to tetrahydrofolate and in the one-carbon metabolism of adenine, guanine, and thymidine. Antifolates are not metabolized in the body but are excreted into the urine and are therefore not useful in patients with renal impairment.

A second group of antimetabolites, *antipurines*, includes 6-mercaptopurine and its imidazole derivative, azathioprine (Imuran). These drugs interfere with multiple sites of purine (adenine and guanine) biosynthesis and the interconversion of purine biosynthesis (adenine and quanine) and the interconversion of purines. Generally effective in acute leukemias, 6-mercaptopurine analogue (a hypoxanthine) is given orally. The circulating leukocyte reduced by chemotherapeutic agents is not specific. Cyclophosphamide primarily reduces recirculating small lymphocytes; 6-mercaptopurine reduces polymorphonuclear leukocytes and large mononuclear cells.

A third group of antimetabolites, the *antipyrimidines*, interferes with biosynthesis of uridine or thymidine. This group includes 6-azauracil, cytarabine, and 5-fluorouracil (5-FU). Cytarabine may compete with deoxycytidine for one or more enzymes and thereby inhibit DNA synthesis. Cytarabine is currently used against acute leukemia. 5-FU is an inhibitor of thymidylate synthase and, consequently, DNA production. It is a widely used drug, effective against colon and breast carcinoma, and significantly palliative in gastrointestinal malignancies. 5-FU is usually administered intravenously; plasma levels vary considerably after oral administration. The primary toxicities of 5-FU are bone marrow suppression, stomatitis, and diarrhea. 5-FU can cause acute and chronic conjunctivitis as well as punctal and canalicular stenosis.

Hormones

The hormone class of chemotherapeutic agents is used in pharmacologic doses 10–100 times the normal physiologic replacement dose to inhibit growth of tumor cells. These compounds include the nonsteroidal antiestrogen tamoxifen, used in progressive prostate carcinoma and breast cancer. The androgens, including testosterone propionate and fluoxymesterone (Halotestin), are useful in metastatic breast cancer and some renal cell carcinomas. The progesterones, including hydroxyprogesterone and medroxyprogesterone acetate (Provera), are useful in adenocarcinoma of the endometrium and occasionally in patients with renal cell or prostatic carcinoma. The corticosteroids such as prednisone are useful in higher doses in acute lymphocytic leukemias, lymphoma, and hypercalcemia of malignancy.

Natural products

Natural products include a wide variety of agents. The most common are vinca alkaloids, podophyllin derivatives, antitumor antibiotics, paclitaxel, and related drugs.

Vinca alkaloids are derived from the periwinkle plant and include vincristine (Oncovin), vinblastine (Velban), and several investigational agents. These agents block incorporation of orotic acid and thymidine into DNA and cause arrest and inhibition of mitosis.

Podophyllin derivatives and semisynthetic plant derivatives arrest cells in the G2 phase. VP-16 (etoposide) and VM-26 (teniposide) are gaining new acceptance in many treatment protocols.

Paclitaxel (Taxol) is a compound originally isolated from the bark of the Pacific yew tree. It has been approved by the FDA to treat breast, ovarian, and lung cancers as well as AIDS-related Kaposi sarcoma. Paclitaxel stops microtubules from breaking down. In normal cell growth, microtubules are formed when a cell starts dividing. Once the cell stops dividing, the microtubules are broken down or destroyed. With paclitaxel, cancer cells become clogged with microtubules and cannot grow and divide.

Antitumor antibiotics are compounds produced by species of *Streptomyces* in culture. These agents interfere with the synthesis of nucleic acid. A partial list includes:

- Anthracyclines (doxorubicin [Adriamycin] and derivatives), which interfere with template function of DNA (a unique side effect is cardiac muscle degeneration leading to cardiomyopathy)
- Bleomycin, which causes DNA-strand scission
- Dactinomycin (actinomycin D), which inhibits DNA-directed RNA synthesis
- Mitomycin, which impairs replication by causing cross-linking between DNA strands

The major dose-limiting toxicity of mitomycin is myelosuppression. Mitomycin has also been implicated as a cause of the hemolytic-uremic syndrome.

Other Approaches

The treatment of cancer in general is evolving rapidly. In some instances, the treatment approaches are entirely new; in others, previously known therapies are used, either individually or in combination, to be more specific and effective. Other treatment approaches include angiogenesis inhibitors and biological therapies.

New conventional approaches

Intraoperative irradiation is a technique wherein a large dose of external radiation is directed at the tumor and surrounding tissue during surgery.

Linear energy transfer radiation makes use of accelerated particles (neutrons, pions, and heavy ions) to destroy cancer cells. These particles deposit more energy along a path they take through tissue than do x-rays or gamma rays.

Radiosensitizers and *radioprotectors* are a new group of drugs developed to make tumor cells more sensitive to radiation or normal cells more resistant to radiation damage, respectively.

Bone marrow transplantation combines aggressive chemotherapy and transplantation techniques. Patients receive either their own previously withdrawn marrow or marrow from a suitable donor after large doses of chemotherapy have destroyed malignant cells to the point of marrow suppression. This approach has been successful against a significant number of tumors, such as breast and medulloblastoma, that failed to respond to all other conventional treatments.

Angiogenesis inhibitors

Angiogenesis is important to the growth and spread of cancers. New blood vessels are critical in the formation of tumors. In animal studies, angiogenesis inhibitors have successfully stopped the formation of new blood vessels, causing the tumor to shrink and die. Currently, various angiogenesis inhibitors are being evaluated in human clinical trials. These studies include patients with cancers of the breast, prostate, brain, pancreas, lung, stomach, ovary, and cervix; some leukemias and lymphomas; and AIDS-related Kaposi sarcoma.

Biological therapies

Biological therapies (sometimes called *immunotherapy, biotherapy,* or *biological response modifier therapy*) uses the immune system, either directly or indirectly, to fight cancer or to lessen the side effects that may be caused by some cancer treatments. Further, cancer may develop when the immune system breaks down or is not functioning adequately. Biological therapies are designed to repair, stimulate, or enhance the immune system's responses.

Cells in the immune system secrete two types of proteins: antibodies and cytokines. Cytokines are substances produced by some immune system cells to communicate with other cells. Types of cytokines include lymphokines, interferons, interleukins, and colony-stimulating factors. Some antibodies and cytokines can be used to treat cancer. These substances are called *biological response modifiers.* Other biological response modifiers include monoclonal antibodies and vaccines.

Interferons are types of cytokines that occur naturally in the body. There are three major types of interferons: interferon-α, interferon-β, and interferon-γ; interferon-α is the type most widely used in cancer treatment. Interferons can improve the way a cancer patient's immune system acts against cancer cells. Furthermore, interferons may act directly on cancer cells by slowing their growth or promoting their development into cells with more normal behavior. Interferons may also stimulate natural killer cells, T cells, and macrophages, boosting the immune system's anticancer function. The FDA has approved the use of interferon-α for the treatment of hairy cell leukemia, melanoma, chronic myeloid leukemia, and AIDS-related Kaposi sarcoma.

Interleukins, like interferons, are cytokines; they occur naturally in the body and can be made in the laboratory. Many interleukins have been identified; interleukin-2 has been the most widely studied in cancer treatment. Interleukin-2 stimulates the growth and activity of many immune cells, such as lymphocytes, that can destroy cancer cells. The FDA has approved interleukin-2 for the treatment of metastatic kidney cancer and metastatic melanoma.

Colony-stimulating factors (sometimes called *hematopoietic growth factors*) usually do not directly affect tumor cells but instead stimulate bone marrow production. Colony-stimulating factors allow doses of anticancer drugs to be increased without increasing the risk of infection or need for transfusion.

Monoclonal antibodies (MOABs) are produced by a single type of cell and are specific for a particular antigen. Researchers are examining ways to create MOABs that are specific to the antigens found on the surface of cancer cells being treated.

MOABs are made by injecting human cancer cells into mice, stimulating an antibody response. The cells producing antibodies are then removed and fused with laboratory-grown cells to create hybrid cells called *hybridomas.* Hybridomas can indefinitely produce large quantities of these MOABs.

MOABs have many potential uses in cancer treatment. One such treatment is to link MOABs to anticancer drugs, radioisotopes, other biological response modifiers, or other toxins. When the antibodies attach to cancer cells, they can deliver these poisons directly to the cells. MOABs carrying radioisotopes may also prove useful in diagnosing certain cancers, such as colorectal, ovarian, and prostate cancer.

Cancer vaccines are being developed to assist the immune system in recognizing cancer cells. These vaccines are designed to be injected after the disease is diagnosed rather than before it develops. They may help the body reject tumors and prevent cancer from recurring. Vaccines are being studied in the treatment of melanomas, lymphomas, and cancers of the kidney, breast, ovaries, prostate, colon, and rectum.

In the future, other biological approaches to cancer therapy may include *genetic profiling* of certain tumors. This may prove more helpful and effective than classifying tumors by their organ of origin. An example of this is the differentiation between those tumors with a normal or an abnormal tumor suppressor gene p53. Tumor cells with normal p53 genes are far more sensitive to chemotherapy than those with mutant p53.

Ophthalmologic Considerations

The eye and its adnexa are frequently involved in systemic malignancies as well as in extraocular malignancies that extend into ocular structures (including local malignancies of skin, bone, and sinuses). Breast and lung cancers frequently metastasize to the eye and are the second most common intraocular tumors in adults. Acute myelogenous and lymphocytic leukemias frequently have uveal and posterior choroidal infiltrates as part of their generalized disease. In children, these manifestations are often signs of central nervous system involvement and suggest a poor prognosis. Although malignant lymphomas do not usually involve the uveal tract, histiocytic lymphoma is one type that often involves the vitreous and presents as uveitis. The retina and choroid may also be involved. Tumors of the eye and adnexa are discussed in several other BCSC books, including Section 4, *Ocular Pathology and Intraocular Tumors;* Section 6, *Pediatric Ophthalmology and Strabismus;* Section 7, *Orbit, Eyelids, and Lacrimal System;* and Section 8, *External Disease and Cornea.*

CHAPTER 12

Behavioral and Neurologic Disorders

Recent Developments

- Neurodegenerative disorders of Alzheimer and Parkinson diseases are linked to several abnormal genes.
- New trials, examining anti-inflammatory drugs and a potential vaccine, offer great new promise for treatment and possible prevention of Alzheimer disease.

Introduction

Since the 1980s began, the World Health Organization (WHO) has focused its efforts on behavioral and neurologic disorders that occur frequently, cause substantial disability, and create a burden on individuals, families, communities, and societies. The WHO approach has been based on epidemiologic evidence: the assessment of disease burden using disability-adjusted life years. This approach has emphasized the public health importance of behavioral and neurologic disorders, which in 1990 accounted for 10.5% of the worldwide disease burden. It is estimated such disorders will account for 15% of disability-adjusted life years in 2030.

In addition to behavioral disorders, the neurologic disorders that significantly affect this disease burden include epilepsy, dementias (in particular, Alzheimer disease), multiple sclerosis, Parkinson disease and other motor system disorders, stroke, pain syndromes, and brain injury.

Behavioral Disorders

Behavioral disorders encompass a wide variety of conditions in which the common factor is disordered functioning of personality. These disturbances range from mild reactions to the events or circumstances of a person's life to debilitating, life-threatening illnesses. Although the practicing ophthalmologist will not be called on to treat mental illness, such disease may profoundly affect the diagnosis and treatment of ocular diseases. In addition, some of the medications used to treat psychiatric disorders have significant ophthalmic side effects. The illnesses and medications discussed below are those most likely to affect the practice of ophthalmology.

Mental Disorders Due to a General Medical Condition

Formerly called *organic mental syndromes*, this category was renamed in DSM-IV. The essential feature of mental disorders due to a general medical condition is a psychological or behavioral abnormality associated with transient or permanent dysfunction of the brain. Causes include any disease, drug, or trauma that directly affects the central nervous system (CNS) and systemic illnesses that indirectly interfere with brain function; Alzheimer disease is included in this category. (Alzheimer disease is discussed at length later in this chapter.) Orientation, memory, and other intellectual functions are impaired. Psychiatric symptoms may occur, including hallucinations, delusions, depression, obsessions, and personality changes.

Patients with a mental disorder due to a general medical condition with or without cognitive impairment are often unable to remember instructions and therefore unable to comply with treatment regimens. Depression, which frequently accompanies the syndrome, can complicate the situation. Medications with CNS side effects, such as β-blockers and carbonic anhydrase inhibitors, must be used with care because these patients are frequently sensitive to these agents. See also discussion of dementia in Chapter 10, Geriatrics.

Schizophrenia

The term *schizophrenia* actually encompasses a group of disorders with similar features. These are some of the most devastating mental illnesses in terms of personal and societal cost. Schizophrenia usually begins when patients are young and continues to a greater or lesser extent throughout their lives. Schizophrenics invariably display thought disturbances, bizarre behavior, and deterioration in their general level of function. Incidence is estimated at 0.5%–1.0% of the population.

The classic manifestations are delusions and hallucinations in a clear sensorium. *Delusions* are disturbances in thought: firmly held beliefs that are untrue. Other thought abnormalities include loosening of associations and tangential thinking. *Hallucinations* are abnormal perceptions, experienced without any actual external stimulus. The patient's affect is often flattened or inappropriate.

Motor disturbances range from uncontrolled, aimless activity to catatonic stupor, in which the patient may be immobile, mute, and unresponsive yet fully conscious. Repetitive, purposeless mannerisms and inability to complete goal-directed tasks are also common.

Treatment involves the use of antipsychotic medications (discussed later), psychosocial support, and hospitalization for acute exacerbations.

Mood Disorders

Also known as *affective disorders,* mood disorders range from appropriate reactions to negative life experiences to severe, recurrent, debilitating illnesses. Common to all of these disorders is depressed mood, elevated mood (mania), or alternations of the two.

The classic term *manic depression* has been replaced by *bipolar disorder,* now used to describe any illness in which mania is present, whether or not depression occurs.

Mania is a period of abnormally and persistently elevated or irritable mood sufficiently severe to cause impairment in social or occupational functioning. It is slightly more common in females and is estimated to affect 0.6%–0.9% of the population. Typical symptoms include euphoria or irritability, grandiosity, decreased need for sleep, increased talkativeness, flight of ideas, and increased goal-directed activity. Lithium is the cornerstone of pharmacologic treatment of bipolar illness and may be used alone or in combination with antipsychotic drugs. Psychotherapy is used as an adjunct.

Major depression is far more common than mania (estimates range from 5% to 9% for women, 2% to 4% for men) and therefore has a greater impact on all aspects of society. Major depression may occur at any age but is most common in the middle-aged and the elderly. Affective changes include a feeling of sadness, emptiness, and nervousness. Thought processes are typically slowed and reflect low self-esteem, pessimism, and feelings of guilt. Social withdrawal and psychomotor retardation are seen, although agitation also occurs. Basic physical functions are impaired, as manifested by sleep disturbances, changes in appetite with associated weight loss or gain, diminished libido, and an inability to experience pleasure *(anhedonia).* Common somatic complaints are fatigue, headache, and other nonspecific symptoms. Up to 15% of seriously depressed patients may commit suicide.

For the nonpsychiatric clinician, depression creates a number of problems. There may be no apparent mood change, the illness being manifested in somatic complaints leading to time-consuming, expensive workups. Conversely, patients known to be depressed may have organic disease overlooked as psychosomatic. Appropriate recommendations for psychotherapeutic intervention may be met with resistance, anger, or denial, disrupting the patient–physician relationship. Compliance with diagnostic and treatment regimens for medical and surgical disorders can be problematic. Drugs with CNS side effects may exacerbate depressive symptoms. Treatment consists of psychotherapy and antidepressant medications. Electroconvulsive therapy is effective in selected cases.

Somatoform Disorders

The essential feature of these disorders is the presence of symptoms that suggest physical disease in the absence of physical findings or a known physiologic mechanism to account for the symptoms. The symptoms in somatoform disorders are considered to be outside the patient's voluntary control. The practicing physician should be aware of these syndromes because encounters with these patients are common.

Several somatoform disorders are recognized. *Conversion disorders* are characterized by temporary and involuntary loss or alteration of physical functioning due to psychosocial stress. Symptoms are typically neurologic and include functional visual loss ("hysterical blindness"). In *somatoform pain disorder,* prolonged, severe pain is the only symptom. Psychotherapy is the primary therapeutic modality.

Somatization disorder is most common in women and consists of multiple somatic complaints. Patients are often histrionic in their description of their symptoms and may have undergone multiple hospitalizations and surgery. The incidence of associated psychiatric illness is high. Treatment is aimed at providing psychological support and minimizing the expenditure of medical resources. Psychotherapy is typically met with resistance and is therefore unsuccessful. Psychopharmacologic treatment of underlying psychiatric disorders may help.

Hypochondriasis is a preoccupation with the fear of having or developing a serious disease. Physical examination fails to support the patient's belief, and reassurance by the examining physician fails to allay the fear. Treatment principles are the same as for somatization disorder. In *body dysmorphic disorder,* the patient believes that his or her body is deformed in the absence of a physical defect or has an exaggerated concern about a mild physical anomaly. This illness is rare, and treatment regimens are not well defined.

Two other conditions that are not actually somatoform disorders bear mentioning here. *Factitious disorders* are characterized by willful production of physical or psychological signs or symptoms in the absence of external incentives. It is thought that these patients feign illness solely because of a psychological need to assume the sick role. Treatment requires discovery of the true nature of the physical illness, a carefully planned confrontation, and psychotherapy. Prognosis for recovery is guarded. *Malingering* is the intentional production of physical or psychological symptoms for the purpose of identifiable secondary gain. Malingering is not considered a primary psychiatric illness.

Ophthalmologists should be familiar with techniques for detecting malingerers who feign loss of vision; such persons are not uncommonly encountered in practice. (See BCSC Section 5, *Neuro-Ophthalmology,* for some of these techniques.)

Substance Abuse Disorders

Substance abuse is one of the major public health problems in the United States. Alcohol-related deaths rank third in frequency behind heart disease and cancer. The cost of illness, death, and crime related to alcohol and drug abuse in the United States has been estimated in the tens of billions of dollars.

Drug dependence is the abuse of a drug causing a threat to physical health, psychological functioning, or the ability to exist within the demands of society. Common to all types of drug dependence is *psychic dependence*—that is, a psychic drive or a feeling of satisfaction requiring periodic or continuous drug administration in order to avoid discomfort, produce pleasure, relieve boredom, or facilitate social interaction. *Physical dependence* occurs when repeated administration of a drug causes an altered physiologic state in the CNS so that sudden cessation of the drug causes an *abstinence syndrome* (a physical illness whose symptoms are determined by the specific drug). *Tolerance* occurs when increasing amounts of a drug are necessary to achieve the same desired effect. The drugs causing dependence fall into several groups, as listed in Table 12-1.

Opiates

Heroin is the most commonly abused opiate in the United States. Diagnosis of heroin use is made by history, and findings may include puncture sites on the skin and miotic pupils. Symptoms of abstinence include restlessness, yawning, rhinorrhea, pupillary mydriasis, hyperthermia (38°–40°C), vomiting, and diarrhea. Withdrawal, although not fatal to people with no other serious illness, can be dangerous in ill or elderly people. A total plan of withdrawal as well as support (economic, social, and psychiatric) must be em-

Table 12-1 Classification of Dependence-Producing Drugs

Class I-Drugs producing both psychic and physical dependence
  A. Opiate type
    1. Morphine group: opium, morphine, diacetylmorphine (heroin), hydromorphone (Dilaudid), codeine, dihydrohydroxycodeinone
    2. Morphinans: oxycodone (Percodan)
    3. Benzomorphans: phenazocine (Prinadol)
    4. Meperidine group: meperidine (Demerol)
    5. Methadone group: methadone, propoxyphene (Darvon)
  B. Alcohol-barbiturate type.
    1. Ethyl alcohol
    2. Barbiturates
    3. Paraldehyde
    4. Chloral hydrate
    5. Meprobamate (Miltown, Equanil)
    6. Piperidinediones: glutethimide, methyprylon (Noludar)
    7. Benzodiazepines: chlordiazepoxide (Librium), diazepam (Valium)
    8. Tertiary carbinols: methylpentynol (Dormison), ethchlorvynol (Placidyl)
  C. Opiate agonist-antagonist type
    1. Nalorphine
    2. Levallorphan
    3. Cyclazocine
    4. Pentazocine (Talwin)
  D. Amphetamine type
    1. dl-amphetamine (Benzedrine), dextroamphetamine (Dexedrine)
    2. Phenmetrazine (Preludin)
    3. Methylphenidate (Ritalin)
    4. Diethylpropion (Tenuate)
    5. Pipradrol (Meratran)
  E. Cocaine type: coca leaf, cocaine

Class II-Drugs producing psychic dependence but not physical dependence
  A. Hallucinogens
    1. Lysergic acid diethylamide (LSD)
    2. Mescaline
    3. Tryptamines: psilocybin, dimethyltryptamine, diethyltryptamine
    4. Hallucinogenic amphetamines
  B. Cannabis type: cannabis leaf (marijuana), hashish
  C. Bromides

ployed to prevent the patient from returning to drug dependence. Because many former heroin abusers are unable to remain drug-free, methadone maintenance is sometimes used.

Methadone maintenance is the most common form of treatment in the United States for heroin dependence. Methadone is absorbed orally, prevents drug craving and abstinence symptoms for 24–36 hours, and causes tolerance (blockage of other opiates). Administered by the government, methadone allows patients to function better in society by freeing them from the need to secure heroin, the mind-altering euphoria of heroin, and IV drug administration. Vocational, educational, and psychiatric rehabilitation services are also available through methadone maintenance programs. Unfortunately, drug-free status is difficult to maintain for long periods; 90% of patients who leave methadone treatment programs will be incarcerated, deeply involved in drugs, readmitted to the program, or dead within 1 year.

Hypnotic drugs

Hypnotic drugs may be used for nonmedical purposes by teenagers and adults. These drugs elevate the threshold of excitation of neurons, thereby resulting in lethargy, ataxia, nystagmus, impaired judgment, and emotional lability. Cessation of the drug causes anxiety, restlessness, convulsions, delusions, and hyperthermia; cessation may even be fatal. Diagnosis of drug abuse is made from history and confirmed by a blood or urine level of the drugs. Hypnotic drug abuse should be suspected in anyone appearing drunk without evidence of alcohol ingestion. Treatment consists of a monitored hospital withdrawal with posthospital support.

Alcohol

Alcohol is by far the most commonly abused drug, owing to its social acceptance and widespread availability. It is estimated that 7% of adults in the United States are alcoholics. Although multiple factors contribute to alcoholism, twin and adoption studies have shown a genetic influence. According to several studies, approximately 25% of fathers and brothers of alcoholics are themselves alcoholics.

Like hypnotic drugs, alcohol depresses the CNS and leads to similar clinical findings; blood levels of ethyl alcohol should be obtained in suspicious cases. An alcoholic patient may experience restlessness, hallucinations, and even seizures 72–96 hours after admission to the hospital (or withdrawal) in the alcohol abstinence syndrome. Treatment consists of a supported, controlled withdrawal using a sedative-hypnotic drug. In addition, the patient needs long-term support such as Alcoholics Anonymous.

Alcohol crosses the placental barrier, and children born to alcoholic mothers may be affected by the fetal alcohol syndrome. Some of the ocular manifestations of this syndrome are blepharophimosis, telecanthus, ptosis, optic nerve hypoplasia or atrophy, and tortuosity of the retinal arteries and veins. (See also BCSC Section 6, *Pediatric Ophthalmology and Strabismus.*)

Amphetamines

Amphetamine-type drugs are sympathomimetic amines that are widely abused. Diagnosis of drug abuse should be suspected in a person who shows paranoid behavior that clears in a few days. Acute use produces euphoria, a heightened sense of effectiveness, tachycardia, and paranoia. Treatment consists of hospital observation until the abstinence syndrome, especially depression, passes.

Cocaine

Cocaine has become an increasingly abused drug in the United States since the mid-1970s. At one time thought not to be addictive, cocaine is now known to cause both psychological and physical dependence.

Cocaine hydrochloride is a white crystal powder derived from coca leaves, which can be taken intranasally or intravenously. Intranasal cocaine has a half-life of less than 90 minutes, its euphoric effects lasting 15–30 minutes. Removal of the hydrochloride salt produces freebase cocaine, an 80% pure alkaloid form of cocaine. "Crack," or "rock," cocaine is a freebase derivative that is smoked, producing intense euphoria within seconds. The widespread availability of inexpensive crack has dramatically increased the scope of the cocaine abuse problem.

The symptoms of cocaine abstinence are not as stereotypical as those of opiate withdrawal. In general, there is a dysphoric state consisting of depression, anhedonia, insomnia, and anxiety lasting about 3 days. As these symptoms wane, cocaine craving persists, often leading to binge cycles at intervals of 3–10 days. If the cycle of abuse can be broken, craving tends to wane over a 3-week period. Symptoms of major depression are common during this period but eventually clear.

Cocaine addiction among pregnant women is a growing problem. Premature labor, abruptio placentae, and fetal asphyxia may occur. "Crack babies" may show intrauterine growth retardation, microcephaly, seizures, sudden infant death syndrome (SIDS), rigidity, developmental delay, and learning disabilities.

Compliance

The term *compliance* refers to a person's behavior as it relates to medical or health advice. Noncompliance is a major problem for both patients and health care professionals. Studies have shown that compliance rates are fairly constant, at about 50%, across all demographic categories (age, gender, socioeconomic class, level of education) and that physicians are unable to accurately estimate patient compliance. In chronic disease states, compliance with treatment regimens also averages about 50%, regardless of the illness or setting. Noncompliance has been linked to an increased number of clinic visits, hospital admissions, emergency room visits, and nursing home admissions. An estimated 125,000 deaths and several hundred thousand hospitalizations are caused annually by noncompliance problems among patients with cardiovascular disease.

Pharmacologic Treatment of Psychiatric Disorders

Antipsychotic Drugs (Major Tranquilizers)

Antipsychotic drugs, or major tranquilizers, are also called *neuroleptics* because of their potential to induce neurologic side effects. The classes of drugs having antipsychotic activity include the phenothiazines, thioxanthenes, butyrophenones, dihydroindolones, dibenzoxazepines, and dibenzodiazepines (Table 12-2).

The major tranquilizers effectively reduce many of the symptoms of acute and chronic psychoses. Their value has been established in reducing fear, panic, hostility, and destructive, antisocial, or withdrawn behavior in patients with schizophrenia, manic reactions, and involutional, senile, organic, and toxic psychoses. Major tranquilizers have allowed many more patients to function outside the walls of psychiatric institutions.

The major tranquilizers are not antianxiety agents and are not used to treat neurotic or existential anxiety. In the management of organic and toxic psychoses, these drugs should be used in small doses and only as an adjunct to treatment of the underlying disorder. These drugs have also found wide use as preoperative and postoperative med-

Table 12-2 Antipsychotic Drugs

Chemical Classification	Drugs
Phenothiazine	
Aliphatic compound	Triflupromazine (Vesprin)
	Chlorpromazine (Thorazine)
Piperidine compound	Mesoridazine (Serentil)
	Thioridazine (Mellaril)
Piperazine compound	Fluphenazine (Permitil, Prolixin)
	Trifluoperazine (Stelazine)
	Perphenazine (Trilafon)
	Prochlorperazine (Compazine)
	Acetophenazine (Tindal)
Thioxanthene	Thiothixene (Navane)
Butyrophenone	Haloperidol (Haldol)
Dihydroindolone	Molindone (Moban)
Dibenzoxazepine	Loxapine (Loxitane)
Dibenzodiazepine	Clozapine (Clozaril)

ications because of their antiemetic effects and potentiation of hypnotics and anesthetic agents.

Although their mechanism of action has not been demonstrated clearly, antipsychotic drugs block the uptake of dopamine by the postsynaptic membranes in the CNS. A wide range of side effects is associated with these agents, including extrapyramidal reactions, drowsiness, orthostatic hypotension, and anticholinergic effects. Less commonly, cholestatic jaundice, blood dyscrasia, photosensitive dermatoses, and sudden death may occur. In addition, ocular side effects include anticholinergic problems, keratopathy, lens pigmentation, and retinal pigmentary degeneration.

Each of the phenothiazines varies from its congeners in the incidence of the different side effects. A particular agent may be selected because of a high or low incidence of a specific side effect. Withdrawal symptoms may occur but usually involve only mild gastrointestinal disturbances. Tardive dyskinesias occur at a rate of 2%–4% per year over the first 7 years of exposure and can worsen on withdrawal after long-term therapy; elderly women constitute the highest risk group.

Antianxiety and Hypnotic Drugs

Benzodiazepines

The benzodiazepines are usually the drugs of choice when an antianxiety, sedative, or hypnotic action is needed. Other indications for selected benzodiazepines include preanesthetic medication, alcohol withdrawal, seizure disorders, spasticity, localized skeletal muscle spasm, and nocturnal myoclonus. The benzodiazepines have distinct advantages over other agents with respect to adverse reactions, abuse or dependence liability, drug interactions, and lethality. The pharmacokinetics of these medications greatly affect their efficacy and adverse reactions and thus influence drug selection (Table 12-3).

Table 12-3 Antianxiety and Hypnotic Drugs

Benzodiazepines
   Compounds with active metabolites
      Chlordiazepoxide (Librium)
      Clorazepate (Tranxene)
      Diazepam (Valium, Valrelease)
      Flurazepam (Dalmane)
      Halazepam (Paxipam)
   Compounds with weakly active, short-lived, or inactive metabolites
      Alprazolam (Xanax)
      Clonazepam (Klonopin)
      Lorazepam (Ativan)
      Midazolam (Versed)
      Oxazepam (Serax)
      Quazepam (Doral)
      Temazepam (Restoril)
      Triazolam (Halcion)
Barbiturates
   Phenobarbital
   Mephobarbital (Mebaral)
   Amobarbital (Amytal)
   Pentobarbital (Nembutal)
   Secobarbital (Seconal)
Nonbenzodiazepine-nonbarbiturates
   Antianxiety agents
      Buspirone (BuSpar)
      Hydroxyzine (Atarax, Vistaril)
      Meprobamate (Equanil, Miltown)
   Hypnotic agents
      Chloral hydrate
      Ethchlorvynol (Placidyl)
      Paraldehyde

All benzodiazepines alleviate the uncomplicated anxiety of generalized anxiety disorder and improve situational anxiety. Some patients with chronic anxiety benefit from long-term administration of these drugs. Such patients must be monitored carefully, however, to ensure the need for continuing medication as well as the continuing efficacy and safety of the drug. Flurazepam, triazolam, and temazepam are used most commonly to treat insomnia, although diazepam, oxazepam, and lorazepam are also effective hypnotic agents.

Daytime or residual sedation (hangover) is the most common initial untoward effect of the benzodiazepines, but it appears to occur less frequently than with the barbiturates. Common dose-related side effects with oral use—dizziness and ataxia, respiratory depression, apnea, and cardiac arrest—have occurred, usually following intravenous administration. Products available in parenteral form, such as diazepam and midazolam, must be administered with careful monitoring and only by personnel trained and equipped to handle cardiorespiratory emergencies.

The abuse potential of benzodiazepines is mild compared with drugs such as pentobarbital, hydromorphone, and cocaine. Nevertheless, long-term administration of these agents can cause physical dependence. Once physical dependence is established, withdrawal reactions may occur if the drugs are discontinued abruptly. Psychological dependence is more common than physical dependence and can occur with any dose. This type of drug reliance is difficult to distinguish from a recurrence of the original anxiety disorder. Consequently, good medical practice demands that these agents be prescribed initially only when a disorder known to respond to such therapy can be diagnosed with reasonable assurance, and their use should be continued only for the shortest time required.

Barbiturates

Derivatives of barbituric acid possess sedative, hypnotic, and anticonvulsant activity. Of the longer-acting barbiturates, phenobarbital and mephobarbital are administered principally for seizure disorders; phenobarbital and butabarbital are also labeled for use as sedatives. The use of barbiturates and these latter compounds as antianxiety agents and sedative-hypnotics has been largely superseded by the benzodiazepines. The benzodiazepines have lower potential for abuse and dependence and a greater therapeutic index.

Side effects with the barbiturate sedative-hypnotics are common and include drowsiness and lethargy, particularly in the elderly or in patients taking large doses; residual sedation is common after hypnotic doses. For these reasons, ambulatory patients should be specifically warned to avoid or be cautious of activities that require mental alertness, judgment, and physical coordination. Allergic reactions, Stevens-Johnson syndrome, and gastrointestinal symptoms are also seen. Paradoxic effects such as restlessness and excitement may occur in some patients, particularly in the elderly and those patients with mental disorder due to a general medical condition. Because barbiturates may aggravate acute intermittent porphyria by inducing the enzymes responsible for porphyrin synthesis, their use is contraindicated in patients with this disease.

Chronic intoxication occurs most commonly with use of the short-acting barbiturates; symptoms are similar to those of alcohol intoxication. Prolonged, uninterrupted use of escalating doses of barbiturates, particularly the short-acting drugs, may result in physical and psychological dependence. Barbiturates also remain one of the leading causes of fatal drug poisoning.

The barbiturates frequently interact with other agents. The dosage of barbiturates must be reduced when they are given with other CNS depressants, such as alcohol, other hypnotic and antianxiety agents, opiate analgesics, antipsychotics, and antihistamines. Barbiturates must be used with caution in patients receiving monoamine oxidase inhibitors because these drugs may potentiate the depressant effects of the barbiturates.

Antidepressants

In patients with major depression, antidepressants usually improve symptoms, increase the chances and rate of recovery, reduce the likelihood of suicide, and help social and occupational rehabilitation. Psychotherapy is the first line of intervention in patients whose depression is based on external or environmental situations such as the loss of a job or family problems.

In general, antidepressants take 3–6 weeks to show significant effect. Most studies find that these drugs can result in mood elevation, improved appetite, better sleep, and increased mental and physical activity. Treatment is usually necessary for 3–6 months after recovery is apparent.

There are two groups of antidepressants: the *heterocyclic antidepressants* and the *monoamine oxidase (MAO) inhibitors* (Table 12-4). In addition to their utility in treating acute depressive episodes, the heterocyclic antidepressants are effective as maintenance therapy in preventing relapses and recurrences of major depressive episodes. Moreover, some heterocyclic compounds are effective in the treatment of panic or phobic disorders.

All heterocyclic compounds are well absorbed orally, extensively metabolized, and slowly eliminated. Because half-lives are prolonged in patients over age 55, the initial dose for older patients may require modification. The initial treatment period is considered to be the 4–8 weeks needed for the patient to become nearly symptom free. Outpatient treatment is usually instituted at the lower dose range and increased gradually if required. An excessive initial dosage regimen can cause a combination of oversedation, orthostatic hypotension, and anticholinergic effects during the first few days; such unpleasant effects can lead to patient noncompliance and, thus, inadequate treatment. Following initial therapy, the treatment is continued approximately 6 months.

A subclass of the heterocyclic antidepressants is the *selective serotonin reuptake inhibitors*, including fluoxetine (Prozac), sertraline (Zoloft), and paroxetine (Paxil). These drugs, which affect levels of serotonin, have fewer side effects than the tricyclic compounds and are therefore better tolerated.

The MAO inhibitors have long been considered second-line drugs in the treatment of mood disorders; however, recognition of their usefulness has increased with refinement of the classification of these disorders and with greater understanding of the need to titrate doses carefully. Nevertheless, the significant risk of hypertensive crisis caused by

---

Table 12-4 Antidepressant Drugs

Heterocyclic antidepressants
Amitriptyline (Elavil)
Bupropion (Wellbutrin)
Desipramine (Norpramin)
Doxepin (Adapin, Sinequan)
Fluoxetine (Prozac)
Imipramine (Tofranil)
Maprotiline (Ludiomil)
Mirtazapine (Remeron)
Nefazodone (Serzone)
Nortriptyline (Aventyl, Pamelor)
Paroxetine (Paxil)
Protriptyline (Vivactil)
Sertraline (Zoloft)
Trazodone (Desyrel)
Trimipramine (Surmontil)
Venlafaxine (Effexor)

Monoamine oxidase (MAO) inhibitors
Isocarboxazid (Marplan)
Phenelzine (Nardil)
Tranylcypromine (Parnate)

interactions between MAO inhibitors and various foods and drugs must be accounted for when they are prescribed.

A common side effect of both groups of drugs is a general anticholinergic action. Cholestatic jaundice, hepatitis, agranulocytosis, and cardiac arrhythmias are uncommon side effects. The MAO inhibitors, when combined with food and beverages of high tyramine content, may produce severe hypertension that can lead to subarachnoid or cerebral hemorrhage. Foods to be avoided include cheese, herring, chicken liver, yeast, and yogurt. Red wine and beer also have high tyramine content.

Because MAO inhibitors prevent catabolism of catecholamines, patients taking these substances have exaggerated responses to drugs containing vasopressors, such as cold remedies, nasal decongestants, and even topical or retrobulbar epinephrine. These drugs may produce seizures, particularly in patients prone to such disorders, including those with a history of severe alcoholism. The MAO inhibitors prolong and intensify the actions of CNS depressants, narcotics, and anticholinergics. Tricyclic antidepressants may also potentiate narcotics.

Lithium carbonate

Lithium carbonate is effective in the treatment of bipolar disorder and in some patients with recurrent unipolar depression. It has a very narrow therapeutic ratio, making close monitoring of plasma levels mandatory. Side effects include renal, thyroid, parathyroid, cardiac, and neurologic toxicity. Weight gain and gastrointestinal upset are common. Toxic plasma levels due to renal dysfunction, concurrent use of diuretics, or overdose can lead to persistent nausea and vomiting, coma, circulatory failure, and death.

Ophthalmologic Considerations

Although behavioral disorders do not directly affect the eye, a number of related issues are important to the ophthalmologist. Noncompliance is a common problem among patients with psychiatric illness, dementia, and depression. Malingering and functional visual loss require a high index of suspicion and special diagnostic skills on the part of the clinician. A number of medications used to treat eye disease, including beta blockers, carbonic anhydrase inhibitors, and oral corticosteroids, may induce or exacerbate depression.

Antipsychotic drugs have several ocular side effects. Corneal and lenticular pigmentations, although not visually significant, are common. Pigmentary retinopathy, which can lead to irreversible blindness, has been reported with prolonged use of several different neuroleptics but is most closely associated with thioridazine (Mellaril). The anticholinergic effects of these drugs can produce pupillary dilation and angle-closure glaucoma in susceptible individuals. Blepharospasm can occur as an extrapyramidal side effect associated with phenothiazine use.

Substance abuse is associated with an increased incidence of ocular trauma. Toxic optic neuropathy is seen in alcoholics, either as a direct effect or related to accompanying malnutrition. Corneal epithelial defects and infectious keratitis have been reported with increasing frequency in otherwise healthy cocaine and crack abusers.

Neurologic Disorders

Parkinson Disease

Parkinson disease, first described by James Parkinson in 1817, belongs to a group of conditions called *motor system disorders*. Parkinson disease is diagnosed in approximately 50,000 Americans each year, with more than half a million Americans affected at any one time. Parkinson disease strikes men and women in almost equal numbers, usually affecting people over the age of 50. The average age of onset is 60 years. In recent years, however, reported cases of "early-onset" Parkinson disease have increased: it is estimated that 5%–10% of patients are now under age 40.

The financial impact on our society caused by this disease is enormous. According to the National Parkinson Foundation, each patient spends an average of $2500 a year for medications. After factoring in office visits, social security payments, nursing home expenditures, and lost income, the total cost to the nation is estimated to exceed $5.6 billion annually.

Etiology

Parkinson disease occurs when neurons in the substantia nigra die or become impaired. Normally, these neurons produce dopamine. Dopamine is a neurotransmitter responsible for transmitting signals between the substantia nigra and the corpus striatum to produce smooth, purposeful muscle activity. Loss of dopamine causes the nerve cells of the striatum to fire out of control, leaving patients unable to direct or control their movements normally. Patients with Parkinson disease have lost 80% or more of dopamine-producing cells in the substantia nigra. The cause of this cell death or impairment is not known, but significant findings raise many possibilities as causes of this disease.

One theory suggests that free radicals may contribute to nerve cell death, thereby leading to Parkinson disease. Another theory suggests that Parkinson disease may occur when either an external or an internal toxin selectively destroys dopaminergic neurons. The theory is based on the fact that there are a number of toxins, such as 1-methyl-4-phenyl-1,2,3,6,-tetrahydropyridine (MPTP) and neuroleptic drugs, known to induce parkinsonian symptoms in humans.

A newer theory explores the role of genetic factors. In 15%–20% of patients, a close relative has experienced parkinsonian symptoms. Several causative genes have been identified. Mutations in the gene for the protein α-synuclein, located on chromosome 4, results in autosomal dominant parkinsonism. A fragment of this protein is also a known constituent of Alzheimer disease plaques, suggesting a shared pathogenic mechanism between Parkinson and Alzheimer diseases.

Yet another theory proposes that Parkinson disease occurs when, for unknown reasons, the normal age-related wearing away of dopamine-producing neurons accelerates in certain individuals. This theory is supported by the knowledge that loss of antioxidative protective mechanisms is associated with both Parkinson disease and increasing age.

Symptoms

Usually, the first symptom of Parkinson disease is tremor of a limb, especially at rest. The tremor often begins on one side of the body, frequently in the hand. Other common symptoms include bradykinesia, akinesia, rigidity, a shuffling gait, and stooped posture. People with Parkinson disease often show reduced facial expression and speak in a soft voice. The disease occasionally causes depression, personality changes, dementia, sleep disturbances, speech impairments, or sexual difficulties.

Treatment

There is currently no cure for Parkinson disease. The main treatment is levodopa (L-dopa). Neurons use L-dopa to make dopamine and replace the brain's diminishing supply.

Dopamine itself cannot be given because it doesn't cross the blood–brain barrier. Although levodopa helps at least three quarters of Parkinson cases, not all symptoms respond equally to the drug. Bradykinesia and rigidity respond best; tremor may be only marginally reduced. Problems with balance and other symptoms may not be alleviated at all. Usually, patients arc given levodopa combined with carbidopa. When added to levodopa, carbidopa delays the conversion of levodopa into dopamine until it reaches the brain, diminishing some of the side effects that often accompany levodopa therapy.

Bromocriptine, pergolide, pramipexole, and ropinirole are four drugs that mimic the role of dopamine in the brain. These drugs can be given alone or in combination with levodopa. They are generally less effective than levodopa in controlling rigidity and bradykinesia. Selegiline (deprenyl) inhibits the activity of the enzyme monoamine oxidase B, which metabolizes dopamine in the brain. Selegiline may delay the need for levodopa or, when given in combination with levodopa, may enhance and prolong the response of levodopa.

Anticholinergics were the main treatment for Parkinson disease before the introduction of levodopa. Their benefit is limited, but anticholinergics may help control tremor and rigidity. Only about half of patients respond to anticholinergics, and their effect is usually short-lived.

Amantidine, an antiviral drug, is often used in the early stages of the disease either alone or in combination with anticholinergics or levodopa. After several months, the effectiveness of amantidine wears off in a third to a half of patients taking it.

Surgical treatment for patients with Parkinson disease used to be common practice. Currently, surgery is reserved for patients in whom medical management has failed. Cryodestruction of the thalamus (cryothalamectomy) and related procedures such as thalamic stimulation are being performed to control severe tremor. Pallidotomy may improve symptoms, possibly by interrupting the neural pathway between the globus pallidus and the striatum of thalamus.

Other new surgical treatments include the implantation of dopamine-producing tissue into the brain as well as stem cell implantation to attempt to replenish the dopamine-producing centers that have been destroyed. These latter two approaches are investigational.

Ophthalmologic considerations

There are numerous ophthalmologic findings in patients with Parkinson disease. These findings can be divided into eyelid disorders and ocular motor abnormalities.

Eyelid disorders include seborrheic dermatitis and blepharitis, apraxia of eyelid opening, lid retraction, decreased blinking, and blepharospasm. Ocular motor abnormalities include convergence insufficiency, limitation of upgaze, hypometric saccades, saccadic ("cogwheel") pursuit, square wave jerks, and oculogyric crisis.

Multiple Sclerosis

See BCSC Section 5, *Neuro-Ophthalmology.*

Epilepsy

Epilepsy is a disorder wherein clusters of neurons in the brain sometimes signal abnormally. The normal pattern of neuronal activity becomes disturbed, causing strange sensations, emotions, and behavior, or sometimes convulsions, muscle spasms, and loss of consciousness. More that 2 million people in the United States—about 1 in 10—have experienced an unprovoked seizure or been diagnosed with epilepsy. In some people, seizures occur only occasionally; in others, hundreds of seizures may occur each day. Epilepsy is a disorder with many possible causes. Any disturbance of normal neuronal activity, including injury, infection, and abnormal brain development, can lead to seizures. Approximately half of all seizures have no known cause. Seizures may develop because of an abnormality in brain wiring, an imbalance of neurotransmitters, or some combination of these factors.

Gamma-aminobutyric acid, an inhibitory neurotransmitter, has been actively investigated and has led to the development of drugs that alter its concentration in the brain. Glutamate, an excitatory neurotransmitter, is also currently being studied for the development of drugs that will affect its level in the brain. Other researchers are studying neuronal cell membranes and neuronal signaling mechanisms, including the study of glial tissue (which affects concentrations of chemicals that bathe neurons). Genetic abnormalities may be important factors contributing to epilepsy. As many as 500 genes could play a role in this disorder.

Several forms of epilepsy have been linked to a defective gene for ion channels, which regulate neuronal signaling. Other abnormal or missing genes that code for specific proteins (cystatin B) or that aid in the degradation of carbohydrates have also been associated with seizure disorders. Genes may affect or increase drug resistance, therefore changing seizure thresholds. Abnormalities in genes that control neuronal development can lead to neuronal dysplasia, which can cause seizures. It is becoming more clear that genetic abnormalities play a role in epilepsy, perhaps increasing a person's susceptibility to seizures that are triggered by an environmental factor.

Epilepsy can result from brain damage caused by numerous disorders. Head injury, prenatal injury, developmental problems, and exposure to lead, carbon monoxide, and other poisons have all been associated with seizures. Brain tumors, alcoholism, and Alzheimer disease frequently lead to epilepsy. Strokes and myocardial infarctions that produce cerebral ischemia may account for as much as 32% of all newly developed epilepsy in the elderly. Meningitis, AIDS, viral encephalitis, and other infectious diseases can lead to epilepsy. Epilepsy can also be part of a set of symptoms in a variety of developmental and metabolic disorders, including cerebral palsy, neurofibromatosis, pyruvate deficiency, tuberous sclerosis, Landau-Kleffner syndrome, and autism.

More than 30 types of seizures have been described. Typically, seizures are divided into two major categories: *partial seizures* and *generalized seizures.* Partial seizures occur in just one part of the brain. About 60% of persons with epilepsy have partial seizures. These seizures are frequently described by the area of the brain in which they originate. Generalized seizures result from abnormal neuronal activity in many parts of the brain. These seizures may cause loss of consciousness, falls, or massive muscle spasms. Not all seizures can be easily defined as either partial or generalized.

Some patients have seizures that begin as partial seizures but then spread to the entire brain. Others may have both types of seizures but with no clear pattern. Just as there are different kinds of seizures, there are many different kinds of epilepsy. Hundreds of disorders have been characterized by a set of symptoms that include epilepsy. Some of the more common forms of epilepsy are:

- *Absence epilepsy,* a condition in which repeated absence seizures cause momentary lapses of consciousness. These seizures almost always begin in childhood or adolescence and are frequently familial, suggesting a genetic cause. Some patients may make purposeless movements during their seizures, such as a jerking arm or rapidly blinking eyes. Others have no noticeable symptoms except for brief periods when they are "out of it." Childhood absence epilepsy usually stops when the child reaches puberty.
- *Psychomotor epilepsy* is another term for recurrent partial seizures, especially seizures of the temporal lobe. The term *psychomotor* refers to the strange sensations, emotions, and behavior seen with these seizures.
- *Temporal lobe epilepsy* is the most common epilepsy syndrome with partial seizures. These seizures are often associated with auras.
- *Frontal lobe epilepsy* usually involves a cluster of short seizures with a sudden onset and termination. There are many subtypes, depending on where in the frontal lobe the seizures originate.
- *Occipital lobe epilepsy* usually begins with visual hallucinations, rapid eye blinking, or other eye-related symptoms. This type of epilepsy otherwise resembles temporal or frontal lobe epilepsy.

Diagnosis

The EEG is the most common diagnostic test for epilepsy. In most patients with epilepsy, the EEG appears abnormal. Magnetoencephalography is an experimental diagnostic technique that detects magnetic signals generated by neurons and allows monitoring of brain activity at different points over time. Although magnetoencephalography is similar in concept to electroencephalography, the former can detect signals from deeper in the brain than an EEG.

Imaging studies including computed tomography, positron emission tomography, and magnetic resonance imaging are useful tools to determine structural abnormalities in the brain that cause epilepsy. Single photon emission computed tomography (SPECT) is a new imaging technique that is sometimes used to locate seizure foci. Magnetic resonance spectroscopy is also a new scan that can detect abnormalities in the brain's biochemical processes.

Treatment

Currently available treatments control seizure activity at least some of the time in 80% of patients with epilepsy. Twenty percent (about 600,000 patients in the United States) experience intractable seizures, and another 400,000 obtain inadequate relief from available treatment. The primary form of treatment for epilepsy is the use of antiepileptic drugs. Patients with newly diagnosed epilepsy are often given carbamazepine, valproate, or phenytoin.

For absence seizures, ethosuximide is often the primary treatment. Other commonly prescribed antiepileptic drugs include clonazepam, phenobarbital, and primidone. In recent years, a number of new drugs have become available. These include tiagabine, lamotrigine, gabapentin, topiramate, levetiracetam, and felbamate, as well as oxcarbazepine, a drug that is similar to carbamazepine but has fewer side effects.

For most patients with epilepsy, seizures can be controlled with one drug at optimal dosage. Combining medications usually amplifies side effects such as fatigue and anorexia; thus, monotherapy is prescribed whenever possible. When medications inadequately control seizures, surgery is a potential option. The most commonly performed surgery for epilepsy is the removal of a seizure focus. This procedure, called *lobectomy* or *lesionectomy*, is appropriate for partial seizures that originate in one area of the brain.

Temporal lobe resection is the most commonly performed type of lobectomy and is successful in 70%–90% of patients. Other surgical procedures for epilepsy include multiple subpial transection, corpus callosotomy, and hemispherectomy.

In 1997, the FDA approved the vagus nerve stimulator for use in patients with seizures poorly controlled by medications. The vagus nerve stimulator is a battery-powered device that is surgically implanted under the skin of the chest and is attached to the vagus nerve in the lower neck. The device delivers short bursts of electrical energy to the brain via the vagus nerve. On average, the device reduces seizures by 20%–40%.

Ophthalmologic considerations

Transient unilateral mydriasis can occur as an expression of minor or major seizure activity, during or after the event. This phenomenon is most common in children. In some patients, the dilated pupil reacts poorly to light.

In children, the eyes may deviate to the side of the dilated pupil. Horizontal or vertical gaze deviations are commonly associated with seizure activity. During the clonic stage of a seizure, some patients experience conjugate, convergence, or monocular nystagmus. Clonic lid retraction has also been described in patients with petit mal or myoclonic seizures.

Stroke

See Chapter 3, Cerebrovascular Disease.

Pain Syndromes

See BCSC Section 5, *Neuro-Ophthalmology.*

Alzheimer Disease

Alzheimer disease (AD) is the most common cause of dementia in people over age 65. AD is an irreversible, progressive disorder that proceeds in stages, gradually destroying memory, reason, judgment, language, and eventually the ability to carry out even the simplest of tasks. AD, the most common neurodegenerative disorder, affects an estimated 4 million people in the United States. After age 65, the percentage of affected people approximately doubles with every decade of life. One recent study found that AD was present in 47.2% of people age 85 and over.

The emotional and financial impact of this disease on individuals, their families, and society is difficult to measure. It is clear, however, that with increasing life expectancy and the demographic impact of the baby boom generation, AD will have an even greater impact in coming years. Currently, 13% of the U.S. population is over the age of 65; by the year 2025, this figure will reach 18%.

AD is estimated to now cost the nation $80–$90 billion a year. Caring for a person with AD is estimated to cost approximately $47,000 per year whether the person lives at home or is in a nursing home. AD is the fourth leading cause of death in adults and is twice as common in women as in men. The pathological hallmarks of the disease are extraneuronal amyloid plaques (fragmented brain cells surrounded by amyloid-family proteins) and intraneuronal neurofibrillary tangles (tangles of filaments largely composed of protein associated with the cytoskeleton). These two findings are associated with neuronal death and decreased levels of the neurotransmitter acetylcholine. Signs of neuronal death first occur in the entorhinal cortex, with eventual extension into the hippocampus (an area essential for memory storage). As the disease progresses, the basal forebrain and eventually the cerebral cortex become involved.

Amyloid plaques

Amyloid plaques are made of protein fragments called *β-amyloid* that are mixed with other proteins. β-amyloid is a chain of 40 or 50 amino acids cleaved from a larger protein called *amyloid precursor protein (APP).*

APP protrudes through the neuronal membrane, partly inside and partly outside the cell, and appears to play a role in membrane growth and survival. This protein is continually replaced by new APP molecules manufactured in the cell. While APP is embedded in the membrane, proteases cleave APP into protein fragments. One protease cleaves APP to form β-amyloid, and another protease cleaves APP in the middle of the amyloid fragment so that β-amyloid cannot be formed.

The β-amyloid formed is of two different lengths, a shorter β-amyloid that is more soluble and aggregates slowly and a longer one that rapidly forms insoluble clumps. β-amyloid aggregates into long filaments outside the cell and, along with fragments of dead and dying neurons and microglia and astrocytes, forms the plaques that are characteristic in AD. The exact mechanism associated with amyloid plaques and neuronal cell death is unclear.

Some think that β-amyloid is toxic to neurons, perhaps by causing inflammation in the brain and/or by generating free radicals. Others have suggested that β-amyloid forms tiny channels in neuronal membranes affecting transport of calcium or potassium, which may cause cell death. Still another study links β-amyloid to reduced choline concentrations in neurons. Because neurons need choline to synthesize acetylcholine, this finding suggests a link between β-amyloid and the death of cholinergic neurons.

Neurofibrillary tangles

Neurofibrillary tangles consist of abnormal collections of twisted fibers found inside nerve cells. The chief component of tangles is one form of a protein called *tau*. Tau proteins are best known for their ability to bind and help stabilize microtubules. In healthy neurons, microtubules are formed like long, parallel railroad tracks with cross-pieces that carry nutrients from the body of the cells down to the ends of the axons.

In cells affected by AD, the healthy structure collapses. In AD, tau is changed chemically, altering its ability to hold microtubules together and causing them to twist into paired helical filaments, like two threads wound around each other. This collapse of the transport system may first result in malfunction in communication between nerve cells and later may lead to neuronal death.

Etiology

The etiology of AD is unknown. It is becoming clear, however, that AD may result from several factors, both genetic and environmental, that may precipitate the cascade of changes causing the disease.

Genetic factors

Two types of AD exist: *familial AD*, which follows a certain inheritance pattern, and *sporadic AD*, in which no inheritance pattern is obvious. AD is further described as *early onset* (occurring in people under age 65) and *late onset* (occurring in over age 65). Early-onset AD is rare (~10%) and generally affects persons 30–60 years of age. Some forms of early-onset AD are inherited and typically progress faster than the more common late-onset forms.

All known familial AD cases have been of early onset, and as many as 50% of familial AD cases are now known to be caused by defects in three genes located on three different chromosomes. These are mutations in the APP gene on chromosome 21; mutations in a gene on chromosome 14 called *presenilin 1;* and mutations in a gene on chromosome 1 called *presenilin 2.* If even one of these three mutations is present in only one of the two genes inherited from the parents, the person inevitably develops that form of early-onset AD. There is no evidence that any of these mutations plays a role in the most common sporadic or nonfamilial form of late-onset AD.

The abnormal APP gene on chromosome 21 leads to increased production of β-amyloid and occurs in about 5% of families affected by early-onset AD. Patients with Down syndrome have trisomy of chromosome 21 and, as they grow older, usually develop plaques and tangles like those found in AD. Mutations in the presenilin genes may lead to the formation of the less soluble long version of β-amyloid and possibly may trigger cellular apoptosis by another unknown mechanism.

Genetics may also play a role in the more common form of late-onset AD. Patients with inheritance of one or two copies of the apolipoprotein E ε4 allele on chromosome 19 have an increased risk of late-onset AD. The APOE protein has many functions, including participation in the transport of cholesterol throughout the body. The APOE gene has three different alleles: APOE ε2, APOE ε3, and APOE ε4. APOE ε3 is the most common in the general population. APOE ε4 occurs in approximately 40% of cases of late-onset AD and is seen in both familial and sporadic forms of the disease.

People who inherit two APOE ε4 genes are eight times more likely to develop AD than those who inherit two of the most common ε3 version. The least common allele, ε2, seems to lower the risk even more. APOE ε4 protein binds rapidly and tightly to β-amyloid; the APOE ε3 protein does not. Normally, β-amyloid is soluble, but when the APOE ε4 protein attaches to it, the amyloid becomes insoluble. APOE ε4 increases deposits of β-amyloid and directly regulates the APP protein from which β-amyloid is formed. Patients with AD and the APOE ε4 gene also have shorter dendrites, limiting the ability of neurons to communicate with other neurons.

Nongenetic factors

Numerous factors have been implicated as playing a role in contributing to the cascade of events that produce AD. Oxidative stress from free radicals may damage cells. Unique characteristics of the brain, including its high rate of metabolism and the long lifespan of its nondividing cells, may make it particularly vulnerable to oxidative stress. Inflammation is another important mechanism that is under intense investigation as a possible cause of AD. Inflammation in the brain increases with age but is more pronounced in patients with AD. Yet another area of interest involves cerebrovascular disease, including small infarcts in specific regions of the brain that accelerate the findings of AD.

Diagnosis

There is no definitive antemortem diagnostic test for AD. Physicians rely on a variety of methods including history, physical examination, laboratory tests, brain scans, and assessments of memory, language skills, and other brain functions.

Several imaging techniques are used, and all may have specific utility in aiding the diagnosis of AD. Positron emission tomography detects changes in glucose metabolism in parts of the brain most affected by AD. Single photon emission computed tomography can be combined with genetic and psychological testing to predict which patients with memory loss will eventually develop AD. Magnetic resonance imaging can be particularly useful in measuring atrophy in the hippocampus, a sign of early AD in patients who demonstrate problems with memory.

Treatment

The FDA has approved two cholinesterase inhibitors for use in AD: tacrine (Cognex), approved in 1993, and donepezil hydrochloride (Aricept), approved in 1996. These drugs do not stop or reverse the disease, but they help some patients for a period ranging from a few months to 2 years. On January 30, 2001, the Alzheimer's Disease Anti-Inflammatory Prevention Trial (ADAPT) was launched to look at the effect of COX-2 inhibitors (naproxen and celecoxib) in preventing AD. This study is scheduled to run for 7 years.

Another exciting therapeutic possibility is an AD vaccine. In mice genetically engineered to develop brain lesions similar to AD, injections of β-amyloid prevented naturally occurring amyloid from accumulating in the brains and eliminated preexisting amyloid plaques. However, at the time of this publication, phase I testing has been suspended because of brain inflammation in some of the human subjects.

Ophthalmologic considerations

AD may present with visual disturbances such as color vision abnormalities, spatial contrast sensitivity disturbance, fixation instability, saccadic latency prolongation with hypometric saccades, and saccadic intrusions during smooth-pursuit eye movements. Patients with AD can also manifest disorders of higher cortical function, such as visual agnosia and surface dyslexia. Defective motion perception (cerebral akinetopsia) has been described, as has Balint syndrome (simultanagnosia, acquired ocular apraxia, and optic ataxia).

American Psychiatric Association. *Diagnostic and Statistical Manual of Mental Disorders.* 4th ed. Washington, DC: American Psychiatric Association; 1994.

Goodwin DW, Guze SB. *Psychiatric Diagnosis.* 4th ed. New York: Oxford University Press; 1989.

Talbott JA, Hales RE, Yudofsky SC, eds. *Textbook of Psychiatry.* Washington, DC: American Psychiatric Press; 1988.

CHAPTER 13

Preventive Medicine

Recent Developments

- Over 95% of all cervical cancers are positive for human papilloma virus (HPV).
- Virtual colonoscopy with high-resolution computed tomography is currently being studied as a screening tool for colon cancer.
- Oseltamivir (Tamiflu) is effective for the treatment and prophylaxis of influenza types A and B.
- Diphtheria-pertussis-tetanus (DPT) vaccine has been replaced recently with the newer vaccine DTaP (diphtheria and tetanus toxoid with acellular pertussis vaccine).
- New childhood immunization recommendations now also include vaccines for hepatitis B, *Haemophilus influenzae* type B, *Pneumococcus,* and *Varicella.*
- New vaccines are now available for meningococcus, Lyme disease, typhoid fever, anthrax, and yellow fever. Other new vaccines are being evaluated for HIV, cholera, respiratory syncytial virus, rabies, herpes simplex type 2, *Pseudomonas,* and plague.

Screening Procedures

The goal of preventive medicine is not only the reduction of premature morbidity and mortality but also the preservation of function and quality of life.

Screening techniques can be used both for research and for practical disease prevention or treatment. Screening for nonresearch purposes is useful if the disease in question is:

- Detectable with some measurable degree of reliability
- Treatable or preventable
- Significant because of its impact (prevalence or severity)
- Progressive
- Generally asymptomatic (or has symptoms a patient might deny or might not recognize)

Screening techniques should not be applied to a certain population until the following concerns have been addressed:

- Sensitivity and specificity of the test

- Convenience and comfort of the test
- Cost of finding a problem
- Cost of not finding a problem

Cost can and should be measured in both economic and human terms, including the cost of suffering, losing function, or dying.

The term *sensitivity* describes how often a test result is positive among persons with a target disease. *Specificity* measures the test's ability to exclude truly negative results. *Relative risk* is the probability of a disease based on a specific finding divided by the probability of that disease in the absence of that specific finding.

Screening can be done as a one-time venture or by the sequential application of screening tests. Initially, a more sensitive test is administered; when appropriate, it is followed by a more specific test (which is often more costly or difficult to use). In judging the predictive value of the screens for an individual patient, the physician should account for the patient's clinical history and current medications.

Cardiovascular Diseases

Hypertension

The consequences of uncontrolled hypertension include significantly increased risk of thrombotic and hemorrhagic stroke, atherosclerotic heart disease, atrial fibrillation, congestive heart failure, left-ventricular hypertrophy, aortic aneurysm and dissection, peripheral vascular disease, and renal failure. About 30% of endstage renal disease is related to hypertension. There are more than 50 million cases of hypertension in the United States, about half of which have been diagnosed and a third of which are being treated in some way. The prevalence of hypertension in developed countries is about 20% of the adult population. Hypertension in childhood is becoming a more widely recognized problem. Hypertension meets all five of the criteria mentioned above for screening: it is detectable, treatable, highly prevalent, progressively damaging, and characteristically asymptomatic until late in its course.

Elevation in either systolic or diastolic blood pressure is associated with increased cardiovascular risk.

Hypertension is defined as systolic blood pressure over 140 mm Hg, diastolic blood pressure over 90 mm Hg, or both. The criteria for the subcategories of mild, moderate, and severe hypertension are listed in Chapter 2. The primary screening method is blood pressure measurement. Abnormal measurements, unless urgently high, should be confirmed on two more occasions. Once hypertension is detected, the cause should be sought to allow appropriate treatment. Regular exercise and dietary modifications such as weight loss, reduction of dietary salt intake, and increased dietary potassium intake may enhance blood pressure normalization. Chapter 2 discusses the pharmacologic treatment of hypertension.

Brown MJ, Haydock S. Pathoaetiology, epidemiology and diagnosis of hypertension. *Drugs.* 2000;59(Suppl 2):1–12.

Kornitzer M, Dramaix M, De Backer G. Epidemiology of risk factors for hypertension: implications for prevention and therapy. *Drugs.* 1999;57:695–712.

Port S, Demer L, Jennrich R, et al. Systolic blood pressure and mortality. *Lancet.* 2000;355:175–180.

Atherosclerotic cardiovascular disease

In the United States, atherosclerosis is responsible for about half of all deaths and for one third of deaths between ages 35 and 65. Three fourths of deaths related to atherosclerosis are from coronary artery disease. Atherosclerosis is the leading cause of permanent disability and accounts for more hospital days than any other illness.

The rationale for early screening emerged with the demonstration that reducing risk factors does reduce the incidence of coronary disease events. Epidemiologic studies demonstrate that each 1% of reduction in total cholesterol produces a 2% reduction in the risk of coronary disease events, including fatal and nonfatal myocardial infarctions. Several studies also confirm that reduction in cholesterol results in reduced cardiovascular morbidity and mortality in patients with previous coronary heart disease.

Established clinical risk factors for coronary artery disease include family history of early-onset coronary disease, increased age, male sex, hypertension, left-ventricular hypertrophy, smoking, diabetes mellitus, physical inactivity, stress, and cocaine abuse. Laboratory risk factors are elevated plasma cholesterol (also elevated LDL cholesterol and low HDL cholesterol levels), elevated plasma homocysteine, and increased C-reactive protein. Patients in the top 20th percentile for risk factors experienced about 50% of the fatal and nonfatal atherosclerotic events. Smoking cessation, lifestyle, and dietary counseling should be an important element of all primary care and preventive care encounters.

Hypertriglyceridemia alone, without elevated cholesterol level, is not associated with a significant incidence of coronary disease; however, the combination of cholesterol and triglyceride elevation confers a greater risk of coronary disease than does cholesterol elevation alone.

Dyslipoproteinemia has become an important concept. We now recognize that excesses or deficiencies of specific lipoproteins and apolipoproteins are more significantly correlated with atherosclerosis than the more general category of lipids. Indeed, screening for cholesterol and triglycerides alone will miss 50% of cases of hyperlipoproteinemia. Therefore, it is valid and important to measure the LDL and HDL cholesterol every 5 years. Total and HDL cholesterol screening is recommended for all patients over age 25. If the level is normal (<200 mg/dL), the screen should be repeated every 5 years. If the level is abnormal, the screen should be repeated with a complete cholesterol profile.

The presence of xanthelasma and corneal arcus, especially in young patients, increases the probability of concomitant dyslipoproteinemia. Although these signs are low in specificity, they are easily detected during a routine eye examination and should prompt a more specific lipid-lipoprotein screening.

Screening for significant coronary artery atherosclerosis is more expensive and time-consuming than screening for associated reversible risk factors. In general, it is reasonable to screen for a history of cardiovascular symptoms and events (chest pain, dyspnea, syncope, arrhythmias, claudication, stroke) and reserve more specific testing (eg, exercise stress testing) for those in increased risk categories. A new diagnostic procedure, electron beam computed tomography, is a rapid, noninvasive, high-resolution imaging study that detects coronary artery calcium as a means of screening asymptomatic patients for coronary atherosclerosis. This technique can detect and even quantitate the presence of coronary atherosclerosis.

Alpert MA. Homocysteine, atherosclerosis, and thrombosis. *South Med J.* 1999;92:858–865.

Caro J, Klittich W, McGuire A, et al. The West of Scotland coronary prevention study: economic benefit analysis of primary prevention with pravastatin. *BMJ.* 1997;315:1577–1582.

Menotti A. Diet, cholesterol and coronary heart disease. A perspective. *Acta Cardiol.* 1999; 54:169–172.

Cancer

In women, the most common cancers are breast, lung, and colorectal. In men, they are lung, prostate, and colorectal. The types of cancer most amenable to screening are cervical cancer, melanoma, breast cancer, urologic cancer, colorectal cancer, and lung cancer. Table 13-1 shows a set of recommendations for early cancer detection.

Cervical cancer

Cervical cancer is the most common gynecologic cancer in patients between the ages of 15 and 34. Overall, about 15,000 cases of invasive cancer of the cervix (about 5000

Table 13-1 American Cancer Society Recommendations for Early Cancer Detection in Asymptomatic Patients

Test or Procedure	Sex	Population Age (Years)	Frequency
Sigmoidoscopy	M, F	>50	After two negative exams 1 year apart, perform every 3-5 years
Stool guaiac slide test	M, F	>50	Annual
Digital rectal exam	M, F	>40	Annual
Papanicolaou test	F	20–65; <20, if sexually active	After two negative exams 1 year apart, perform at least every 3 years
Pelvic examination	F	20–40	Every 3 years
		>40	Annual
Endometrial tissue sample	F	Women at high risk* and at menopause	At menopause
Breast self-examination	F	>20	Monthly
Breast physical examination	F	20–40	Every 3 years
		>40	Annual
Mammography	F	35–40	Baseline
		40–49	Every 1–2 years
		>50	Annual
Chest x-ray			Not recommended
Sputum cytology			Not recommended
Health counseling and cancer checkup**	M, F	>20	Every 3 years
	M, F	>40	Annual

* History of infertility, obesity, failure to ovulate, abnormal uterine bleeding, or estrogen therapy.
** To include examination for cancers of the thyroid, testis, prostate, ovary, lymph nodes, oral region, and skin.

resulting in death) and 45,000 cases of carcinoma in situ occur each year in the United States. Cervical cancer is the eighth most common cause of cancer mortality in the United States. The risk factors for cervical cancer are the number of lifetime sexual partners, the presence of high-risk serotypes of HPV, low socioeconomic status, positive smoking history, and a history of other sexually transmitted diseases. Over 95% of all cervical cancers are positive for HPV. Early detection and appropriate treatment markedly reduce the morbidity and mortality from invasive cancer of the cervix. Cervical cancer is asymptomatic when it occurs in situ, and the most effective screening technique remains the Papanicolaou smear ("Pap test").

Breast cancer

Breast cancer is the most common malignancy in women and the most common cause of death in women over age 40. The overall incidence of breast cancer in the United States is 10%–12%; 50% of these patients are curable. About 180,000 new cases of breast cancer and over 44,000 related deaths are reported annually in the United States alone. Over 75% of all breast cancers are cured with current therapy.

The importance of specific screening is increased by the presence of known risk factors, all of which are identifiable by history: (1) first-degree relative with breast cancer, (2) prior breast cancer, (3) nulliparity, (4) first pregnancy after age 30, and (5) early menarche or late menopause. Additional risk factors are elevated serum estrogen levels, elevated testosterone levels, high-fat diet, obesity, and sedentary lifestyle. Fibrocystic disease is not a risk factor unless there is demonstrated hyperplasia or atypia on biopsy. Hormone replacement therapy with estrogen and progesterone was associated with an increased risk of invasive breast cancer and abnormal mammograms in the Women's Health Initiative randomized trial.

About 42% of breast cancers detectable by mammography are not detectable by physical examination alone, and one third of those found by mammographic screening are noninvasive or less than 1 cm in size if invasive. Because mammograms can yield false-negative results, the best detection strategy involves a physical examination plus mammography, with fine-needle aspiration or biopsy if either reveals an abnormality. Mammograms have been shown to be safe as well as effective, with current low-dose radiation not inducing added cancer risk. Mammographic screening should be performed yearly in women beyond age 50. Between the ages of 40 and 50, mammography should be a patient–physician decision. A woman should undergo mammographic screening until at least age 70.

Urologic cancer

The prostate, bladder, kidney, and testes yield about 16% of new cancer cases per year, with most of the common malignancies in middle-aged and older men. About 150,000 new cases of prostate cancer and 40,000 related deaths occur each year in the United States. Screening remains controversial, but preliminary estimates suggest that screening can reduce mortality. Prostate and testicular cancer can be detected early by digital examination of the prostate, serum prostate-specific antigen (PSA) measurements, and physical examination of the testes. It is now generally accepted that PSA should be measured yearly in men over age 50 with over 10 years of life expectancy. For patients with a family history of prostate cancer, screening should begin at age 40 or earlier. PSA levels over 10 ng/mL strongly suggest metastatic disease; levels under 4 ng/mL usually suggest benign hypertrophy or a normal prostate. A trend of increasing PSA levels is an even more sensitive indicator of prostate cancer than an individual elevated PSA level.

Lung cancer

Lung cancer is the leading form of cancer in adults. Among male patients with lung cancer, 93% are smokers. The number and percentage of cases in women have risen with the increased incidence of smoking in women. In one study of lung cancer, 40% of cases were detected by chest radiography and 60% were detected by symptoms. The usefulness of radiographic and sputum cytologic screening is generally considered to be low, but some studies have suggested that annual chest radiography may reduce morbidity and mortality.

Gastrointestinal cancer

(Colorectal carcinoma is discussed later.) Risk factors for esophageal cancer are excessive alcohol and cigarette use, accounting for perhaps 80%–90% of esophageal cancers. Treatment has poor results; thus, prevention or elimination of the risk factors is worthwhile.

Gastric cancer appears to be associated with certain geographic areas, high ingestion of nitrates, loss of gastric acidity, and blood type A. Pancreatic cancer is two to three times more common in heavy smokers, and hepatocellular cancer is more common in persons with preexisting liver disease, especially cirrhosis.

Colorectal cancer

Colorectal cancer is a major killer in Western society, second only to lung cancer in incidence and mortality. The cumulative lifetime probability of developing colon cancer is roughly 6%, with a 3% probability of dying from it. The chance for survival 5 years after diagnosis remains only 40%, despite the optimistic theory that early detection would lead to curative surgery. Potentially modifiable risk factors such as fiber and fat intake are important in primary prevention.

Most authorities accept the theory that colorectal cancer develops from an initially benign polyp in a mitotic process that occurs over 5–10 years. Supportive evidence shows that many operative specimens containing colon cancer have at least one adenoma and that invasive cancer frequently occurs in close proximity to adenomatous tissue. Histologic studies have shown that growth of adenomas is associated with increasing cellular atypia. This theory is supported by the malignant potential of adenomas in familial polyposis; furthermore, patients who refuse removal of polyps frequently develop cancer at the same site and at other sites in their colon.

Studies to date lack the necessary longevity to prove definitively that polyp removal prevents carcinoma. Yet colonoscopic removal or ablation of all polyps has become the standard of care where facilities and trained personnel are available.

A national polyp study is under way to define the biology of these tumors, to identify factors that seem to promote invasive carcinoma, and to clarify whether early removal prevents invasive cancer. A recent study reported characteristics associated with high-grade dysplasia in colorectal adenomas. The major independent risk factors were adenoma size and extent of the villous component in the adenoma. Increasing age was associated with increased risk for high-grade dysplasia. Gender was not an independent factor.

Increased dietary fiber and reduced dietary fat intake have been associated with reduced risk of colorectal cancer. Some studies have suggested that regular use of nonsteroidal anti-inflammatory drugs is correlated with reduced risk of colorectal cancer. Also, calcium supplementation is associated with a moderate reduction in the risk of recurrent colorectal adenomas.

Detection must be improved with more widespread use of screening studies such as Hemoccult slides, flexible sigmoidoscopy, barium enema, and colonoscopy, with aggressive follow-up of positive cases. It is estimated that widespread adoption of these recommendations could reduce the mortality rate of colorectal cancer by more than 50%.

Periodic sigmoidoscopy (every 3 years) and annual digital rectal examination with fecal occult blood testing have been recommended in asymptomatic adults older than 50 years. Recommendations remain controversial because of a lack of randomized trials. Sigmoidoscopy offers good specificity but misses proximal cancers. Nevertheless, several case-control studies have demonstrated a 50%–70% reduction in the risk of colorectal cancer in patients screened with sigmoidoscopy. Similarly, fecal occult blood testing every 2 years has been shown to decrease the mortality rate of colon cancer by up to 40%.

The sensitivity of the barium enema is the main disadvantage. Historically, this test has been ineffective in examination of the rectum. Double-contrast or air-contrast barium enema is more sensitive but is still not the standard examination in many radiology departments.

Colonoscopy as a screening test for asymptomatic patients over age 50 has been gaining popularity. When results are negative, the test is repeated every 10 years in low-risk patients. Colonoscopy is thought to be about twice as sensitive as barium enema for detection of colon cancers. Also, many of the lesions discovered with colonoscopy would not be detected with sigmoidoscopy. Yearly colonoscopy has been advocated in populations at very high risk, such as patients with familial polyposis and first-degree relatives of patients with colon cancer. The disadvantages of colonoscopy are the increased cost, the number of trained personnel required, and the risks of intravenous sedation and colonic perforation (approximately 0.2%). Virtual colonoscopy with high-resolution computed tomography is currently being evaluated as a screening tool, but this modality does not yet offer the image resolution of actual colonoscopy.

Melanoma

Melanoma is the most deadly form of skin cancer, and its incidence is increasing faster than that of all other cancers. In the United States, about 1 in 75 persons will develop melanoma during their lifetime. Over 44,000 new cases and over 7000 related deaths are reported per year in the United States. Most melanomas probably arise from dysplastic nevi. Risk factors for melanoma include history of melanoma or atypical moles, presence of over 75–100 moles, positive melanoma family history, history of previous nonmelanoma skin cancer, giant congenital nevus (over 20 cm), xeroderma pigmentosum, treatment with UVA and psoralens, frequent tanning with UVA light, and a history of three or more severe (blistering) sunburns. Other, less significant risk factors are light complexion of the hair and eyes, inability to tan, freckles, proximity to the equator, and having an indoor occupation with outdoor hobbies.

Ultraviolet damage probably causes most melanomas. Intense intermittent exposures are directly related to melanoma, whereas other skin cancers are more associated with cumulative exposure. Ultraviolet radiation causes DNA damage, which is usually corrected by DNA repair enzymes. These DNA repair processes decrease with increasing age. The features of a pigmented lesion that are suggestive of melanoma can be remembered by the *ABCDE* mnemonic: *a*symmetrical lesions, *b*order (irregular), *c*olor (variable), *d*iameter (over 6 mm), and *e*levation. A lesion with any of these characteristics is suspicious for melanoma. Other suspicious characteristics are pruritus, bleeding, changing morphology, and new lesions or scalp lesions. Everyone should perform self skin examinations every 1 or 2 months, and suspicious lesions require referral and possible biopsy. Sun avoidance and use of sun blockers can reduce the risk of melanoma and other skin cancers.

Berwick M, Halpern A. Melanoma epidemiology. *Curr Opin Oncol.* 1997;9:178–182.

Bond JH. Screening guidelines for colorectal cancer. *Am J Med.* 1999;106:7S–10S.

Chlebowski RT, Hendrix SL, Langer RD, et al. Influence of estrogen plus progestin on breast cancer and mammography in healthy postmenopausal women: the Women's Health Initiative Randomized Trial. *JAMA.* 2003;289:3243–3253.

Coley CM, Barry MJ, Fleming C, et al. Early detection of prostate cancer. Part I: Prior probability and effectiveness of tests. *Ann Intern Med.* 1997;126:394–406.

Glasziou P, Irwig L. The quality and interpretation of mammographic screening trials for women ages 40–49. *J Natl Cancer Inst Monogr.* 1997;22:73–77.

Inadomi JM, Sonnenberg A. The impact of colorectal cancer screening on life expectancy. *Gastrointest Endosc.* 2000;51:517–523.

Lieberman DA, Weiss DG, Bond JH, et al. Use of colonoscopy to screen asymptomatic adults for colorectal cancer. Veterans Affairs Cooperative Study Group 380. *N Engl J Med.* 2000; 343:162–168.

Nanda K, McCrory DC, Myers ER, et al. Accuracy of the Papanicolaou test in screening for and follow-up of cervical cytologic abnormalities: a systematic review. *Ann Intern Med.* 2000;132:810–819.

Strauss GM, Gleason RE, Sugarbaker DJ. Chest X-ray screening improves outcome in lung cancer. A reappraisal of randomized trials on lung cancer screening. *Chest.* 1995; 107(Suppl):270S–279S.

Winawer SJ, Stewart ET, Zauber AG, et al. A comparison of colonoscopy and double-contrast barium enema for surveillance after polypectomy. National Polyp Study Work Group. *N Engl J Med.* 2000;342:1766–1772.

Ylitalo N, Sorensen P, Josefsson AM, et al. Consistent high viral load of human papillomavirus 16 and risk of cervical carcinoma in situ: a nested case-control. *Lancet.* 2000;355:2194–2198.

Metabolic Diseases

Diabetes

The prevalence of diabetes mellitus (DM) is difficult to determine accurately because many cases remain undiagnosed until patients experience significant symptoms. Also, prevalence rates differ according to race, age, and sex. Prevalence in the United States is estimated to be about 1%. Insulin-dependent DM accounts for one fourth of cases. Blood glucose screening is recommended for anyone over age 45. Persons at higher risk for type 2 DM should be screened earlier, including patients with symptoms suggestive of DM, obese patients, pregnant women, those with a positive family history of DM, patients on long-term corticosteroids, blacks, and Native Americans.

A random fasting blood glucose test is very sensitive for detecting DM but not specific. A fasting glucose level of 126 mg/dL or higher on two separate occasions or a positive glucose tolerance test result is diagnostic of DM. Hemoglobin A_{1c} levels provide additional helpful screening information regarding a patient's long-term glycemic status.

Thyroid diseases

The prevalence of abnormal thyroid test results is high, particularly in older persons. Up to 15% of women over age 60 have asymptomatic elevated thyroid-stimulating hormone levels or low T_4 levels. A low percentage of such persons progress to clinical hypothyroidism. Although no clinical trials justify widespread screening, it would be reasonable to test older women. The availability of the newer ultrasensitive thyroid-stimulating hormone tests has simplified screening for thyroid disease.

Infectious Diseases

The major public health screening efforts in the United States have been for tuberculosis and sexually transmitted diseases. Hepatitis screening is used primarily for blood donation rather than for general population screening.

Tuberculosis

The prevalence of tuberculosis has recently increased in the United States, reversing decades of steady decline. High-incidence clustering occurs in certain subgroups: HIV-infected patients; inner city, economically disadvantaged males; nursing-home residents (3.5% incidence of skin test results converting to positive); health care workers, including physicians; people over age 50; recent immigrant groups; drug- and alcohol-dependent groups; and patients who have undergone gastrectomy and who have debilitating diseases. Tuberculosis skin testing should be performed in these high-risk groups. Such testing is sensitive, although interpretation of results may be complicated by coinfection with HIV. Positive results should prompt chest radiography and consideration of chemoprophylaxis. Some experts advocate routine skin testing of all people younger than 35 years at the time of routine health examination (for detection as well as for baseline data). The Occupational Safety and Health Administration requires annual tuberculosis skin testing of all health care workers. Although the BCG vaccine seems to reduce the mortality of childhood tuberculosis in developing countries, the vaccine does not significantly affect the 90% of cases that occur in adults. Several candidate vaccines for tuberculosis are currently being developed, including subunit, DNA, microbial vector, and live attenuated vaccines.

Syphilis

Syphilis is almost always transmitted sexually; congenital disease transmitted in utero is now rare. In fact, the incidence of congenital syphilis has dropped 90% since the 1940s because of required premarital screening and pregnancy screening.

Latent, untreated cases of syphilis in which the primary or secondary mucocutaneous lesion is no longer present can be detected only by screening. It is important to detect early latent disease: in about 25% of cases, infectious mucocutaneous lesions re-emerge spontaneously in the first 2 years. Late latent disease should be detected and treated because of the long-term destructive effects on the central nervous system, the aorta, and the skeletal system.

Screening is generally performed with the more sensitive, but less specific, nontreponemal antigen tests (VDRL, RPR). Positive results are then confirmed with treponemal antigen tests (FTA-ABS, MHA-TP, HATTS), which are more expensive.

Immunization

The development of immunization as a means of preventing the spread of infectious disease began in 1796, when Edward Jenner injected cowpox virus, which causes a mild disease, into a child to prevent smallpox, a severe, potentially fatal illness. Immunization today still relies on Jenner's inoculation methods in protecting against disease. There are two types: active and passive.

In *active immunization,* the recipient develops an acquired immune response to inactivated or killed viruses, viral subtractions, bacterial toxoids or antigens, or synthetic vaccines. Once the immune response to a particular pathogen has developed, it protects the host against infection. The persistence of acquired immunity depends on the perpetuation of cell strains responsive to the target antigenic stimulus, and booster inoculations may be required for certain immunogens.

In general, live inactivated vaccines produce longer-lasting immunity; however, they are contraindicated in immunocompromised persons or pregnant women because the pathogen can potentially replicate in the host. Ideally, active immunization should be completed before exposure; however, life-saving postexposure immunity can be developed through combining active and passive immunization.

The current Recommended Childhood Immunization Schedule for the year 2001, developed by the American Academy of Pediatrics Committee on Infectious Diseases, is summarized in Table 13-2.

Passive immunization depends on the transfer of immunoglobulin in serum from a host with active immunity to a susceptible host. Passive immunity does not result in active immunity and sometimes even blocks the development of active immunity. Passive immunity is short-lived and without immune memory; however, it confers immediate protection on the recipient who has been exposed to the pathogen. Pooled human globulin, antitoxins, or human globulin with high antibody titers for specific diseases are the usual products available for passive immunization.

Immunization should be avoided in persons who have allergic reactions to the vaccine or its components. Idiopathic autoantibody or cross-reacting antibody development

Table 13-2 Recommended Childhood Immunization Schedule

Age	Immunizations
Birth	HepB #1
2 mo	DTaP #1, HiB #1, IPV #1, PCV #1, HepB #2
4 mo	DTaP #2, HiB #2, IPV #2, PCV #2
6 mo	DTaP #3, HiB #3, IPV #3, PCV #3, HepB #3 (HepB #3 must be given at least 2 mo after HepB #2)
12–15 mo	HepB #3 (if not given at 6 mo) HiB #4 (booster) IPV (or OPV) #4, MMR #1, PCV #4 Varivax (if no chickenpox by 12 mo of age)
15–18 mo	DTaP #4 HepB #3 (if not previously given) IPV (or OPV) #4 (if not given at 12–15 mo) PCV (if not previously given)
4–6 yr	DTaP #5, MMR #2, IPV (or OPV) #5
11–12 yr	Td MMR #3 (booster; if not given at age 4–6 yr) Varivax (if not previously immunized, and if no reliable history of chickenpox)
14–16 yr	Td (if not given at 11–12 yr) Check anti-HBV titers: consider HepB booster

DTaP = diphtheria/tetanus/acellular pertussis vaccine; HepB = hepatitis B virus vaccine; HiB = *Haemophilus influenzae* type B conjugate vaccine; IPV = inactivated polio vaccine; MMR = measles/mumps/rubella; OPV = oral polio vaccine; PCV = pneumococcal conjugated vaccine; Td = tetanus and diphtheria toxoid vaccine; Varivax = live attenuated *Varicella* vaccine

Additional recommendations:
PCV is also recommended for children with chronic illnesses between 2 and 5 yr of age.
Hepatitis A vaccine is recommended for children over 2 yr of age and adolescents living in endemic areas or in contact with infected patients.
Give a Td booster every 10 yr, sooner if severe traumatic wound occurs.

(Adapted from Committee on infectious diseases. American Academy of Pediatrics. Recommended childhood immunization schedule-United States, January-December, 2001. *Pediatrics.* 2001;107:202–204.)

may occur after vaccination, resulting in systemic disease such as Guillain-Barré syndrome, a rare but devastating complication of vaccination. Immunization should be avoided during a febrile illness. Multidose immunization schedules that are interrupted can be resumed; however, doses given outside the schedule should not be counted toward completion of the vaccination sequence.

Hepatitis B

Approximately 100,000 symptomatic cases of hepatitis B occur annually in the United States. Between 6% and 10% of adult patients with hepatitis B become carriers. Chronic active hepatitis occurs in 25% of carriers. Of those patients with chronic active disease, 20% will die of cirrhosis and 5% will die of hepatocellular carcinoma.

The two available recombinant vaccines based on hepatitis B virus (HBV) surface antigen are Energix-B and Recombivax HB. HBV vaccine is usually administered in three sessions, with the second and third occurring 1 and 6 months after the initial injection in adults. On this regimen, 90% of recipients develop protective antibody levels for at least 3 years. The recombinant vaccine can also be given on an accelerated dosing schedule. This schedule requires vaccination at 0, 1, and 2 months followed by a booster dose at 12 months. Antibody levels greater than 10 mIU/mL are considered to be adequate protection. Booster injections are advised for persons whose antibody levels are less than 10 mIU/mL. Approximately 3%–4% of healthy persons lack the immune response gene needed to produce antibodies after receiving the vaccine. Repeat vaccination results in the development of protective antibodies in 50% of the nonresponders. Vaccines are also available for hepatitis A and are being developed for hepatitis C and E.

Vaccination before exposure is recommended and cost effective for all infants and children and in certain high-risk groups: health care workers, hemodialysis patients, residents and staff of institutions for the retarded, household and sexual contacts of chronic carriers of hepatitis B, hemophiliacs, users of illicit injectable drugs, prison inmates, sexually active homosexual men, and HIV-positive patients. Vaccination can be combined with passive immunization for postexposure prophylaxis without affecting the development of active immunity.

Postexposure prophylaxis with hepatitis B immune globulin should be considered when there is perinatal exposure of an infant born to a carrier, accidental percutaneous or permucosal exposure to blood positive for HBV surface antigen, or sexual exposure (within 14 days) to a carrier of hepatitis B. Hepatitis B immune globulin should be given as soon as possible after exposure in a single intramuscular dose of 0.06 mL/kg body weight; the recombinant HBV vaccine should be concurrently administered in an accelerated dosing schedule.

Lamivudine (Epivir) is a nucleoside analogue inhibitor of reverse transcriptase and was initially developed for the treatment of HIV infection. It has also been found to be very effective against HBV and is now considered to be the drug of choice for the treatment of patients with chronic HBV infection.

Influenza

Although influenza is usually a self-limited disease with rare sequelae, it can be associated with severe morbidity and mortality in elderly persons or those with chronic diseases. Influenza vaccines produce long-lasting immunity. However, antigenic shifts, primarily in type A rather than type B influenza virus, necessitate yearly reformulation of the vaccine to contain the antigens of strains considered most likely to cause disease. Protection is correlated with the development of antihemagglutinin and antineuraminidase antibodies, which decrease the patient's susceptibility and the severity of the disease. The influenza vaccine is as effective in HIVpositive patients as it is in HIV-negative patients, regardless of CD4 T cell counts. Annual vaccination is recommended for adults and children with chronic diseases requiring medical care, immunosuppressed patients (including HIV-infected patients), nursing home residents, children who require long-term aspirin therapy (in whom influenza could lead to Reye syndrome), persons over age 65, and medical personnel with extensive contact with high-risk patients. The vaccine is well tolerated, and there has been no increased risk of neurologic complications with the vaccines administered after 1991. Influenza vaccine should not be administered to persons with anaphylactic hypersensitivity to eggs or to pregnant women in their first trimester. A trivalent intranasal influenza vaccine (FluMist) is available and provides protection against type A and type B influenza virus. Newer antiviral agents, such as zanamivir (Relenza) and oseltamivir, are active against influenza types A and B. These drugs are effective for the treatment of influenza infection as well as the prophylactic treatment of the contacts of infected persons.

Varicella-Zoster

Varivax, the approved varicella zoster vaccine, is recommended for immunocompetent patients older than 12 months with no history of previous varicella infection. For patients older than 12 years, two doses of vaccine are given 4–8 weeks apart. Also, health care workers who have not been exposed to chickenpox should be vaccinated. Varivax is safe and provides immunity for up to 20 years.

Measles

Vaccination has dramatically reduced the incidence of measles, along with associated encephalitis, mental retardation, and mortality. Introduced in 1963, the initial vaccine was an inactivated virus that did not provide a long duration of protection; therefore, many young adults are at risk for measles, which is more severe as an adult disease. Vaccination before age 1 with any form of vaccine is ineffective because maternal antibodies block the development of immunity. In 1967, a live attenuated vaccine that causes long-lasting immunity was introduced. Vaccination with the attenuated strain should be routine not only at age 15 months but also for persons born between 1957 and 1967 who were neither vaccinated nor infected and for persons who received the inactivated viral vaccine. Individuals born before 1957 are considered immune by virtue of natural infection. For persons who cannot have the vaccine (which should be given within 72 hours of exposure), postexposure prophylaxis with immune globulin should be considered within 6 days. The vaccine is contraindicated for persons with hypersensitivity to eggs. Measles-mumps-rubella (MMR) vaccination is recommended for all children and is usually given at about age 15 months and again between ages 4 and 6 years.

Mumps

Reported cases of mumps in the United States have decreased steadily since the introduction of live mumps vaccine in 1967. Although mumps is generally self-limited, meningeal signs may appear in up to 15% of cases and orchitis in up to 20% of clinical cases in postpubertal males. Other possible complications include permanent deafness and pancreatitis. Mumps vaccination is indicated in all children and all susceptible adults, particularly postpubertal males.

Rubella

Rubella immunization is intended to prevent fetal infection and consequent congenital rubella syndrome, which can occur in up to 80% of fetuses of mothers infected during the first trimester of pregnancy. The number of reported cases of rubella in the United States has decreased steadily from more than 56,000 in 1969, the year rubella vaccine was licensed, to 954 cases in 1983. A single subcutaneously administered dose of live, attenuated rubella vaccine provides long-term (probably lifetime) immunity in approximately 95% of persons vaccinated.

Rubella vaccine is recommended for adults, particularly women, unless proof of immunity is available (documented rubella vaccination on or after the first birthday or a positive serologic test result) or the vaccine is specifically contraindicated. Rubella vaccine should be given at least 14 days before administration of immune globulin or deferred for 3 months after administration. Because of the theoretical risk to the fetus, women of childbearing age should receive the vaccine only if they are not pregnant. A new nonreplicating rubella virus DNA vaccine is being evaluated and may offer a safer alternative for pregnant patients.

Polio

Before the introduction of the first polio vaccine in 1955, polio caused thousands of cases of paralysis. Despite widespread immunization with oral vaccine in 1962, there has been a steady decline in polio immunization and a growing number of susceptible persons. Although the incidence of polio is low, the possibility of large-scale outbreaks increases as the number of susceptible persons increases. There are two forms of the vaccine: an oral form that is a live attenuated virus (OPV, Sabin vaccine) and a subcutaneous injectable form of killed virus (IPV, Salk vaccine). Vaccine-associated paralytic poliomyelitis has been associated more with the OPV than the IPV. Therefore, the American Academy of Pediatrics has recommended that the IPV be administered for all four vaccinations in the series, or for the first two of the series. Either IPV or OPV can be used for the last two vaccinations of the series. OPV is contraindicated in pregnant women, who should only receive the killed virus vaccine (IPV).

Tetanus and Diphtheria

The combined tetanus and diphtheria toxoid vaccine (Td) is highly effective. It is used for both primary and booster immunization of adults. The pediatric vaccine, diphtheria-pertussis-tetanus (DPT), has been the standard vaccine for years but has been replaced recently with the newer vaccine DTaP (diphtheria and tetanus toxoids with acellular pertussis vaccine). Now, DTaP is the preferred vaccine formulation for all doses in the immunization series. These vaccines should not be given to adults because of the risk of adverse neurologic reactions among adults to the pertussis component. All young adults should have completed a primary series of tetanus and diphtheria toxoids. Persons who have completed a primary series of tetanus and diphtheria immunization should receive a booster dose every 10 years. If serious doubt exists about the completion of a primary series of immunization, two doses of 0.5 mL of the combined toxoids should be given intramuscularly at monthly intervals, followed by a third dose 6–10 months later. Thereafter, a booster dose of 0.5 mL should be given at 10-year intervals.

In wound management for tetanus, previously immunized persons with severe wounds should receive a booster if more than 5 years have elapsed since the last injection. The management of previously unimmunized patients with severe wounds should include tetanus immune globulin as well as Td. Though tetanus is uncommon, more than

60% of cases occur in persons older than 60. Older adults should be given a single booster at age 65.

Pneumococcal Pneumonia

Pneumococcal pneumonia is the most serious and prevalent of the community-acquired respiratory infections. Although pneumococcal disease affects children and adults, the incidence of pneumococcal pneumonia increases over the age of 40. Pneumococci that are resistant to penicillin have emerged since 1974. The mortality rate from bacteremic pneumococcal infection exceeds 25% despite treatment with antibiotics.

The current unconjugated pneumococcal vaccine contains polysaccharide antigens from 23 of the types of pneumococci most commonly found in bacteremic pneumococcal disease. The 23-valent vaccine has been designed to induce a protective level of serum antibodies in immunocompetent adults. The vaccine is highly effective in healthy young adults, but its effectiveness in the elderly and the infirm has not been precisely determined. However, the vaccine is well tolerated and it is recommended for the elderly, for patients who have cardiac or respiratory disease, and for other patients who are at high risk for pneumococcal infection, including those with sickle cell disease, splenic dysfunction, renal and hepatic disease, or immunodeficiency. The pneumococcal vaccine is given subcutaneously or intramuscularly as a 0.5 mL dose. In most circumstances, persons who have previously received the 14-valent vaccine should not be revaccinated with the 23-valent vaccine because it may be associated with increased local and systemic reactions. The duration of protection afforded by primary vaccination with pneumococcal vaccine seems to be 9 years or more. Persons who received pneumococcal vaccine before age 65 should be reimmunized at 65 if more than 6 years have passed since the initial vaccination.

A new conjugated heptavalent pneumococcal vaccine (Prevnar) is now approved and recommended for all children under age 5. It is administered in four intramuscular doses at 2, 4, 6, and 12–15 months of age. The vaccine provides coverage for about 80% of the invasive pneumococcal disease in children in the United States. The conjugated pneumococcal vaccine is recommended for all infants under age 2 and for all children with chronic cardiopulmonary disorders or immune suppression between ages 2 and 5.

Haemophilus influenzae

A vaccine against *H influenzae* type B (HiB vaccine) has been endorsed by the American Academy of Pediatrics and the Immunization Practices Advisory Committee. They have recommended that the vaccine be given to all children before age 24 months. The vaccine has significantly reduced infections caused by encapsulated *H influenzae* type B, which previously affected 1 in every 200 children in the United States during the first 5 years of life. Approximately 60% of these infections were meningitis, amounting to about 10,000 cases each year. The type B capsule enhances the invasive potential of *H influenzae*. These encapsulated strains may result in life-threatening bacteremic infections. A critical factor that determines an individual's susceptibility to systemic *H influenzae* type B infection is the presence or absence of serum antibodies to capsule antigens. Thus, the induction of serum antibodies by immunization with HiB vaccine is a reasonable strategy.

The vaccine significantly reduces the risk of contracting systemic *H influenzae* type B infection and is protective in reducing the incidence of epiglottitis, meningitis, and orbital cellulitis. The majority of children who develop these *H influenzae* type B infections are older than 2 years. The vaccine is estimated to be 90% effective when given before age 24 months. HiB is one of the safest vaccine products approved for use in children. A new combination vaccine (HiB-DTaP), which includes HiB conjugate vaccine and DTaP, is now available. It is effective and safe and offers the increased convenience of fewer injections for pediatric immunization.

Meningococcus

A polysaccharide vaccine for the prevention of meningococcal meningitis is available and is recommended for use in military personnel, college students living in dormitories, travelers to endemic areas, close contacts of infected patients, new outbreaks, and high-risk patients, especially splenectomized and complement deficient patients. The vaccine is about 85% effective in preventing the spread of group C meningococcal infections. The vaccine is used primarily in controlling spread of the disease and is generally not given as a routine immunization.

New and Future Vaccines

New vaccines are now available for Lyme disease, typhoid fever *(Salmonella typhi)*, anthrax, and yellow fever. Additional vaccines are now undergoing clinical trials for HIV, cholera, *Campylobacter, Clostridium difficile,* respiratory syncytial virus, Ebola virus, cytomegalovirus, rabies, viral encephalitis, herpes simplex type 2, Epstein-Barr virus, *Pseudomonas aeruginosa, Helicobacter pylori, Staphylococcus, Streptococcus,* HPV, parainfluenza virus, leishmaniasis, and plague.

Passive immunization with human hyperimmune globulin is currently available to treat or prevent rabies, tetanus, respiratory syncytial virus, cytomegalovirus, hepatitis A, hepatitis B, hepatitis C, herpes virus, and varicella zoster infections.

Considering the worldwide impact of many other infectious diseases, there is considerable interest in developing new vaccines for the organisms that cause tuberculosis, AIDS, malaria, gonorrhea, syphilis, toxigenic *Escherichia coli* infection, leprosy, trachoma, and others. It is hoped that ongoing research will lead to safe and effective vaccines for many or all of these illnesses.

Assad S, Francis A. Over a decade of experience with a yeast recombinant hepatitis B vaccine. *Vaccine.* 1999;18:57–67.

Butler JC, Shapiro ED, Carlone GM. Pneumococcal vaccines: history, current status, and future directions. *Am J Med.* 1999;107:69S–76S.

Centers for Disease Control and Prevention. Update: influenza activity—United States and worldwide, 1999–2000 season, and composition of the 2000–01 influenza vaccine. *MMWR.* 2000;49:375–381.

Chartrand SA. Varicella vaccine. *Pediatr Clin North Am.* 2000;47:373–394.

Committee on infectious diseases. American Academy of Pediatrics. Recommended Childhood Immunization Schedule—United States, January–December, 2001. *Pediatrics.* 2001; 107:202–204.

Galazka AM, Robertson SE, Kraigher A. Mumps and mumps vaccine: a global review. *Bull WHO.* 1999;77:3–14.

Meltzer MI, Dennis DT, Orloski KA. 1999 cost-effectiveness of a vaccine against Lyme disease in humans. *Emerging Infect Dis.* 1999;5:1–8.

Poliomyelitis prevention: revised recommendations for use of inactivated and live oral poliovirus vaccines. American Academy of Pediatrics Committee on Infectious Diseases. *Pediatrics.* 1999;103:171–172.

Pollard AJ, Levin M. Vaccines for prevention of meningococcal disease. *Pediatr Infect Dis J.* 2000;19:333–344.

Pougatcheva SO, Abernathy ES, Vzorov AN, et al. Development of a rubella virus DNA vaccine. *Vaccine.* 1999;17:2104–2112.

Welliver R, Monto AS, Carewicz O, et al. Effectiveness of oseltamivir in preventing influenza in household contacts. A randomized controlled trial. *JAMA.* 2001;285:748–754.

CHAPTER 14

Medical Emergencies

Recent Developments

- Adult basic life support rescuers should "phone first" for unresponsive adults. *Exceptions:* "phone fast" (provide CPR first) for adult victims of submersion, trauma, and drug intoxication.
- Patients with suspected stroke merit the same priorities for dispatch as patients with acute myocardial infarction or major trauma.
- Victims of suspected ischemic stroke should be transported to a facility capable of initiating fibrinolytic therapy within 1 hour of arrival unless that facility is more than 30 minutes away by ground ambulance.

Introduction

Although only occasionally called upon to manage a patient in acute distress, the ophthalmologist must be aware of the diagnostic and therapeutic steps necessary for proper care of these emergencies. Infrequent use of these techniques makes periodic review of life-support techniques particularly important. The American Red Cross and the American Heart Association both offer courses in, and periodic review of, basic life support and advanced cardiac life support (ACLS).

Cardiopulmonary Arrest

Cardiopulmonary resuscitation (CPR) is intended to rescue patients with acute circulatory failure, respiratory failure, or both. The most important determinant of short- and long-term neurologically intact survival is the interval from the onset of the arrest to the restoration of effective spontaneous circulatory and respiratory function. Numerous studies have demonstrated that early defibrillation is the most important factor influencing survival and the minimization of sequelae. The following sequences have been developed to optimize treatment and are useful guidelines for most patients. They do not preclude other measures that may be indicated for individual patients, however. The most crucial aspects of treatment are contained in the mnemonic *ABC*— *a*irway maintenance, *b*reathing, and *c*irculation.

Following are the steps to perform in an encounter with an unconscious patient:

1. Determine unresponsiveness. Attempt to arouse the patient by shaking the shoulders and saying, "Are you OK?" Do not shake the head or neck unless trauma to this area has been ruled out.

2. Activate the EMS system if there is no response (911 where available). Rescuers should "phone first" for unresponsive adults. *Exceptions:* "phone fast" (provide CPR first) for adult victims of submersion, trauma, and drug intoxication. Be prepared to give the location and nature of the emergency and condition of the victim.

3. Position the victim supine on a firm, flat surface. Patients with suspected stroke should be rapidly transported to a hospital capable of initiating fibrinolytic therapy within 1 hour of arrival unless that facility is more than 30 minutes away by ground ambulance. These patients merit the same priorities for dispatch as patients with acute myocardial infarction or major trauma.

4. Open the airway. The head-tilt, chin-lift maneuver is preferred because it is most likely to provide a good airway opening; the jaw thrust and the neck lift are alternative maneuvers. The rescuer can use the chin lift to tilt the head backward by applying firm pressure to the forehead while placing the fingers of the other hand under the chin, supporting the mandible. The modified jaw thrust should be used if a neck injury is suspected.

5. Determine breathlessness. If spontaneous respiration is not present, gently pinch the nose closed with the index finger and thumb of the hand that is on the forehead. Make a tight seal over the patient's mouth and ventilate twice with slow, full breaths (1.5–2.0 seconds each). A 2 second pause should be observed between breaths. Slow breaths result in less gastric distension.

   Health care professionals should be proficient in the use of barrier devices for basic life support. A face shield can help prevent transmission of most infections and exposure to HIV in saliva. (One such device is the Microshield from Medical Devices International.) The mouth-to-nose technique is recommended when it is impossible to ventilate through the victim's mouth. Masks are more effective than face shields in delivering adequate ventilation. Features can include a non-rebreathing (one-way) valve, an extension tube to eliminate close proximity, low resistance, a bacterial filter, transparency, and ease in maintaining a seal over the mouth (eg, the Seal-Easy Mask from Respironics). Alternative airway devices (eg, laryngeal mask airway and the esophageal-tracheal Combitube) may be acceptable when rescuers are trained in their use.

6. Determine presence or absence of pulse. Palpate the carotid pulse for at least 5 seconds to ensure that a pulse is not missed because of bradycardia.

7. Call for help again. If a carotid pulse is present, rescue breathing should be continued at a rate of 10–12 ventilations per minute. If there is no pulse, begin chest compressions.

8. To ensure good hand placement for chest compressions, the heel of one hand should be placed at the midsternal region with the bottom of the hand 1–2 fingerbreadths above the xiphoid process.

9. The recommended cardiac compression rate is 100 per minute in order to maximize cardiac output. Cardiac output varies, but on average, 30% of normal cardiac output can be expected with CPR. The depth of chest compression is critical; optimal compressions are 1.0–1.5 inches for children and 1.5–2.0 inches for adults. Duration of chest compression should be at least 50% of the total duration of the cycle.

10. For one- and two-rescuer CPR, 15 compressions should be performed before the victim is ventilated twice when the victim's airway is unprotected. About 3–5 seconds should be taken for two ventilations, and there should be a pause between ventilations.

11. The rescuer responsible for airway management should assess the adequacy of compressions by periodically palpating for the carotid pulse. Once the patient is intubated, ventilations are continued at a rate of 12–15 per minute, without pausing for compressions. The rescuer should stop and check for return of pulse and spontaneous breathing every few minutes.

12. CPR is most effective when started immediately after cardiac arrest. If cardiac arrest has persisted for more than 10 minutes, CPR is unlikely to restore the victim's central nervous system (CNS) to prearrest status. If there is any question about the exact duration of cardiac arrest, the victim should be given the benefit of the doubt and resuscitation should be started. In sharp contrast with cardiac arrest in adults, most causes of cardiopulmonary arrest in infants and children (younger than 8 years) are related to airway or ventilation problems rather than sudden cardiac arrest. In these victims, rescue support (especially rescue breathing) is essential and should be attempted first before activation of the EMS system (if the rescuer is trained).

The following adjuncts are helpful in CPR and are suggested components for a medical emergency tray, crash cart, or tackle box:

- Oxygen, to enhance tissue oxygenation and to prevent or ameliorate a hypoxic state.
- Airways, adult and child, oral and nasal, to be used on unconscious or sedated patients.
- A barrier device such as a face shield or mask-to-mouth unit to prevent disease transmission. Both can be used with supplemental oxygen and are especially useful if the rescuer is unfamiliar in the use of a standard bag-valve device (eg, Ambu Bag), which should also be included as standard equipment to help secure the airway. Alternative airway devices may also be acceptable when appropriate (see No. 5 above).
- Intravenous drugs (Table 14-1)
- Intravenous solutions: 5% dextrose and water, D5 lactated Ringer's, normal saline
- Syringes (1, 5, and 10 mL), hypodermic needles (20, 22, and 25 gauge), and venous catheters
- A suction apparatus, tourniquet, taped tongue blade, and tape
- Laryngoscope and endotracheal tubes (adult and child)

Table 14-1   Medications Used in Acute Medical Emergencies

Drugs	Indications	Adult Dose (IV)	Adverse Effects
Epinephrine (1:1000)	Anaphylaxis	0.3–0.5 mg subcutaneously every 5 minutes	Tachycardia, hypertension
Epinephrine (1:10,000)	Asystole, ventricular fibrillation, EMD	Bolus 0.5–1.0 mg every 5 minutes	Hypertension in excess doses
Lidocaine	PVCs, ventricular tachycardia, ventricular fibrillation	Bolus 1.0 mg/kg with subsequent doses of 0.5 mg/kg to a maximum total dose of 3.0 mg/kg	Focal and grand mal seizures in excess doses
Atropine	Bradycardia, EMD, asystole	Bolus 0.5–1.0 mg every 5 minutes	Induced ventricular fibrillation, ventricular tachycardia, or supraventricular tachycardia
Diphenhydramine HCl (Benadryl)	Anaphylaxis and anaphylactoid reactions	10–20 mg	Drowsiness
Diazepam (Valium)	Seizures	5–10 mg	Sedation
Hydrocortisone sodium succinate (Solu-Cortef)	Anaphylaxis and anaphylactoid reactions	500 mg every 6 hours	Adrenal-pituitary axis suppression
Sodium bicarbonate	Severe metabolic acidosis	Bolus 1 mEq/kg	Hypernatremia, hypocalcemia, and metabolic alkalosis
Calcium chloride (ampule of 10% solution)	Acute hyperkalemia and hypocalcemia, calcium-channel blocker toxicity	2–4 mg/kg	Bradycardia
Aminophylline	Bronchospasm	6 mg/kg (loading dose)	Tachycardia
Glucose (D 50)	Profound hypoglycemia	Bolus 10 ml	Hyperglycemia

In the absence of a 911 community emergency phone system, it is essential to have the phone number of the local paramedic emergency squad posted near all office telephones.

Basic life support also outlines methods for aiding choking victims, including the Heimlich maneuver and appropriate manual techniques for removing foreign bodies from the oral pharynx. Epigastric thrusts should be attempted; up to 10–12 thrusts may be necessary. Thereafter, ventilation should be attempted. If these efforts are unsuccessful, the mouth should be cleared with a finger sweep and ventilation attempted again. Transtracheal ventilation by means of cricothyrotomy may be necessary.

In addition to basic CPR, the American Heart Association has established guidelines and procedures for ACLS. ACLS includes intubations, defibrillation, cardioversion, pacemaker placement, administration of drugs and fluids, and communication with ambulance and hospital systems. Protocols and algorithms have been established in critical cardiac care for ventricular fibrillation, ventricular tachycardia, asystole, electrical-mechanical dissociation, premature ventricular contractions, atrial tachycardia, and bradycardia. The provider of ACLS must precisely understand the actions, indications, doses, and adverse effects of the cardiac drugs used in the specific protocols. Except in dire emergencies, these drugs should be administered to treat cardiac arrhythmias *only* by physicians who use them routinely.

Because of the comprehensive and changing nature of ACLS algorithms, these procedures are beyond the scope of this chapter.

Shock

Shock is a state of generalized inadequacy of tissue perfusion that leads to impaired cellular metabolism and—if uncorrected—progresses to multiple organ failure and death. The clinical syndrome is usually characterized by an altered sensorium, relative hypotension, tachycardia, tachypnea, oliguria, metabolic acidosis, weak or absent pulse, pallor, diaphoresis, and cool skin (however, the skin may be warm in septic shock).

Classification

Shock is classified according to the four primary pathophysiologic mechanisms involved:

- Oligemic or hypovolemic (eg, hemorrhage, diabetic ketoacidosis, burns, or sequestration)
- Cardiogenic (eg, myocardial infarction or arrhythmia)
- Obstructive (eg, pericardial tamponade, pulmonary embolus, or tension pneumothorax)
- Distributive, characterized by maldistribution of the vascular volume secondary to altered vasomotor tone (eg, sepsis, anaphylaxis, spinal cord insult, beriberi, or an arteriovenous fistula)

The type of shock can often be determined by history, physical examination, and appropriate diagnostic tests. Regardless of the event that precipitated the state of shock, microcirculatory failure is the common factor that eventually leads to death in advanced shock. Ventilatory failure appears to be the most significant factor in the morbidity and mortality of shock, with subsequent hypoxemia and metabolic acidosis leading to many complications.

If one rules out vasovagal syncope (by virtue of its short duration and knowledge of the situations that produce this condition), the basic life-support measures for the initial emergency care of the unconscious patient are similar. The most important aspects of treatment are the ABCs, the same principles used in CPR.

Failure of respiratory gas exchange is the most frequent single cause of death in patients with shock. One must first rule out respiratory obstruction. Oxygen is then given by mask, and if respiratory movements are shallow, mechanical ventilation is necessary. If laryngeal edema is present, as with anaphylaxis, endotracheal intubation (if possible), tracheotomy, or cricothyrotomy is indicated. Respiratory obstruction can be assumed if there is stridor with respiratory movements or if cyanosis persists even when adequate ventilatory techniques have been applied. A conscious patient in distress who cannot speak but is developing cyanosis may be choking on food or a foreign body; the Heimlich maneuver has been shown to be an effective means of treatment for the "cafe coronary."

Assessment

The vital signs must be monitored. Tachycardia, tachypnea, arrhythmia, hypothermia, and hypotension are the hallmarks of shock. Decreased pulse pressure is often an early sign of shock, and systolic pressures of less than 90 mm Hg are often associated with vital organ hypoperfusion. Blood pressure, however, is not always a reliable indicator of tissue perfusion. The following tests and procedures are useful:

- Arterial blood gases
- Electrocardiogram (ECG)
- Pulmonary artery (Swan-Ganz) catheter monitoring
- Complete blood count: a low hematocrit may indicate blood loss; a high hematocrit may indicate intravascular volume depletion.
- Serum electrolytes and creatinine
- Renal function: oliguria, increased urinary osmolarity, and decreased urinary sodium are signs of tissue hypoperfusion.

Treatment

Treatment of shock is often complex; specific guidelines are beyond the scope of this text. General guidelines for the treatment of shock are as follows:

- The patient should be positioned with the legs elevated.
- Supplemental oxygen should be administered to enhance tissue oxygenation. Mechanical ventilation may be necessary to maintain the PO_2 and to prevent respiratory acidosis.
- Volume expansion with an IV infusion is of primary importance in maintaining circulation. Initially, a crystalloid solution (ie, normal saline or Ringer's lactate) should be administered rapidly.
- Sodium bicarbonate, given intravenously over 5–10 minutes, is indicated for correction of severe metabolic acidosis. The dosage should be titrated according to arterial blood gas results.
- Vasopressor drugs (norepinephrine bitartrate or dopamine) may be needed for augmentation of cardiac output and perfusion of vital organs after an adequate circulating volume is established.
- Antibiotic therapy should be initiated promptly if sepsis is suspected.

Anaphylaxis

One specific cause of shock that requires immediate and specific therapy is anaphylaxis. *Anaphylaxis* is an acute allergic reaction following antigen exposure in a previously sensitized person. It is usually mediated by immunoglobulin E antibodies and involves release of chemical mediators from mast cells and basophils. *Anaphylactoid reactions*, which are more common yet less severe, are the result of direct release of these chemical mediators triggered by nonantigenic agents. Anaphylaxis or anaphylactoid reactions may occur after exposure to pollen, drugs, foreign serum, insect stings, diagnostic agents such as iodinated contrast materials or fluorescein, vaccines, local anesthetics, and food products. The most important parameter for prediction of such an attack is a history of a previous allergic reaction to any other drug or possible antigen. Unfortunately, a history of known sensitivity may not always be elicited.

Anaphylaxis is particularly important to the ophthalmologist, in view of the increasing number of surgical procedures and fluorescein angiograms being performed in the office setting. It is estimated that allergic reactions to fluorescein (including urticaria) occur in up to 1% of all angiograms. In a recent survey, the overall risk of a severe reaction was 1 in 1900 patients, including a risk of respiratory compromise in 1 in 3800 subjects. Any patient developing diaphoresis, apprehension, pallor, a rapid and weak pulse, or any combination thereof after administration of a drug should be considered to have an allergic reaction until proven otherwise. The diagnosis is certain if there is associated generalized itching, urticaria, angioedema of the skin, dyspnea, wheezing, or arrhythmia. This process may lead rapidly to loss of consciousness, shock, cardiac arrest, coma, or death. Once an acute allergic reaction is suspected, prompt treatment is indicated.

- Epinephrine (0.3–0.5 mL of 1:1000 injected subcutaneously or intramuscularly in a limb opposite to the antigenic agent injection site is usually effective.
- Intravenous volume expansion may be needed to restore and maintain tissue perfusion.
- Oxygen should be administered to all patients in respiratory distress.
- Tracheostomy or cricothyrotomy is indicated for laryngeal edema unresponsive to the above methods or when oral intubation cannot be performed.
- Hydrocortisone should be administered for serious or prolonged reactions. When given early, corticosteroids help control possible long-term sequelae. Antihistamines are also helpful in slowing or halting the ongoing allergic response but are of limited value in acute anaphylaxis.
- All patients with anaphylaxis or anaphylactoid reactions should be observed for at least 6 hours.

In cases of mild allergic reactions, the physician can give 10–50 mg of diphenhydramine (Benadryl) orally or intramuscularly and observe the patient closely to determine whether further treatment is necessary. Pretreating high-risk patients with an antihistamine, corticosteroids, or both prior to a fluorescein angiogram may reduce the risk of an allergic reaction. In all cases of anaphylaxis, supportive treatment should be maintained until the emergency medical team arrives.

Personal emergency kits containing epinephrine are available for patients with a known history of anaphylaxis to use while awaiting medical help. The kits are designed to allow self-treatment by the patient or administration by a family member or an informed bystander. The Ana-Kit contains a syringe and needle preloaded with 0.6 mL of 1:1000 epinephrine. The physician who prescribes this kit must give detailed instructions concerning the use of the device. The EpiPen or EpiPen Jr contains a spring-loaded automatic injector, which does not permit graduated doses to be given but automatically injects 0.3 mg of epinephrine (0.15 mg in the junior version) when the device is triggered by pressure on the thigh. The epinephrine ampules contained in these self-treatment kits have a limited shelf life. They should be replaced prior to the expiration date or if the solution becomes discolored.

Guidelines 2000 for Cardiopulmonary Resuscitation and Emergency Cardiac Care. The American Heart Association in collaboration with the International Liaison Committee on Resuscitation. *Circulation.* 2000;102(suppl I).

Lipson BK, Yannuzzi LA. Complications of intravenous fluorescein injections. *Int Ophthalmol Clin.* 1989;29:200.

Roth CS, Weaver DT, eds. *Pocket Manual of Emergency Medical Therapy.* 4th ed. Toronto: Decker; 1987.

Seizures and Status Epilepticus

A *seizure* is a paroxysmal episode of abnormal electrical activity in the brain resulting in involuntary transient neurologic, motor activity, behavioral, or autonomic dysfunction. Seizures can present with many different clinical manifestations, but most fit into the categories of simple-partial, complex-partial, or generalized tonic-clonic.

As in the treatment of all medical emergencies, the first consideration is airway maintenance. This becomes particularly important if the seizure progresses to status epilepticus. *Status epilepticus* is defined as a prolonged seizure or multiple seizures without intervening periods of normal consciousness. Status epilepticus, like seizures, may have a local onset with secondary generalization or be generalized from onset. A seizure is considered status epilepticus when it lasts for 30 minutes or longer. Status epilepticus is often found concomitantly with hyperthermia, acidosis, hypoxia, tachycardia, hypercapnia, and mydriasis and, if persistent, may be associated with irreversible brain injury. Status epilepticus that is completely stopped within 2 hours usually has relatively minor morbidity compared with episodes lasting longer than 2 hours.

Major causes of seizures and status epilepticus include:

- Drug withdrawal, such as from anticonvulsants, benzodiazepines, barbiturates, or alcohol
- Metabolic abnormalities, such as hypoglycemia, hyponatremia, hypocalcemia, or hypomagnesemia
- Conditions that affect the CNS, such as infection, trauma, stroke, hypoxia, ischemia, or sleep deprivation
- Toxic levels of various drugs

In management, it is important not only to stop the seizure activity but also to identify and treat the underlying cause. A general treatment protocol is outlined below.

1. Note time of seizure onset. Monitor airway, vital signs, and ECG.

2. Establish IV line. Position patient on side to allow gravity drainage of saliva. Insert oral airway if possible. Some experts advocate using a washcloth or taped tongue blade as a bite block.
3. Draw blood immediately and check glucose, electrolytes, calcium, magnesium, sodium, and toxicology screen.
4. Give 50 mL of 50% dextrose IV push (or 1 mL/kg).
5. Administer a benzodiazepine such as diazepam (Valium) or lorazepam (Ativan) slowly by IV line, titrated to an effective dose, usually 5.0 mg/min to a total dose of 0.5 mg/kg.
6. Proceed immediately to administer phenytoin (or fosphenytoin) intravenously. Monitor pulse, blood pressure, and ECG. Watch especially for hypotension.
7. If seizures continue for 20 minutes, administer a loading dose of phenobarbital.
8. Emergency medical management of seizures is best left to physicians who perform this routinely. Activation of the emergency response (911) team is indicated in all cases of acute seizure onset.

Toxic Reactions to Local Anesthetics and Other Agents

Toxic overdose is an additional cause of unconsciousness or of acute distress in a conscious patient, and it must be considered whenever the patient is undergoing a procedure that requires local anesthesia. Table 14-2 lists commonly used local anesthetics with their maximum safe dose.

Reactions following the administration of local anesthetics are almost always toxic and only rarely allergic. A high blood level of local anesthetic can be produced by the following: too large a dose, unusually rapid absorption (including inadvertent IV administration), and unusually slow detoxification or elimination (especially in liver disease). Hypersensitivity (ie, decreased patient tolerance) and idiosyncratic reactions are rare, but they may occur with local anesthetic agents, as with any drug. Although true allergic or anaphylactic reactions are also rare, they may occur, particularly with agents belonging to the aminoester class.

Toxic reactions cause overstimulation of the CNS, which may lead to excitement, restlessness, apprehension, disorientation, tremors, and convulsions (cerebral cortex effects) as well as nausea and vomiting (medulla effects). Cardiac effects initially include

Table 14-2 Maximum Recommended Local Anesthetic Doses

Agent	Commercially Available Concentrations (%) 1% = 10 mg/cc	Plain Solutions (mg)	Epinephrine-Containing Solutions (mg)
Chloroprocaine	1.0, 2.0, 3.0	800	1000
Lidocaine	0.5, 1.0, 1.5, 2.0, 4.0, 5.0	300	500
Mepivacaine (Carbocaine)	1.0, 1.5, 2.0	300	225
Bupivacaine	0.25, 0.5, 0.75	175	225
Tetracaine	1.0	100	100

tachycardia and hypertension. Ultimately, however, depression of the CNS and cardio-vascular systems occurs, which may result in sleepiness and coma (cerebral cortex effects) as well as in irregular respirations, sighing, dyspnea, and respiratory arrest (medulla effects). Cardiac effects of CNS depression are bradycardia and hypotension.

Injected local anesthetic agents can also produce a direct toxic effect on muscle tissue. In the case of retrobulbar injections, this can result initially in muscle weakness, which in some patients is followed by muscle contracture. Extraocular motility can be affected, resulting in diplopia (usually hypertropia) that may require surgical revision. Recent evidence suggests that hyaluronidase may be partially protective by allowing more rapid diffusion of the anesthetic agent following injection.

Signs of cortical stimulation require immediate treatment, before progressive changes to cortical and medullary function and cardiac depression occur. Increased metabolic activity of the CNS and poor ventilatory exchange lead to cerebral hypoxia. Treatment consists of oxygenation, supportive airway care, and titrated IV administration of midazolam, which is used to suppress cortical stimulation. Respiratory stimulants are to be avoided because the medullary respiratory center has already been stimulated by the local anesthetic and these drugs lead to eventual respiratory depression.

In cases of toxic overdose, other emergency procedures include suctioning if vomiting occurs and use of taped tongue blade if convulsions develop. If shock develops, the appropriate drugs can be administered by IV infusion.

The addition of *epinephrine* to the local anesthetic can also cause adverse reactions. Epinephrine can produce symptoms similar to early CNS stimulation by local anesthetic, such as anxiety, restlessness, tremor, hypertension, and tachycardia. Unlike local anesthetics, however, epinephrine does not produce convulsions or bradycardia as the toxic reaction proceeds. Oxygen is useful in the treatment of epinephrine overdoses.

A recent study looked at the effect of intraocular epinephrine irrigation at a concentration that maintained pupillary dilation during routine extracapsular cataract surgery. The study found no additional risk of significant interval changes in either arterial blood pressure or heart rate in patients with or without preexisting hypertension.

The administration of retrobulbar *bupivacaine* has been associated with respiratory arrest. This reaction may be caused by intra-arterial injection of the local anesthetic, with retrograde flow to the cerebral circulation. It could also result from puncture of the dural sheath of the optic nerve during retrobulbar block, with diffusion of the local anesthetic along the subdural space in the midbrain. A large prospective study comparing retrobulbar injection of 0.75% bupivacaine plus 2.0% lidocaine to 0.75% bupivacaine plus 4.0% lidocaine found that those patients receiving 4.0% lidocaine mixed with bupivacaine had an almost nine times greater risk of respiratory arrest than the patients receiving 2.0% lidocaine mixed with bupivacaine. (See also Chapter 15, Perioperative Management in Ocular Surgery, for further discussion of reactions to local anesthetics.)

The use of *edrophonium chloride* (Tensilon) in the diagnosis of myasthenia gravis can have toxic side effects. The signs and symptoms result from cholinergic stimulation and may include nausea, vomiting, diarrhea, sweating, increased bronchial and salivary secretions, muscle fasciculations and weakness, and bradycardia. Some of these signs may be transient and self-limited because of the very short half-life of IV edrophonium. Whenever a Tensilon test is to be performed, a syringe containing 0.5 mg of atropine sulfate must be immediately available. (Some physicians routinely pretreat all patients undergoing Tensilon testing with atropine.)

If signs of excess cholinergic stimulation occur, 0.4–0.5 mg of atropine sulfate should be administered intravenously. This dose may be repeated every 3–10 minutes if necessary. The total dose of atropine necessary to counteract the toxic effects is seldom more than 2 mg. If toxic signs progress, the treatment described above for toxic overdose may be necessary.

Brown SM, Brooks SE, Mazow ML, et al. Cluster of diplopia cases after periocular anesthesia without hyaluronidase. *J Cataract Refract Surg.* 1999;1245–1249.

Capo H, Guyton DL. Ipsilateral hypertropia after cataract surgery. *Ophthalmology.* 1996; 103:721–730.

Wittpenn JR, Rapoza P, Sternberg P, et al. Respiratory arrest following retrobulbar anesthesia. *Ophthalmology.* 1986;93:867–870.

Yamaguchi H, Matsumoto Y. Stability of blood pressure and heart rate during intraocular epinephrine irrigation. *Ann Ophthalmol.* 1988;20:58–60.

Ocular Side Effects of Systemic Medications

Because of the development of compartmentalized medical specialties and the proliferation of specific therapeutic agents, patients frequently have multiple simultaneous drug regimens. Often, no single physician (among the several to whom a patient may relate) is aware of all of the drugs the patient is taking. The clinical problem is compounded by several factors. For example, physicians are often not aware of what other drugs a patient uses or might not be familiar with agents used outside of their specialty. In addition, the interaction may affect a bodily system not usually monitored by a given specialist. Finally, the patient might not associate a symptom with a particular drug if that symptom is not related to the system for which the drug was given. For example, the association between ophthalmic epinephrine therapy and cardiac arrhythmia might not be readily apparent to the patient. Conversely, the commonly prescribed erectile dysfunction agent sildenafil (Viagra) has been noted to block photoreceptor signals, causing electroretinographic changes, visual disturbances, and increased light sensitivity. The spectrum of systemic side effects with commonly used ophthalmic drugs is covered extensively elsewhere in this series (see BCSC Section 9, *Intraocular Inflammation and Uveitis,* and Section 10, *Glaucoma*). From the opposite perspective, the ocular side effects of several commonly prescribed systemic medications are presented in Table 14-3. Drug interactions must always be suspected in patients on multiple topical and systemic agents.

The ophthalmologist can minimize adverse effects from multiple drug therapy by doing the following:

- Maintain a high level of suspicion for drug interactions.
- Question the patient closely about other drug therapy and general symptoms.
- Encourage all patients to carry a card listing the drugs they use.
- Keep in close communication with the patient's primary physician.
- Consult with a clinical pharmacologist or internist whenever a question of drug interaction arises.

- Unrecognized adverse effects of topical or systemic medications should be reported to the National Registry of Drug-Induced Ocular Side Effects:

Joan Randall, MPH
Casey Eye Institute
Oregon Health Sciences University
3375 S.W. Terwilliger Blvd.
Portland, OR 97201-4197
Phone: 503-494-5686
Fax: 503-494-6864

Doran M. When good drugs go bad. *EyeNet.* 2001;5:43–48.

Fraunfelder FT, Fraunfelder FW. *Drug-Induced Ocular Side Effects.* 5th ed. Boston: Butterworth Heinemann; 2001.

Table 14-3 Potential Ocular Effects of Popular Drugs

Drug	Side Effects
Antibiotics	
Cefaclor (Ceclor)	Mild inflammation of ocular surface (rare); eyelid problems; nystagmus; visual hallucinations
Cefuroxime axetil (Ceftin)	Mild inflammation of ocular surface (rare)
Ciprofloxacin (Cipro)	Eyelid problems; exacerbation of myasthenia; visual sensations
Minocycline (Dynacin, Minocin)	Papilledema secondary to pseudotumor cerebri; transient myopia; blue-gray, dark blue, or brownish pigmentation of the sclera; hyperpigmentation of eyelids or conjunctiva; diplopia
Rifampin (Rifadin and others)	Conjunctival hyperemia; exudative conjunctivitis; increased lacrimation
Antidepressants/Anxiolytics	
Alprazolam (Xanax)	Diplopia; decreased or blurred vision; decreased accommodation; abnormal extraocular muscle movements; allergic conjunctivitis
Fluoxetine (Prozac)	Blurred vision; photophobia; mydriasis; dry eye; conjunctivitis; diplopia
Imipramine (Tofranil)	Decreased vision; decreased accommodation; slight mydriasis; photosensitivity
Analgesics, Anti-Inflammatory Agents	
Aspirin	Transient blurred vision; transient myopia; hypersensitivity reactions
Ibuprofen (Advil)	Blurred vision; decreased vision; diplopia; photosensitivity; dry eyes; decrease in color vision; optic or retrobulbar neuritis
Naproxen (Anaprox, Aleve)	Decreased vision; changes in color vision; optic or retrobulbar neuritis; papilledema secondary to pseudotumor cerebri; photosensitivity; corneal opacities
Piroxicam (Feldene)	Decreased vision; photosensitivity

(Continued)

Asthma, Allergy Drugs

Corticosteroids (general) — Decreased vision; posterior subcapsular cataracts; increased IOP

Antihistamines (general) — Decreased vision; may induce or aggravate dry eye; pupillary changes; decreased accommodation; blurred vision; decreased mucoid or lacrimal secretions; diplopia

Cardiovascular Drugs

Amiodarone (Cordarone, Pacerone) — Photophobia; blurred vision; corneal opacities; subcapsular lens opacities; optic neuropathy

β-Blockers (general) — Decreased vision; visual hallucinations; decreased IOP; decreased lacrimation

Calcium channel blockers — Decreased or blurred vision; periorbital edema; ocular irritation (general)

Captopril/enalapril (Vaseretic) — Angioedema of the eye and orbit; conjunctivitis; decreased vision

Digitalis glycosides — Decreased vision; color vision defects; glare phenomenon; flickering vision

Diuretics (thiazide-type) — Decreased vision; myopia; color vision abnormalities; retinal edema

Flecainide (Tambocor) — Blurred vision; decreased vision; decreased accommodation; abnormal visual sensations; decreased depth perception; nystagmus

Warfarin (Coumadin) — Retinal hemorrhages in susceptible persons; hyphema; allergic reactions; conjunctivitis; lacrimation; decreased vision

Hormones, Hormone-Related Drugs

Clomiphene (Clomid and others) — Visual sensations; decreased vision; mydriasis; visual field constriction; photophobia; diplopia

Danazol (Danocrine) — Decreased vision; diplopia; papilledema secondary to pseudotumor cerebri; visual field defects

Estradiol (general) — Decreased vision; retinal vascular disorders; papilledema secondary to pseudotumor cerebri; fluctuations of corneal curvature and corneal steepening; color vision abnormalities

Leuprolide (Lupron) — Blurred vision; papilledema secondary to pseudotumor cerebri; retinal hemorrhage and branch vein occlusion; eye pain; lid edema

Oral contraceptives (general) — Decreased vision; retinal vascular disorders; papilledema secondary to pseudotumor cerebri; color vision abnormalities

Tamoxifen (Nolvadex) — Decreased vision; corneal opacities; retinal edema or hemorrhage; optic disc swelling; retinopathy; decreased color vision; possible optic neuritis or neuropathy

---

(From Doran M. When good drugs go bad. *EyeNet.* 2001;5:43–48.)

CHAPTER 15

Perioperative Management in Ocular Surgery

Recent Development

- Preoperative medical tests for patients undergoing cataract surgery *may* not reduce perioperative morbidity and mortality.

Preoperative Evaluation

Adult Patients

All patients undergoing eye surgery require a thorough history and physical examination. Current general guidelines for preoperative testing in asymptomatic patients scheduled for elective surgery are given in Table 15-1. Some authors also advocate chest radiography in smokers and in any patient with cardiac or pulmonary disease if general anesthesia is anticipated.

However, a recent study by Schein and coworkers has questioned the value of routine preoperative medical testing before cataract surgery. The investigators randomly assigned 19,557 elective cataract operations to be preceded or not preceded by a standard battery of medical tests (ECG, complete blood count, and measurement of serum levels of electrolytes, urea nitrogen, creatinine, and glucose). Adverse medical events and interventions were recorded on the day of surgery and during the 7 days after surgery. The study demonstrated no significant differences between the no-testing group and the testing group in the rates of intraoperative and postoperative events. Furthermore, no benefit of routine preoperative medical testing was found when the analysis was stratified according to age, sex, race, coexisting illness, American Society of Anesthesiologists risk class (Table 15-2), or self-reported health status. The investigators stated that most abnormalities in laboratory value can be predicted from the patient history and findings on physical examination; moreover, laboratory abnormalities, when discovered, rarely lead to changes in perioperative management. Therefore, despite the fact that most patients who undergo cataract surgery are over age 65 and the prevalence of coexisting illnesses in this patient population is high, perioperative morbidity and mortality are not reduced by routine preoperative medical testing. The authors concluded that tests should only be ordered when the history or physical examination indicate the need for a test

Table 15-1 Preoperative Test Recommendations in Asymptomatic Patients Scheduled for Elective Operations

| Age | General Anesthesia | | Sedation for MAC and Regional Technique (Men and Women) | Nerve Block (Local) (Men and Women) |
	Men	Women		
<40 yr	None	Hb or Hct Pregnancy test?	None	None
40–50 yr	ECG	Hb or Hct Pregnancy test?	None	None
50–64 yr	Hb or Hct ECG	Hb or Hct ECG Pregnancy test?	Hb or Hct*	None
65–74 yr	Hb or Hct ECG Creatinine/BUN Glucose	Hb or Hct ECG Creatinine/BUN Glucose	Hb or Hct* ECG[†]	Hb or Hct*
>74 yr	Hb or Hct ECG Creatinine/BUN Glucose Chest radiograph?	Hb or Hct ECG Creatinine/BUN Glucose Chest radiograph?	Hb and Hct* ECG Creatinine/BUN* Glucose*	Hb and Hct* ECG

MAC, monitored anesthesia care; Hb, hemoglobin; Hct, hematocrit; ECG, electrocardiogram; BUN, blood urea nitrogen.
* Within 6 months.
[†] Within 12 months.

(Modified from Roizen M, Cohn S. Preoperative evaluation for elective sugery: what laboratory tests are needed? In: Stoelting RT, Barash PG, Gallagher TJ, eds. *Advances in Anesthesia.* Chicago: Mosby-Year Book; 1993:25–43, with permission.)

Table 15-2 American Society of Anesthesiologists Physical Status Classification

Class I	A normal healthy patient
Class II	A patient with mild systemic disease (eg, controlled chronic obstructive pulmonary disease [COPD], hypertension, diabetes mellitus, prior myocardial infarction)
Class III	A patient with severe systemic disease that is not incapacitating (moderate to severe COPD, coronary artery disease with angina)
Class IV	A patient with severe systemic disease that is a constant threat to life (marked congestive heart failure, unstable angina)
Class V	A moribund patient not expected to survive without the operation

even if surgery had not been planned (eg, ECG for new or worsening angina). The authors suggested extrapolating these recommendations to similar populations of patients scheduled to undergo other procedures that are associated with similar surgical risk and in which local anesthesia with intravenous sedation is used.

Schein OD, Katz J, Bass EB, et al. The value of routine preoperative medical testing before cataract surgery. Study of Medical Testing for Cataract Surgery. *N Engl J Med.* 2000;342:168–175.

If laboratory evaluation reveals marked elevations of fasting blood glucose (>300 mg/dL) or the discovery of new-onset diabetes at the time of glucose screening, elective eye surgery should be delayed because the sequelae of an unexpected neurologic event during the perioperative period is worse in patients with hyperglycemia.

Preoperative ECG findings that pose problems and require further evaluation are apparently "new" onset of atrial fibrillation, "new" ST-T segment changes that suggest ischemia, or "new" myocardial infarction, premature ventricular contractions, or severe bradycardia or heart block. When the preoperative ECG shows ST-T segment changes, the ECG should be compared with an old ECG if possible. Changes in an asymptomatic patient are less ominous than changes in a patient with chest pain. In patients with a history of myocardial infarction, elective surgery should be postponed for 6 months, when the incidence of reinfarction decreases.

Pediatric Patients

Different considerations apply to pediatric eye patients. There is no evidence that abnormalities in a complete blood count affect the choice of anesthetic management for asymptomatic children. In general, if the child is healthy and does not chronically take prescribed medications, no laboratory tests are necessary even for general anesthesia. However, a family history of sickle trait or sickle disease is significant because some aspects of anesthetic management will change in these patients. Bleeding time or routine urinalysis is unnecessary in the healthy child and only serves to traumatize the patient.

The issue of elective eye surgery in children with an upper respiratory infection is controversial. A child who is already ill will feel even worse after surgery, and the significance of a postoperative fever may be difficult to interpret. Furthermore, contaminated nasal discharge could possibly enter the ocular area. If a child has a fever above 101°F, has purulent nasal discharge, or appears systemically ill, a bacterial lower respiratory infection should be considered. This circumstance argues for a delay to avoid increased risk of laryngospasm and bronchospasm with general anesthesia. However, in the absence of such findings—such as a child who appears well except for a runny nose—many anesthesiologists elect to proceed.

Specific Preoperative Concerns

Obstructive pulmonary disease

Chronic obstructive pulmonary disease can pose a distinct problem in ophthalmic surgery. Cessation of smoking is extremely helpful in reducing intra- and postoperative coughing. Preoperative bronchopulmonary care with chest physiotherapy can decrease the susceptibility to infection and improve air exchange. General anesthesia may be preferred over local anesthesia because the anesthesiologist may have better control over tracheal bronchial secretions and the cough reflex. (See also Chapter 6, Pulmonary Diseases.)

Malignant hyperthermia

Malignant hyperthermia (MH), which is discussed later and at greater length under Intraoperative Complications, is a serious intraoperative complication triggered by certain anesthetic agents. MH can be fatal if diagnosis and treatment are delayed. MH can occur as an isolated case or as a dominantly inherited disorder with incomplete penetrance. Physical disorders associated with MH include strabismus, muscular dystrophy, and congenital ptosis. The incidence is reported variously as between 1:6000 and 1:30,000 and is generally thought to be higher in children. MH can occur in all age groups, however.

The preoperative personal and family history is helpful in determining whether the patient is at risk for MH. Patients with a history of masseter muscle rigidity after the administration of succinylcholine may be at risk for MH. If the patient or other family members have a history of sudden onset of tachycardia, breathing problems, or high fever during anesthesia or a history of ventricular arrhythmias or cardiac failure during anesthesia, the diagnosis of MH should be considered.

Muscle biopsy with in vitro halothane and caffeine contraction testing is the most specific test to confirm the clinical diagnosis. Patients with a history that is unconfirmed but suspicious for MH or a relative with MH should undergo testing to detect susceptibility. Creatine kinase measurement is not reliable. Although levels are elevated in up to two thirds of patients with MH, normal results have no predictive value.

MH occurs most commonly with the use of succinylcholine, often combined with an inhalation anesthetic such as halothane. Safer agents include nitrous oxide, barbiturates, narcoleptics, antipyretics, nondepolarizing muscle relaxants, propofol, and droperidol. However, even the stress of having surgery itself can trigger MH.

Latex allergy

Latex allergy is a condition that has caused growing concern in the last few years. The overall prevalence of latex allergy has not been determined, but certain populations appear to be at particular risk for reactions. Health care workers and hospital employees can experience progressive sensitization to latex because of repeated occupational exposure. This sensitivity is accentuated if the health care worker has a history of atopy. Certain medical populations also are at significant risk for latex allergy and anaphylaxis, including patients with myelodysplasia or spina bifida and those who have undergone repeated urinary catheterization or frequent surgical procedures. A cross-reactivity with bananas, avocados, mangoes, and chestnuts has been demonstrated, and allergies to these foods have also been associated with latex allergy. Other implicated foods include apricots, celery, figs, grapes, papayas, passion fruit, peaches, and pineapples. A history of reactivity to balloons also suggests a latex allergy.

Any patient suspected of having latex allergy should be referred to an allergist, and the surgery should be delayed until this concern can be evaluated. The entire operating room environment must be changed to care for the patient allergic to latex. Furthermore, the allergic patient should be the first case of the day in that particular operating room.

Local anesthetic allergies

A patient reporting an allergy to all the "-caines" might actually have experienced an intravascular injection of epinephrine, a vasovagal attack, or even a panic attack rather than a true allergic reaction. True allergic reactions occur but account for less than 1% of all local anesthetic reactions. A true allergic reaction to a -caine medication includes wheezing, urticaria, and respiratory distress. A history of sweating, tachycardia, headache, or hypertension suggests intravascular injection of epinephrine. However, an overdose of local anesthetic produces tinnitus, a bad taste in the mouth, or CNS changes such as confusion, slurred speech, or respiratory arrest. An overdose is unlikely in ophthalmic anesthesia given the relatively small volumes used.

A true allergy to local anesthetics is more likely with the ester derivatives such as procaine, tetracaine, chloroprocaine, and benzocaine. An allergy can even occur to the preservative Paraben, which is widely used in multidose vials of local anesthetics, as well as in other medicines, cosmetics, and foods.

If a patient is suspected of having a true allergy to local anesthetics, preoperative skin testing by appropriate personnel with adequate monitoring and resuscitation equipment nearby is recommended. If the patient proves to have true ester allergy, *amides* (lidocaine, bupivacaine, or mepivacaine) can be used as an alternative. Conversely, if the patient has a true allergy to amides, an ester-type of anesthetic can be used, such as chloroprocaine or tetracaine. Preservative-free agents are also available. (Allergic or toxic reactions to local anesthetics are discussed more fully under the later heading, Intraoperative Complications, and in Chapter 14, Medical Emergencies.)

Preoperative Fasting

Questions often arise as to how long the patient must be kept on NPO status before surgery. A pediatric patient who is kept on NPO status for 10–12 hours preoperatively may become hypotensive as a result of dehydration. It has been shown that use of clear liquids orally up to 2 hours prior to surgery does not lead to any higher incidence of aspiration or other gastrointestinal complications of general anesthesia or local anesthesia.

The purpose of preoperative fasting is to reduce the particulate matter in the stomach and to lower the gastric fluid volume and acidity in case aspiration of stomach contents occurs. Diabetics, particularly those with autonomic neuropathy, are at risk for gastroparesis. Pregnant patients have a higher-than-normal risk of aspiration. Additionally, patients with known gastroesophageal reflux and those with peptic ulcer disease may also have some increased risk of aspiration.

Oral administration of an H_2 blocker such as *ranitidine* or *famotidine* 2–4 hours prior to surgery reduces the percentage of patients with low gastric pH or high gastric volume. *Metoclopramide* or *cisapride* (restricted access in the United States) also promotes intestinal motility and decreases reflux; these drugs are especially useful in a nonfasting patient who requires urgent surgery. (See Table 15-3 for selected perioperative medications.)

Management of Concurrent Medications

In general, medication regimens should not be interrupted if possible. Treatments for asthma, hypertension, angina, and congestive heart failure should be continued throughout the day of surgery. However, as will be discussed, diabetic patients require modification of glucose management. The following are guidelines, although individual practice can vary from locality to locality.

Table 15-3 Selected Perioperative Medications

Name (Generic and Brand)	Uses
Metoclopramide (Reglan)	Relief of gastric paresis, reduction of gastroesophageal reflux, perioperative antiemetic
Cisapride (Propulsid)	Reduction of gastroesophageal reflux
Midazolam (Versed)	Preoperative sedation
Propofol (Diprivan)	Preoperative sedation/general anesthesia
Diazepam (Valium)	Preoperative sedation
Alfentanil (Alfenta)	Analgesic/anesthetic
Fentanyl citrate (Sublimaze)	Analgesic/anesthetic
Methohexital (Brevital Sodium)	Analgesic/anesthetic
Sufentanil (Sufenta)	Analgesic/anesthetic
Ondansetron (Zofran)	Postoperative antiemetic
Ketorolac (Toradol)	Postoperative analgesic

Antihypertensive medications should be continued until the time of surgery to avoid rebound hypertensive crises and the risk of end-organ damage associated with uncontrolled hypertension (specifically myocardial ischemic diseases). Such medications include clonidine (both dermal patch and orally administered), beta blockers, and angiotensin-converting enzyme inhibitors. Oral antihypertensive medications can be taken with a sip of water the day of surgery whether or not the patient is on NPO status.

Digoxin can be withheld the day of surgery for many patients, given its long half-life. However, if a patient is receiving digoxin to control the ventricular response to atrial fibrillation, it is important to be sure that the resting heart rate is appropriate on the morning of surgery; digoxin should be given if the resting heart rate is more than 90 beats per minute.

Anticonvulsant medications should be administered (with sips of water) on the patient's usual schedule because stress and particularly general anesthesia can lower the seizure threshold.

Thyroid medications can be held the day of surgery given their long half-life.

The patient who has taken *systemic corticosteroids* for more than 1 month within the previous 6 months before surgery is customarily "covered" with the equivalent of 300 mg/day of hydrocortisone perioperatively. At the start of the procedure, 100 mg is given intravenously, an additional 100 mg is given at the end of the procedure, and the last 100 mg is administered 6 hours after the end of surgery. Lower doses can be administered for procedures associated with minimal physiologic stress, in the range of 25–30 mg of hydrocortisone intravenously in the first 24 hours after surgery.

In general, *antimicrobial prophylaxis* of bacterial endocarditis in patients with cardiac valvular disease is not necessary for ocular surgery. An exception to this guideline is when there is a chance of exposure to pathogens in the upper respiratory system, such as during dacryocystorhinostomy, orbital surgery, or incision and drainage of infected tissue. Prophylaxis is not recommended for elective oral endotracheal intubation. Mitral valve prolapse without valvular regurgitation is not an indication for prophylaxis.

If a patient does require prophylactic antibiotic treatment for prevention of endocarditis, either the intravenous or the oral route can be used, depending on the situation.

IV *ampicillin* or oral *amoxicillin* can be used. In case of penicillin allergy or intolerance, *clindamycin* or *azithromycin (Zithromax)* can be substituted. For children, consultation with the patient's pediatrician or anesthesiologist should be considered.

As previously mentioned, *management of blood glucose* is important to avoid CNS dysfunction. Whenever possible, insulin-dependent patients should undergo surgery early in the day to allow for postoperative insulin management. Successful perioperative glucose management depends on careful monitoring, and no single regimen works for all patients. Perioperative management of blood glucose during a brief surgical procedure in the *diet-controlled diabetic* generally involves only monitoring of blood glucose immediately perioperatively and every 3 hours until oral intake is resumed.

For cases of relatively well-controlled insulin-requiring diabetes with reasonable glucose control (<250 mg/dL), one option is to hold all short-acting insulin and give half the intermediate- or long-acting insulin the morning of the surgery. It is imperative to provide close preoperative, intraoperative, and postoperative glucose and electrolyte monitoring. Additionally, careful titration of a dextrose 5% in water drip with an initial intravenous rate of 75 mL/hour should prevent hypoglycemia or hyperglycemia. Blood glucose should be monitored hourly and the infusion rate adjusted to maintain glucose at 100–200 mg/dL. Alternatively, for patients who are on insulin and undergoing procedures shorter than 2 hours, the "no insulin, no glucose" regimen works well preoperatively on the morning of surgery. Perioperative monitoring of blood glucose before, during, and after surgery is important. The availability of one-touch monitoring makes such measurements very easy, even in the operating room. During the procedure, intravenous solutions without dextrose (lactated Ringer's or saline) are given. After the surgical procedure, the patient should receive a portion (usually one half or one third) of the usual insulin dose, once oral intake is established. If a procedure lasts more than 2 hours, insulin may have to be given as an infusion of at least 4 units per hour, with monitoring of the blood glucose level every 30–60 minutes. The anesthesiologist and primary care physician should be involved in managing the blood glucose level in such patients.

Oral hypoglycemic medications are usually withheld the day of surgery. These medications have a relatively long duration of action, which could lead to hypoglycemia late in the day if the patient's oral caloric intake is inadequate.

It may be desirable to discontinue diuretics on the day of surgery. A patient under local anesthesia may become uncomfortable from a full bladder caused by a preoperative dose of diuretic. A patient undergoing general anesthesia who continues diuretic use on the morning of surgery may become hypotensive because of intravascular volume depletion prior to surgery.

Drugs that interfere with platelet function should be discontinued, if possible. Aspirin irreversibly acetylates platelet cyclooxygenase. Because cyclooxygenase is not regenerated in the circulation within the lifespan of the platelet, and because this enzyme is essential for the aggregation of platelets, one aspirin may affect platelet function for a week. All other drugs that inhibit platelet function (eg, vitamin E, indomethacin, sulfinpyrazone, dipyridamole, tricyclic antidepressant drugs, phenothiazines, furosemide, steroids) do not inhibit cyclooxygenase function irreversibly; these drugs disturb platelet function for only 24–48 hours. Usually it takes approximately 8 days for platelet function to entirely return to normal after aspirin administration; however, platelet function may become adequate a day or two earlier. If emergency surgery is needed before the 8 day aspirin waiting period or the 2 day period for other drugs has elapsed, consultation with an internist or hematologist, platelet transfusions, or both may be advisable.

The management of anticoagulation in the perioperative setting must be individualized because the risk of thrombosis and the strength of the indication for anticoagulation varies greatly. Therefore, no single regimen satisfies all patient needs and consultation with an internist, family practitioner, or hematologist is advisable. In most patients, warfarin should be stopped 5 days before surgery and the prothrombin time should be checked. As the international normalized ratio level drops below 2.0, heparin therapy with either IV unfractionated heparin or subcutaneous low-molecular-weight heparin should be started and dosed to maintain adequate anticoagulation. Intravenous heparin is discontinued approximately 12 hours prior to surgery and restarted 24 hours after surgery. Low-molecular-weight heparin can be discontinued 12–24 hours prior to surgery and restarted on the first postoperative day. If gastrointestinal function is normal, warfarin may be restarted on the day of surgery. Heparin may be discontinued once therapeutic warfarin levels have been reached.

Nicotinic acid should be discontinued before general anesthesia because it can cause an exaggerated hypotensive response from vasodilation. It is generally taught that *monoamine oxidase (MAO) inhibitors* should be discontinued 2–3 weeks before elective surgery because these medications are associated with an exaggerated hypertensive response to systemically released vasopressors during general anesthesia. In addition, the ephedrine or dopamine that is sometimes needed to increase blood pressure intraoperatively can cause marked elevation in blood pressure in patients who are on MAO inhibitors. The administration of meperidine to patients who are taking MAO inhibitors can result in hyperpyrexia, muscle rigidity, seizures, coma, hypotension, and respiratory depression, probably in response to an increase in cerebral serotonin occurring secondary to MAO inhibition. Nevertheless, there is some debate as to whether MAO inhibitors need to be discontinued in that anesthetic techniques with vasoactive medications other than ephedrine and dopamine can be used to avoid the chance of hypertension or sympathetic stimulation. This is an issue best discussed with the anesthesiologist.

Though echothiophate iodide eyedrops are rarely used today, their use affects the choice of muscle relaxant prior to endotracheal intubations. Ideally, the drops should be stopped 3 weeks before the elective surgery to allow recovery of the cholinesterase enzyme system. However, if echothiophate iodide must be continued, succinylcholine cannot be used during intubations. Alternative medications are available in such cases.

Preoperative Sedation

Preoperative sedation is an important part of comfortable regional or general anesthesia in a patient undergoing elective surgery. Anxiolytics such as midazolam can be given intramuscularly (1–4 mg) 30–60 minutes before the procedure or intravenously (0.5–2.0 mg) 2–3 minutes before the stimulus of the anesthetic block. Midazolam is a more appropriate sedative than diazepam for outpatient surgery because its elimination half-life is 2–4 hours; diazepam's half-life is 20–40 hours. Midazolam can also be reversed with flumazenil. Careful IV titration of sedatives and narcotics is important in the elderly to avoid oversedation or respiratory depression.

Alfentanil can be given intravenously in titrated doses with appropriate anesthesia monitoring. Its peak effect occurs in 1–2 minutes and lasts 10–20 minutes. *Fentanyl citrate,* which has a peak effect in 3–5 minutes and lasts about 30 minutes, is also given in titrated doses for ophthalmic monitored anesthesia. The effects of narcotics can be reversed with the antagonist *naloxone,* given intravenously. The duration of naloxone reversal is 1 hour or less.

Thiopental sodium, given in increments every 30 seconds, can be used to ensure amnesia and hypnosis for regional anesthesia or local infiltration of anesthetic agents. It should be remembered that too rapid or too large a dose can depress hemodynamics and respiration. *Methohexital* can be similarly used in increments given intravenously every 20–30 seconds.

Propofol is a drug with unique properties of rapid hypnosis and a tendency to produce bradycardia, but it has rapid clearance with very little hangover. It must be given through a large-bore vein or administered after a lidocaine flush of the IV line to avoid significant burning on administration. Propofol is a lipid-based medication that supports rapid bacterial growth at room temperature. Indeed, extrinsically contaminated propofol has been associated with postoperative infections including endogenous endophthalmitis. It is therefore imperative that hospital personnel involved in the preparation, handling, and administration of this drug adhere to strict aseptic technique during its use.

Preoperative sedation for children can include midazolam or methohexital.

Intraoperative Complications

Adverse Reactions to Local Anesthesia

Screening for possible allergies to local anesthetic agents was discussed as part of preoperative evaluation. Other types of adverse reactions are discussed below.

Local anesthetic injection into the retrobulbar space can lead to apnea, respiratory arrest, and cranial nerve palsies on the side being injected or even on the opposite side. Anatomic studies of the position of the retrobulbar needle in relation to the optic nerve when the adducted or supraducted position of the eye is used during injection show that it is possible to inject anesthetic into the subdural space with a standard Atkinson-type needle. Cases of cranial nerve palsies in association with respiratory difficulties represent actual brain stem anesthesia from injection of the anesthetic agent into the subdural space, with subsequent diffusion into the circulating cerebrospinal fluid.

Several suggestions have been made to avoid such complications, including changing the traditional positioning of the eye during the retrobulbar anesthetic injection so that the nerve is rotated away from the track of the needle—for example, by having the patient look straight ahead. Using less sharp, nondisposable retrobulbar needles less than 1¼ inch long also reduces the chance of perforating the optic nerve sheath. Although one series implicated the concentration of anesthetic as the cause of respiratory arrest, it is more likely that a larger volume and, therefore, a larger total dose of anesthetic was delivered to the brain stem through an inadvertent subdural injection. The peribulbar technique was devised, in part, to avoid such complications. If apnea, respiratory arrest, or cranial neuropathies occur after a retrobulbar injection, the patient's airway must be supported with mask ventilation. Intubation and mechanical ventilation may be necessary. Apnea seldom lasts more than 30–50 minutes, but it is important that experienced medical personnel stabilize the patient's condition during this time.

Respiratory distress and dysphagia can result from the Nadbath block, an injection into the stylomastoid foramen that is used to provide facial akinesia. These complications occur when the anesthetic agent is injected deeply into the area of the facial nerve as it exits the stylomastoid foramen, and the anesthetic bathes cranial nerves IX, X, and XI as they exit the jugular foramen. This leads to paralysis of these nerves, and the patient becomes dysphagic, begins to cough or has a hoarse voice, and may develop stridor or severe respiratory insufficiency. These complications tend to occur in thin persons, in whom it is easier to bury the needle deeply. Management of the respiratory distress requires suctioning the pharynx, positioning the patient on his or her side, and supplementing the patient's inspired gases with oxygen or even intubation. This complication can be avoided by use of a short hypodermic needle, advancing it only part way into the area to be injected, and injecting a small volume ($<$3 mL).

Anesthetic toxicity can occur when high concentrations of anesthetic agent are given. For example, if 4% lidocaine is used for a peribulbar injection, the total volume that can be safely given to a 70 kg patient is limited to 8 mL. A smaller patient would be able to tolerate no more than 5 mL of 4% lidocaine without risking complications of systemic toxicity, including confusion, cardiac arrhythmias, and respiratory depression.

Seizures have occurred from the intra-arterial injection of local anesthetic agent into the ophthalmic artery. Such seizures are instantaneous with injection; supportive measures should include airway maintenance and blood pressure support. These seizures are of short duration.

Malignant Hyperthermia

As discussed earlier in this chapter, preoperative evaluation can help to identify some patients who are at risk for MH. Nevertheless, such preoperative screening is not infallible, and the surgeon should be prepared to respond to this complication.

MH is a disorder of calcium binding by the sarcoplasmic reticulum of skeletal muscles. In the presence of an anesthetic triggering agent, unbound intracellular calcium increases, which stimulates muscle contracture. This increased metabolism outstrips oxygen delivery, and anaerobic metabolism develops with the production of lactate and subsequent massive acidosis. Hyperthermia thus results from the hypermetabolic state.

The earliest signs of MH include tachycardia that is greater than expected for the patient's anesthetic and surgical status and elevated end-tidal carbon dioxide level when the patient is monitored by capnography. Labile blood pressure, tachypnea, sweating, muscle rigidity, blotchy discoloration of skin, cyanosis, and dark urine all signal progression of the disorder. Temperature elevation, which can reach extremely high levels, is a relatively late sign. Ultimately, respiratory and metabolic acidosis, hyperkalemia, hypercalcemia, myoglobinuria, and renal failure can occur, as can disseminated intravascular coagulation and death.

Although volatile anesthetics such as halothane, enflurane, isoflurane, and intravenous succinylcholine are all known to trigger MH, haloperidol, trimeprazine, and promethazine also can cause MH.

If a surgeon wishes to avoid the use of succinylcholine, a laryngeal mask airway can be considered for strabismus surgery in adults if muscle relaxation is not otherwise required. The use of the laryngeal mask airway reduces the soreness and irritation of the throat that occurs after oral endotracheal intubation.

MH is treated as a medical emergency (see Table 15-4 for the treatment protocol). The Malignant Hyperthermia Association of the United States staffs a 24-hour hotline to advise medical personnel on the diagnosis and treatment of MH at (800) 644-9737.

Postoperative Care

The use of balanced general anesthesia—in which small amounts of several different types of medications are titrated to avoid the side effects of a large dose of any one type—has been effective in reducing prolonged anesthesia and prolonged recovery time. Neuromuscular blocking agents of short duration (12 minutes for mivacurium and 30 minutes for atracurium and vecuronium) administered with an infusion pump allow the anesthesiologist to fine-tune the degree of neuromuscular blockade during balanced anesthesia.

The shorter-acting narcotics such as sufentanil have potencies up to 1000 times that of morphine. These agents help provide short-term stability of hemodynamics during intensive stimulation without the cost of prolonged excessive sedation postoperatively.

Table 15-4 Malignant Hyperthermia Protocol

1. Stop the triggering agents immediately, and conclude surgery as soon as possible.
2. Hyperventilate with 100% oxygen at high flow rates.
3. Administer:
   a. Dantrolene: 2–3 mg/kg initial bolus with increments up to 10 mg/kg total. Continue to administer dantrolene until symptoms are controlled. Occasionally, a dose greater than 10 mg/kg may be needed.
   b. Sodium bicarbonate: 1–2 mEq/kg increments guided by arterial pH and pCO_2. Bicarbonate will combat hyperkalemia by driving potassium into cells.
4. Actively cool patient:
   a. If needed, IV iced saline (not Ringer's lactate) 15 mL/kg q 10 minutes × 3. Monitor closely.
   b. Lavage stomach, bladder, rectum, and peritoneal and thoracic cavities with iced saline.
   c. Surface cool with ice and hypothermia blanket.
5. Maintain urine output. If needed, administer mannitol 0.25 g/kg IV, furosemide 1 mg/kg IV (up to 4 doses each). Urine output greater than 2 mL/kg/hr may help prevent subsequent renal failure.
6. Calcium channel blockers *should not* be given when dantrolene is administered, as hyperkalemia and myocardial depression may occur.
7. Insulin for hyperkalemia: Add 10 units of regular insulin to 50 mL of 50% glucose and titrate to control hyperkalemia. Monitor blood glucose and potassium levels.
8. Postoperatively: Continue dantrolene 1 mg/kg IV q 6 hours × 72 hours to prevent recurrence. Lethal recurrences of MH may occur. Observe in an intensive care unit.
9. For expert medical advice and further medical evaluation, call the MHaus MH hotline consultant at (800) 644–9737. For nonemergency professional or patient information, call (800) 986–4287.

Using such agents immediately before intubation as part of an anesthetic induction has become nearly universal.

Management of postoperative nausea and vomiting after general anesthesia has become easier with more powerful antinausea medications such as ondansetron and metoclopramide. Ondansetron and metoclopramide do not cause sedation as droperidol does, thus speeding recovery of the patient in same-day surgery settings.

Postoperative pain can be prophylactically treated during the procedure with IV ketorolac in a 30–60 mg dose or with small titrated doses of IV fentanyl in the range of 50–100 µg. Because of the reported gastrointestinal complications of higher doses of ketorolac, patients over the age of 60 should receive no more than 30 mg of IV ketorolac, total. Longer-acting narcotics, such as morphine or meperidine, can delay the patient's discharge because of excessive sedation. Also, there is evidence that IV ketorolac, because of its pain-reducing qualities, can reduce the amount of postoperative nausea and vomiting in patients undergoing strabismus surgery and other procedures requiring general anesthetic. There is no evidence that this particular nonsteroidal anti-inflammatory drug increases postoperative bleeding during ophthalmic surgery.

Bennett SN, McNeil MM, Bland LA, et al. Postoperative infections traced to the contamination of an intravenous anesthetic, propofol. *N Engl J Med.* 1995;333(3):147–154.

Everett LL, Kallar SK. Current status of treatment to prevent aspiration in outpatients. *Anesthesiol Clin North Am.* 1996;14:679–693.

Haberkern CM, Lecky JH. Preoperative assessment and the anesthesia clinic. *Anesthesiol Clin North Am.* 1996;14:609–630.

Kay MC, Kay J. Complications of anesthesia for ocular surgery. In: *Ophthalmic Surgery Complications: Prevention and Management.* Philadelphia: Lippincott; 1995.

Miller RD, ed. *Anesthesia.* 5th ed. Philadelphia: Churchill Livingstone; 1999.

Van Norman G. Preoperative management of common minor medical issues in the outpatient setting. *Anesthesiol Clin North Am.* 1996;14:655–677.

CHAPTER 16

Epidemiology and Statistics

The role of clinical research is vital in establishing a standard of care for patients. Such research is best performed using an interdisciplinary approach that combines the efforts of the clinician, statistician, and epidemiologist from the conception of the study through data analyses and interpretation. The choice of study design depends on the research questions to be answered, the population available, and the resources and effort to be expended. If a study finds a statistical association, it may be considered valid after alternative explanations—such as chance, bias, and confounding—have been ruled out. Furthermore, the association may be more credible if it is a consistent finding in other studies.

This chapter aims to provide a general overview of the different types of epidemiologic studies and the more common statistical tests and terms used in clinical research. We hope this discussion will stimulate interested investigators to further explore the field of epidemiologic research. More importantly, the chapter is intended to encourage the clinician to critically review the results of clinical research.

Epidemiology: Definition and Design Strategies

Epidemiology is defined as the study of the occurrence of disease in human populations. Epidemiologic methodology, a powerful tool for clinical research, can be broadly categorized into either descriptive or analytic components. *Descriptive epidemiology,* employed by practitioners for centuries, is the practice of describing the symptoms and quantifying the occurrence of disease. Information is gathered on the distribution of a disease with respect to what part of the population gets the disease, when they get it, and where the disease occurs. This knowledge allows the development of hypotheses concerning the etiology and treatment of the disease. Such hypotheses can be analytically tested via appropriate epidemiologic study designs. Thus, *analytic epidemiology* evaluates factors that may cause or prevent disease by testing the hypotheses generated from descriptive studies.

The analysis of data collected systematically in epidemiologic studies includes determining whether a statistical association exists between the presence or absence of a factor and the disease *(observational studies)* or whether a difference exists between "treated" and "control" groups *(experimental studies).* If a statistical association is observed, it is important to rule out alternative explanations such as luck of the draw *(chance)*, systematic errors in collecting or interpreting the data *(bias)*, or the effects of other associated variables *(confounding).*

Various types of epidemiologic studies are used in clinical research (Table 16-1). As stated earlier, choosing a type depends on the question to be answered, the population available, and the resources and effort to be expended. The various epidemiologic approaches to clinical research, their strengths and weaknesses, and the appropriate situation in which to use each are summarized in Table 16-2.

Hennekens CH, Buring JE. *Epidemiology in Medicine.* Boston: Little Brown; 1987.

Rothman K. *Modern Epidemiology.* Philadelphia: Lippincott-Raven; 1998.

Epidemiologic research design strategies can be categorized as descriptive or analytic. *Descriptive studies* are concerned with the distribution of the disease in relation to person, time, and place. Such descriptive data provide information valuable to health care providers and administrators for developing effective prevention and education programs as well as for allocating appropriate resources. Furthermore, such data are useful in the formulation of hypotheses that may be tested in analytic studies. In *analytic studies,* the investigator designs a direct comparison to determine whether the risk of disease is different for persons exposed or not exposed to a factor of interest. The appropriate use of a comparison group allows for testing epidemiologic hypotheses. Depending on the role of the investigator, analytic studies are further divided into observational (the investigator observes the outcome in subjects with self-selected factors) and experimental, or *interventional,* studies (the investigator purposely manipulates factors that might influence the outcome).

Descriptive Studies

Case reports and case series

A *case report* is the simplest type of descriptive study. A *case series* is a systematic grouping of case reports. These descriptive studies organize information concerning a new disease or raise suspicion about the possible influence of a particular factor or treatment on the disease. Further formulation of hypotheses may then lead to the design of analytic studies to test these hypotheses.

An example of a case report is the initial description of acute uveitis with retinal periarteritis and detachment. Subsequent case series of such patients have established the defined syndrome of acute retinal necrosis. From this knowledge, an etiologic factor such as herpes zoster has been implicated.

Case series of untreated patients with available follow-up data have also been used to define the natural history of a disease. This process, however, has its limitations: many published case series do not have clearly defined eligibility and exclusion criteria, and follow-up is often incomplete in a sizable proportion of patients. A successful case series that illustrates the natural history of a disease is the natural history portion of the Diabetic Retinopathy Vitrectomy Study. This study was designed to assess the risk of visual loss in persons with a specified level of severe diabetic retinopathy. It was considered necessary to ascertain the natural history prior to considering a clinical trial of vitrectomy with retinopathy this severe. Patients with the defined degree of severe diabetic retinopathy were entered into the study and examined at regular visits. This study demonstrated that eyes with specific characteristics of severe diabetic retinopathy are at high risk for severe

Table 16-1   Clinical Research Designs: Types of Studies

	Observational				Experimental
	Case Reports/Series, Natural History	Surveys (Population Based)	Cohort Studies	Studies of Cases and Controls	Clinical Trials
Object*	Diagnostic characteristics, complications, limited natural history, etiology	Prevalence, association between disease and factor (etiology)	Incidence, association between disease and factor (etiology)	Association between disease and factor (etiology)	Evaluation of therapy, diagnostic procedures, preventive measures
Information sought for study analysis*	Variable	Previous and present risk factors, disease status at the time of the survey	Follow-up for development of disease	Disease status, previous and present risk factors	Occurrence for the defined outcome following randomized treatment, complications of therapy
Use of old records*	Possible	Possible	Possible	Possible	No
Dependent on patient's memory*	Possible	For historical questions	Not usually	Usually	No
Study groups	Persons with disease	Total population	Persons with and without factor	Diseased (cases) and not diseased (controls)	Treated and controls
Sample size (depends on likelihood of disease outcome)*	Variable	Large	Large	Small	Variable (depending on treatment efficacy and likelihood of "events" in the controls)
Risk estimate	Absolute and relative risk of developing complications	Absolute and relative risk of having disease	Absolute and relative risk of developing disease	Relative risk of developing disease	Risks and benefits of therapy

* This is usual; variations are possible.

Table 16-2 Strengths and Weaknesses of Clinical Research Designs

Design	Strengths	Weaknesses
Case report or series	Description of a new aspect of an old disease, or description of clinical characteristics of a new disease	Cannot assess the effects of treatment or risk factor without a concurrent control group
Cohort studies	Useful for common diseases, especially with respect to outcomes; internal comparison group present	Generally requires large sample size and lengthy follow-up; costly in terms of time and money
Case-control studies	Suitable for rare diseases and for studying a variety of risk factors; efficient in use of time and money	Subject to bias (selection bias of cases and controls and information bias)
Clinical trial	Randomization of subjects to treatment provides concurrent controls who are comparable to the treated group in every aspect except for treatment. This comparison group is essential in the assessment of therapeutic effects.	Costly in terms of money and time; potential for loss to follow-up

visual loss. These characteristics, found in a descriptive study, were then used to develop major eligibility criteria for entry into a randomized clinical trial (analytic design strategy) to evaluate the beneficial effects of vitrectomy in such eyes.

In a series of patients who underwent decompression for ischemic optic neuropathy, the results suggested a possible beneficial effect. However, a randomized, controlled, clinical trial found that decompression was not only ineffective but possibly harmful. This illustrates how the case series may be important in identifying a potential risk factor and generating a hypothesis, but the association of the specific factor with disease remains unproven until analytical assessment is conducted.

> Culbertson WW, Blumenkranz MS, Haines H, et al. The acute retinal necrosis syndrome. Part 2: Histopathology and etiology. *Ophthalmology*. 1982;89:1317–1325.
>
> Diabetic Retinopathy Vitrectomy Study Research Group. Two-year course of visual acuity in severe proliferative diabetic retinopathy with conventional management. *Ophthalmology*. 1985;92:492–502.
>
> Ischemic Optic Neuropathy Decompression Trial Research Group. Optic nerve decompression surgery for nonarteritic anterior ischemic optic neuropathy (NAION) is not effective and may be harmful. *JAMA*. 1995;273:625–632.

Surveys

Surveys measure the *prevalence* of a disease—that is, the number of cases of a disease present in a defined population at a specified time. In addition, information on the characteristics of the disease as well as on characteristics of the population may be used to study possible associations between the disease and various risk factors. However, this type of study can only demonstrate associations and not impute cause and effect because the risk factor found may be the cause of the disease or the result of the disease, or it may simply coexist with the disease. Associations may be used to formulate hypotheses to be tested by analytic studies.

Because surveys are based on population, they require either the examination of each person in the population or everyone in a specifically defined subgroup. To the extent that some persons may not be available for examination, the accuracy of the prevalence estimate is diminished. Other factors limiting the success of a survey are the techniques used to identify the population to be studied and the methods used to motivate those selected to participate in the examination process or interview.

An example of a successful cross-sectional survey is the Wisconsin Epidemiologic Study of Diabetic Retinopathy. Attempts were made to identify all known diabetic persons in several counties in southern Wisconsin. A random sample of this group was then selected, and efforts were made to examine each of the identified persons. The main goal of this study was to determine the prevalence of various types of retinopathy in this population of diabetic persons and to identify risk factors, such as the degree of hyperglycemia or hypertension, which might be associated with more severe retinopathy.

If the goal of a survey is to determine disease prevalence for a general population rather than for a segment of the population (such as diabetics), the sample to be examined must be drawn from the overall population. The Health and Nutrition Examination Survey and the Visual Acuity Impairment Study, both performed in cooperation with the United States Bureau of the Census, are examples of population-based studies. As noted earlier, the success of a survey depends on appropriately identifying a representative sampling of the population to be studied and motivating the selected persons to participate in the study.

Another population-based study is the Baltimore Eye Survey. This study compared the prevalence of primary open-angle glaucoma between black residents and white residents of east Baltimore. Previous clinical studies had supported a growing acceptance that blacks were at a higher risk for glaucoma than whites, and the Baltimore Eye Survey confirmed this clinical impression. Using comprehensive examination techniques in population-based samples of blacks and whites, researchers found the rate of primary open-angle glaucoma in black Americans to be four to five times higher than in whites. The comprehensive examination techniques maximized the sensitivity and specificity of the diagnosis of primary open-angle glaucoma.

Additional population-based studies of chronic age-related eye diseases include the Beaver Dam Eye Study (Wisconsin), the Rotterdam Study (the Netherlands), and the Blue Mountain Eye Study (Australia). Important information regarding the prevalence of disorders such as age-related cataract and age-related macular degeneration (AMD) are collected in these well-conducted surveys. The prevalence data appear to be similar in these studies of different populations.

Attebo K, Mitchell P, Smith W. Visual acuity and the cause of vision loss in Australia. The Blue Mountain Eye Study. *Ophthalmology.* 1996;103:357–364.

Ganley J, Roberts J. Eye conditions and related need for medical care among persons 1–74 years of age. *United States: Vital and Health Statistics,* Series 11, No 2287. Washington, DC: Department of Health and Human Services Pub No 83-1678.

Klaver CC, Wolfs RC, Vinglerling JR, et al. Age-specific prevalence and causes of blindness and visual impairment in an older population: the Rotterdam Study. *Arch Ophthalmol.* 1998;116:653–658.

Klein R, Klein BEK, Moss SE, et al. The relationship of age-related maculopathy, cataract, and glaucoma to visual acuity. The Beaver Dam Eye Study. *Invest Ophthalmol Vis Sci.* 1995; 36:183–191.

Klein R, Klein BEK, Moss SE, et al. The Wisconsin Epidemiologic Study of Diabetic Retinopathy. II. Prevalence and risk of diabetic retinopathy when age at diagnosis is less than 30 years. *Arch Ophthalmol.* 1984;102:520–526.

Klein R, Klein BEK, Moss SE, et al. The Wisconsin Epidemiologic Study of Diabetic Retinopathy. III. Prevalence and risk of diabetic retinopathy when age at diagnosis is 30 or more years. *Arch Ophthalmol.* 1984;102:527–532.

Tielsch JM, Sommer A, Katz J, et al. Racial variations in the prevalence of primary open-angle glaucoma. The Baltimore Eye Survey. *JAMA.* 1991;266:369–374.

Visual Acuity Impairment Survey Pilot Study. *Biometry & Epidemiology.* National Eye Institute/National Institutes of Health, Department of Health and Human Services. Washington, DC: US Government Printing Office; 1984.

Analytic Design

Observational

Analytic studies can be experimental or observational. There are two basic types of observational analytic studies: cohort and case-control.

Cohort studies In cohort, or follow-up, studies, persons who are initially free of the disease under study are followed over a period of time, during which some subjects develop the disease. Groups are defined at study entry on the basis of the presence or absence of exposure to possible risk factors. Examples could be those who are hypertensive versus those who are not, or those with elevated hemoglobin A_{1c} versus those with less elevated hemoglobin A_{1c}.

The analysis of data from cohort studies results in a calculation of the incidence of the disease in the cohort. The number of new cases observed during the specified period of follow-up is divided by the number of persons at risk for the disease. The incidence in the group with a positive exposure or with a specific risk factor divided by the incidence in the group without the risk factor is called the *relative risk*, which is a primary statistic used to assess whether the risk factor is associated with the disease. When the relative risk is significantly greater than 1.0, the factor is thought to be associated with the development of the disease; when the relative risk is significantly less than 1.0, the factor is associated with not developing the disease.

Because all persons in a cohort study are disease free at the outset of the study, the researcher can document that exposure to a risk factor predated development of the disease. However, cohort studies require following large numbers of persons over long periods to observe an adequate number of cases developing the disease. The cost in terms of money and time is a major drawback of the cohort study. In addition, because persons must be followed for long periods, even as long as decades, there is a great potential for introducing bias as a result of losses in follow-up. This study design is best suited for a relatively common disease that can be expected to develop in a large proportion of the study group during the follow-up period.

An early and important example of a cohort study is the Framingham Heart Study: 5209 residents of Framingham, Massachusetts, between the ages of 30 and 62 (at the beginning of the study), were followed every 2 years to assess a wide variety of possible cardiovascular risk factors such as hypertension, cigarette smoking, and blood cholesterol levels. The subjects were all initially free of cardiovascular disease. Over the next 35 years, all cardiovascular events were ascertained, and incidence rates and relative risks were calculated. For example, among persons with diastolic blood pressure (at first examination) of 90 mm Hg or greater, the incidence rate of myocardial infarction, adjusted for age and sex, was several times the rate among persons with diastolic blood pressure that was less than 90 mm Hg. This was one of the earliest studies to demonstrate the association between cardiovascular disease and hypertension.

An example of a cohort study concerning eye diseases is the Wisconsin Epidemiologic Study of Diabetic Retinopathy (already mentioned). Persons in whom diabetes mellitus was diagnosed in the original survey were reexamined 4 years and then 10 years later. The objectives of this cohort study were to examine the incidence and progression of diabetic retinopathy and to determine the relationships between incidence and progression of diabetic retinopathy and risk factors. Of patients in whom diabetes mellitus was diagnosed at age 30 or older who were free of retinopathy at the baseline examination, 47% of insulin users and 34% of nonusers had developed retinopathy by the 4 year visit.

Other studies have shown that the most potent risk variable for prevalence and incidence of diabetic retinopathy is the duration of diabetes. In the Wisconsin cohort study, this characteristic was found to be an important predictor during the 4 years of observation, but it did not have a consistent linear effect on the rate of development or on the rate of progression. A likely explanation is the increasing rates of mortality in older patients. As stated earlier, this cohort study was composed of subjects whose diagnosis of diabetes mellitus was made at age 30 or older. Because 25% had died during the 4-year interval, only 72% of this group of patients participated in the follow-up visit. In the study of patients with onset of diabetes at a younger age, 82% participated in the follow-up examination. Death accounted for the majority of the nonparticipation rate in this cohort study. Nevertheless, the incidence and progression rates for diabetic retinopathy provided important information for future studies (ie, clinical trials) and for planners of health care.

This study was further extended to include 10 and 14 years of follow-up, showing an increase in the incidence of clinically significant diabetic eye disease. A number of risk factors (systemic or ocular risk factors) were also analyzed for association with diabetic retinopathy. These data are important for planning future clinical trials and for health care administrators who allocate resources for these conditions.

The Framingham Study. An Epidemiological Investigation of Cardiovascular Disease. Department of Health, Education & Welfare (National Institutes of Health). Washington, DC: US Government Printing Office; 1975. Pub No 74-478.

Klein R, Klein BEK, Moss SE, et al. The Wisconsin Epidemiologic Study of Diabetic Retinopathy. IX. Four-year incidence and progression of diabetic retinopathy when age at diagnosis is less than 30 years. *Arch Ophthalmol.* 1989;107:237–243.

Klein R, Klein BEK, Moss SE, et al. The Wisconsin Epidemiologic Study of Diabetic Retinopathy. X. Four-year incidence and progression of diabetic retinopathy when age at diagnosis is 30 years or more. *Arch Ophthalmol.* 1989;107:244–249.

Klein R, Klein BEK, Moss SE, et al. The Wisconsin Epidemiologic Study of Diabetic Retinopathy. XIV. Ten-year incidence and progression of diabetic retinopathy. *Arch Ophthalmol.* 1994;112:1217–1228.

Moss SE, Klein R, Klein BEK. Ten-year incidence of visual loss in a diabetic population. *Ophthalmology.* 1994;101:1061–1070.

Studies of cases and controls In a case-control study, sometimes referred to as a *retrospective study*, subjects are selected on the basis of the presence (case) or absence (control) of disease. The two groups are then compared with respect to the proportion having a particular characteristic or exposure factor. A statistic called the *odds ratio* is calculated from the data, based on the presence or absence of the exposure factor among the cases and the controls. The odds ratio is similar to the relative risk calculated in a cohort study. If statistically the odds ratio is significantly greater or less than 1.0, the factor is said to be either positively or negatively associated with the disease. If the odds ratio is not significantly different from 1.0, there is no evidence that the factor and the disease are associated.

A type of case-control study that determines the presence or absence of a risk factor at the time of the examination is called a *cross-sectional study*. Both case-control and cross-sectional studies use cases and controls. They differ in that within the case-control study format an effort is made to ascertain that the exposure to the suspected risk factor (eg, history of cigarette smoking) predated the onset of the disease; in the cross-sectional format, the factor and the disease coexist (eg, current cigarette smoking regardless of past history, or the measurement of current blood pressure or serum cholesterol). Often, retrospective and cross-sectional elements are combined in a single study of cases and controls.

A study of AMD by Hyman and coworkers (1983) is one example of a study of cases and controls. Patients with AMD were identified at 34 ophthalmologists' offices. An equal number of age- and sex-matched controls were also selected from the same offices. Presence or absence of AMD was documented by retinal photographs. Historical information—such as family history of AMD, history of various medical problems, and exposure to a number of environmental risk factors—was ascertained. In addition, present conditions such as refractive errors, current blood pressure, handgrip strength, and iris color were collected in the cross-sectional aspect. A positive association was found between several of the factors studied and the presence of AMD. A subsequent study of cases and controls by Hyman and associates found an association between hypertension and AMD; this risk factor was not found in the initial case-control study. Another case-control study, performed as a nested study within a cohort study at baseline, confirmed the association of hypertension with AMD.

Hyman L, Lilienfield AM, Ferris FL III, et al. Senile macular degeneration: a case-control study. *Am J Epidemiol.* 1983;118:213–227.

Hyman L, Schachat AP, He Q, et al. Hypertension, cardiovascular disease, and age-related macular degeneration. *Arch Ophthalmol.* 2000;118:351–358.

A disadvantage of the case-control study is the difficulty of establishing the temporal relationship between an exposure factor and a disease, despite efforts to ascertain risk factors that might have predated the disease. Iris color, for example, is a risk factor that can be assessed after disease diagnosis but that almost certainly predated the development of the disease. In contrast, intraocular pressure (IOP) could well be modified by the presence of a disease and cannot be assumed to have been the same prior to the development of the disease. An effective way to minimize such problems is the selection of cases prospectively as they occur *(incident cases)*. An example of such a technique is a case-control study of the relative risk of ulcerative keratitis among users of soft contact lenses. Cases were defined to be soft contact lens users with newly diagnosed ulcerative keratitis who were evaluated at six university ophthalmologic centers between November 1986 and November 1987. The use of these incident cases provided advantages in that the risk factors examined in the study were more likely to be related to the development of the disease and not to the duration of the disease once it had developed (ie, prognosis). In addition, the use of incident cases minimized the time between the development of the condition and the interview, which provided more accurate reporting of the information on prior exposures.

Schein OD, Glynn RJ, Poggio EC, et al. The relative risk of ulcerative keratitis among users of daily-wear and extended-wear soft contact lenses: a case-control study. Microbial Keratitis Study Group. *N Engl J Med.* 1989;321:773–778.

Of all the analytic studies, the case-control study has the greatest potential for bias, especially in the selection of cases and controls. It is important to consider possible sources of bias prior to starting a case-control study. In the study of risk factors for cataract (The Lens Opacities Case-Control Study), cases were not selected from patients undergoing cataract surgery because the reasons that lead to patient selection and referral for surgery may cause biases that are difficult to assess. In addition, the selection of controls for such cases may be difficult. The cases and controls for the cataract study were selected from the same general eye services of outpatient clinics in order to increase comparability on socioeconomic, demographic, health care utilization, and other factors. Misclassification of these cases and controls was minimized by a system of lens classification based on clinical examination and centralized grading of lens photographs. Among the factors found to be associated with less extensive lens opacities were use of multivitamins and dietary intake of antioxidant vitamins. This association was further tested and confirmed by adjusting for age, sex, race, and education. This finding demonstrates an association of vitamin use and lens opacities; because of possible biases or confounding, however, the finding does not necessarily imply that decreased intake of antioxidant vitamins potentially causes cataracts, nor does it follow that the disease process is prevented or retarded by the use of such vitamins. A randomized clinical trial must be designed to address such questions.

Leske MC, Chylack LT Jr, Wu SY, et al. The Lens Opacities Case-Control Study. Risk factors for cataract. *Arch Ophthalmol.* 1991;109:244–251.

In the Eye Disease Case-Control Study, patients with high serum levels of carotenoids had a reduced rate of neovascular AMD compared with patients with low serum levels of carotenoids. This association was statistically significant at the level of $P < .0001$. However, this association does not imply a causal relationship of carotenoids to AMD.

Again, the only way to prove that antioxidants may play an etiologic role in AMD is by assessing them in a randomized controlled clinical trial. The Age-Related Eye Disease Study is such a study designed to evaluate the role of antioxidants and minerals in the treatment of both AMD and cataract. Thus far, the results of the randomized portion of the natural history study of the Age-Related Eye Disease Study indeed show a significant beneficial effect of treatment with antioxidant vitamins (vitamin C, 500 mg; vitamin E, 440 IU; beta carotene, 15 mg or 25,000 IU) and minerals (zinc oxide, 80 mg, and cupric oxide, 2 mg) for the treatment of age-related macular degeneration. At 5 years of follow-up, the risk of developing advanced AMD was reduced by 25% and the risk of vision loss of 15 or more letters on the logMAR visual acuity chart was reduced by 19% by the combination treatment of vitamins and minerals compared with placebo controls. Previous epidemiologic studies showed a strong protective effect of vitamins for lens opacities, but in this randomized, controlled clinical trial, no treatment effect, neither beneficial nor harmful, was found for the treatment of cataracts. This is a good example of the power of the controlled clinical trial to evaluate the causal relationship of factors determined in epidemiologic studies.

Age-Related Eye Disease Study Group: Design Paper: The Age-Related Eye Disease Study (AREDS): Design Implications. AREDS Report No. 1. *Control Clin Trials.* 1999;20:573–600.

Age-Related Eye Disease Study Research Group. A randomized, placebo-controlled, clinical trial of high-dose supplementation with vitamins C and E, beta carotene, and zinc for age-related macular degeneration and vision loss. *Arch Ophthalmol.* 2001;119:1417–1436.

Age-Related Eye Disease Study Research Group. A randomized, placebo-controlled, clinical trial of high-dose supplementation with vitamins C and E, beta carotene, and zinc for age-related cataract and vision loss. *Arch Ophthalmol.* 2001;119:1439–1452.

Age-Related Eye Disease Study Research Group. Risk factors associated with age-related macular degeneration. A case-control study in the Age-Related Eye Disease Study: Age-Related Eye Disease Study Report No. 3. *Ophthalmology.* 2000;107:2224–2232.

Eye Disease Case-Control Study Group. Antioxidant status and neovascular age-related macular degeneration. *Arch Ophthalmol.* 1993:111:104–109.

When potential sources of bias in selection of cases and controls and in the ascertainment of historical information are recognized and minimized in both the design and the analysis of the study, case-control studies are a valuable tool in clinical research. Unlike cohort studies, case-control studies are efficient in terms of time and expense. This design is suitable for studying rare diseases. It is also useful in testing a variety of exposure factors among the diseased and controls, making it particularly suitable for early investigations of the risk factors of a disease.

Experimental, or interventional, study (clinical trial)

The experimental, or interventional, study is a prospective study in which the investigator assigns the exposure factor or the treatment. This type of study is also known as a *clinical trial.* It is defined as a prospective study comparing the effect and value of interventions against a control in human subjects. Rarely does the introduction of a new therapy or procedure produce such unequivocal results as that of penicillin in the treatment of pneumococcal pneumonia. More often, the effects of therapy are much smaller but still clinically important and significant. Observational studies may fail to demonstrate such a beneficial effect, whereas randomized clinical trials reveal the strongest epidemiologic evidence of the beneficial effect.

Friedman LM, Furberg CD, DeMets DL. *Fundamentals of Clinical Trials.* 3rd ed. St Louis: Mosby; 1996.

Meinert CL, Tonascia S. *Clinical Trials. Design, Conduct, and Analysis.* New York: Oxford University Press; 1986.

In a clinical trial, the researcher generally selects a study population that is at high risk for the outcome or response variable. Eligibility criteria for inclusion in the study must be clearly defined at the beginning of the study. Treatment, which should be standardized, is ideally allocated by randomization, which helps to ensure that the treatment groups are similar to the control group in all respects except for treatment. Data from baseline and subsequent visits must be collected systematically, preferably by trained personnel. The response or outcome variable that is to be measured must also be clearly defined. To prevent bias, the outcome variable should be objectively assessed by someone who is unaware of the treatment assignment.

Sample size calculations must be performed in the initial development phase of all analytic studies, but they are particularly important in a clinical trial. A trial must have a sufficiently large sample size to have adequate statistical power to detect differences between groups considered to be of clinical interest. These calculations are essential to planning a clinical trial. (Sample size calculations and power are explained later in this chapter.)

During follow-up, the proportion of individuals in each study group who experience the predetermined outcome is calculated and the effects of the intervention are compared. Monitoring of noncompliance and adverse side effects is important. The problem of loss to follow-up must be addressed when the selection of the study population and the nature of the intervention are being considered because a high follow-up rate is essential to the success of the study.

Analysis of clinical trials is similar to that of cohort studies, wherein the comparison is between the rates of the outcome of interest in the treated (exposed) group(s) and the corresponding rates in the control (unexposed) group. As a result of randomization, the comparison groups are likely to be similar in all aspects other than treatment. A crucial initial step in analysis involves comparing the groups to ensure that important baseline characteristics are indeed balanced. Once subjects are randomized to a particular group, they will remain in that group for analysis, regardless of whether they drop out or become noncompliant ("once randomized, always analyzed"). It is important to minimize noncompliance and drop-out rates and to attempt to ascertain complete information.

The disadvantage of interventional studies is the enormous cost in expense and time. However, carefully designed clinical trials, involving adequate numbers of randomized subjects, provide the most powerful epidemiologic evidence of the effects of an intervention.

One example of an interventional study in ophthalmology is the Diabetic Retinopathy Study (DRS), a randomized, controlled clinical trial to evaluate photocoagulation treatment for proliferative diabetic retinopathy. (This study is also discussed in BCSC Section 12, *Retina and Vitreous.*) Between 1972 and 1975, 1758 patients were enrolled and follow-up was continued until 1979. Eligible patients had proliferative diabetic retinopathy in at least one eye or severe nonproliferative retinopathy in both eyes and visual acuity of 20/100 or better in each eye. One eye was randomized to immediate photocoagulation with either xenon arc or argon laser photocoagulation; the fellow untreated eye acted as the control. At 4 month intervals, an examiner who was not aware of the treatment status of the eyes obtained best-corrected visual acuity. The primary outcome variable measured was "severe visual loss," defined as visual acuity of less than 5/200 at two or more consecutively completed follow-up visits.

In 1976, a change of protocol was implemented because the incidence of severe visual loss in the treated eyes was reduced by 50% or more compared with the control eyes. At this change of protocol, eyes with certain characteristics were observed to be at particularly high risk for severe visual loss. The data and safety monitoring committee recommended that treatment no longer be withheld from eyes with high-risk characteristics that had initially been randomized to no treatment. Thus, the DRS, a randomized controlled clinical trial, successfully demonstrated the efficacy of photocoagulation in the treatment of proliferative diabetic retinopathy and identified a high-risk group of persons with diabetes for whom photocoagulation was indicated.

Adverse side effects, such as visual field loss and persistent decrease of visual acuity associated with argon and xenon photocoagulation, were also carefully documented in the DRS. The rates of adverse side effects for these two different types of treatments were also compared; the xenon group was found to have higher rates of harmful effects.

The subsequent clinical trial of treatment of diabetic retinopathy, the Early Treatment Diabetic Retinopathy Study (ETDRS), evaluated the timing of photocoagulation during the course of diabetic retinopathy, the efficacy of photocoagulation for diabetic macular edema, and the role of aspirin in altering the course of diabetic retinopathy. (This study is discussed in BCSC Section 12, *Retina and Vitreous.*)

The aspirin portion of the ETDRS consisted of randomly assigning each patient to 650 mg of aspirin or placebo. Compliance with study medication was assessed with laboratory studies such as serum thromboxane B_2 and urine salicylate levels at annual visits and with counts of pills and patient interviews at each clinic visit. The results of these tests showed that 80% of the patients were taking prescribed study medications, a compliance level similar to that reported for other trials of aspirin. The primary endpoint for assessing the effect of aspirin on the course of diabetic retinopathy was the development of high-risk proliferative retinopathy. The relative risk of high-risk proliferative retinopathy for patients assigned to aspirin compared with patients assigned to placebo is 0.97 with a 99% confidence interval of 0.85–1.11. Thus, there was no difference between the treated and the untreated group because the confidence interval included 1.0.

The power of this study to detect a 25% treatment effect as estimated during the design phase of the study was 99%, given the sample size and projected event rates of 40%. After adjustments were made for noncompliance with study medications and the actual outcome rates, the study had power to detect a 25% treatment effect. When negative results of a clinical trial are presented, it is important to report the study's power to detect the proposed clinical difference. (Confidence interval and power are discussed at greater length later in the chapter.)

The Diabetes Control and Complications Trial (DCCT) was another important clinical trial of diabetic retinopathy. The DCCT evaluated the role of intensive management and control of hyperglycemia in preventing the development or progression of diabetic retinopathy. Previous observational studies in humans and animal studies of experimental models of diabetes suggested that intensive treatment of hyperglycemia was important in preventing the progression of diabetic retinopathy. Only through this randomized, controlled clinical trial were the beneficial effects of intensive treatment of hyperglycemia proven. Intensive treatment reduced the incidence of development and progression of diabetic retinopathy, loss of vision, and the need for photocoagulation. Intensive management of hyperglycemia also significantly reduced other secondary endpoints, including diabetic nephropathy, neuropathy, and macrovascular diseases. The DCCT provided important guidelines for the treatment of complications for persons with type 1 diabetes mellitus. (Again, this trial is also discussed in BCSC Section 12, *Retina and Vitreous.*)

The importance of glycemic control is emphasized by the long-term follow-up of this population of subjects with type 1 diabetes enrolled in the DCCT. Four years following the end of the clinical trial, an epidemiologic study, the Epidemiology of Diabetes Interventions and Complications Research, documented that reduction of the risk of progression of diabetic retinopathy and nephropathy with type 1 diabetes continued to be as much as 72%–87%. Again, careful follow-up is needed to obtain such important information.

Another landmark study of glycemic control in patients with type 2 diabetes, the United Kingdom Prospective Diabetes Study, showed that intensive therapy to control glucose also reduced the rates of microvascular complications of diabetes—namely, diabetic retinopathy, nephropathy, and neuropathy—in this older population. Furthermore, a subset of patients was randomized to tight versus standard treatment of elevated blood pressure. A modest reduction of the blood pressure compared with the standard treatment showed that the rate of progression of diabetic retinopathy was decreased by as much as 37%. Previous observational studies did not show a consistent association of diabetic retinopathy with hypertension, but this randomized clinical trial established the importance of controlling hypertension in terms of the progression of diabetic retinopathy.

Another clinical trial in ophthalmology evaluated the common use of corticosteroids to treat optic neuritis. (This trial is discussed in BCSC Section 5, *Neuro-Ophthalmology.*) The following research questions were posed by the investigators:

- Does treatment with either oral prednisone or intravenous methylprednisolone improve visual outcome in acute optic neuritis?
- Does either treatment speed the recovery of vision?
- What are the complications of treatment in relation to its efficacy?

Visual field, the primary measure of outcome, was graded in a masked fashion by a central reading center. Best-corrected visual acuity was obtained by technicians who were unaware of the treatment assignment. Results of this clinical trial showed that intravenous methylprednisolone followed by oral prednisone accelerated the recovery of visual loss from optic neuritis and resulted in slightly better vision at 6 months. However, oral prednisone alone actually increased the risk of new episodes of optic neuritis. These findings were somewhat surprising because a mail survey performed in 1986 of ophthalmologists and neurologists in Michigan and Florida indicated that 65% of the ophthalmologists and 90% of the neurologists prescribed corticosteroids for optic neuritis.

As mentioned, the case-control study can provide valuable information about the possible association of certain risk factors with the disease being studied, but such observational studies cannot provide conclusive data as to the causal role of the risk factor. An example of this is seen in the Alpha-Tocopherol, Beta Carotene Cancer Prevention Study, sponsored by the National Institutes of Health (NIH) and performed in Finland. Rates of lung cancer were higher in patients with lower serum levels of both vitamin E and beta carotene at baseline (a nested case-control evaluation). However, when these patients were randomly assigned the two antioxidants and followed for 5–8 years, no beneficial effect in reducing the rates of lung cancer was found in the treated group. In fact, the patients receiving beta carotene had increased rates of lung cancer and mortality. This was similar to the results of another large NIH-sponsored study of vitamin E and vitamin A treatment to prevent lung cancer, the Carotene and Retinol Efficacy Trial. The results of these two studies emphasize the need for randomized controlled clinical trials to evaluate the validity of associations seen in observational studies such as the case-control studies.

The Alpha-Tocopherol, Beta Carotene Cancer Prevention Study Group. The effect of vitamin E and beta carotene on the incidence of lung cancer and other cancers in male smokers. *N Engl J Med.* 1994;330:1029–1235.

Beck RW, Cleary PA, Anderson MM, et al. A randomized, controlled trial of corticosteroids in the treatment of acute optic neuritis. *N Engl J Med.* 1992;326:581–588.

The Diabetes Control and Complications Trial Research Group. The effect of intensive treatment of diabetes on the development and progression of long-term complications in insulin-dependent diabetes mellitus. *N Engl J Med.* 1993;329:977–986.

The Diabetes Control and Complications Trial/Epidemiology of Diabetes Interventions and Complications Research Group. Retinopathy and nephropathy in patients with type 1 diabetes four years after a trial of intensive therapy. *N Engl J Med.* 2000;342:381–389.

The Early Treatment Diabetic Retinopathy Study Research Group. Effects of aspirin treatment on diabetic retinopathy. ETDRS Report Number 8. *Ophthalmology.* 1991;98:757–765.

Omenn GS, Goodman GE, Thornquist MD, et al. Effects of a combination of beta carotene and vitamin A on lung cancer and cardiovascular disease. *N Engl J Med.* 1996;334:1150–1155.

UK Prospective Diabetes Study Group. Intensive blood-glucose control with sulphonylureas or insulin compared with conventional treatment and risk of complications in patients with Type 2 diabetes (UKPDS 33). *Lancet.* 1998;352:837–853.

UK Prospective Diabetes Study Group. Tight blood pressure control and risk of macrovascular and microvascular complications in type 2 diabetes: UKPDS 38. *BMJ.* 1998;317:703–713.

Statistical Terminology

To critically review the medical literature, the reader should understand the more commonly used statistical terms and methods.

Mean

The mean (arithmetic mean) is one of the most widely used and understood ways of describing the average, or central, tendency of a set of data. The sum of values of a set of individual observations is divided by the number of values. For example, the mean age for cataract extraction is 65.7 years.

Median

The median has the connotation of the "middlemost" or "most central" value of a set of numbers; it is the value that divides the set so that one half is smaller and one half is larger. With an odd number of observations, the median is directly ascertainable. With an even number of items, there are two central values; by convention, the arithmetic mean of these two central values is designated the median.

Mode

The mode is a conceptually useful term, but often it is not calculated explicitly. The mode is the observation that occurs with the greatest frequency. The mode of a frequency distribution has the connotation of a "typical" or representative value, a location in the distribution at which there is maximal clustering. In this application, if a frequency distribution is symmetrical (a bell curve), the mode, the median, and the mean coincide. However, in a skewed distribution, the mean is pulled away from the mode toward the extreme values. If more than one mode appears, the frequency distribution is described as *multimodal.* If there are two modes, the frequency distribution is called *bimodal.* Bimodal distributions would result, for example, by merging the weight data for men and women. Often, the observation of a bimodal distribution suggests that two different "causes" are present and that two distinct distributions should be recognized.

Distribution

A *normal curve, normal distribution,* or *gaussian distribution* describes a symmetrical distribution (eg, mean, median, and mode are the same) of great utility in statistics. The graph of the normal distribution forms a bell-shaped curve, symmetrical around an ordinate erected at the mean (which, of course, lies at the center of the distribution). If the total area under the graph of a normal curve is equal to 1.0, one half of the area (representing probability) lies to the left or right of the mean and the probability is 0.5 that a value will fall below or above the mean (μ).

Variance and standard deviation

Although the central tendency, as measured by the various averages already discussed, is an important descriptive characteristic of statistical data, it is not the only measure required to completely specify the distribution of observations. The most common probability distribution encountered in medical literature is the normal distribution. Although the specification of the normal distribution's average or mean is important, some measure of the spread of the observations must also be given. The most commonly used measures of an average dispersion from some measure of central tendency are the variance and the standard deviation:

$$\sigma = \left[\frac{\Sigma (x - \mu)^2}{(N - 1)} \right]^{1/2}$$

The *standard deviation* (σ) of a normal distribution may be used with the mean to indicate the percentage of items that fall within specified ranges. The following relationships apply for a population of observations that form a normal distribution:

μ (mean) + σ includes 68.3% of all items
μ (mean) + 2σ includes 95.5% of all items
μ (mean) + 3σ includes 99.7% of all items

For populations with normal distribution, 5% of values lie at least 1.96 standard deviations (σ) away from the mean. This concept is important because it is the basis for many statistical tests. Because the curve is symmetrical, 2.5% of the population is at this distance either above or below the mean. The variance of a distribution is the square of its standard deviation, σ^2.

The variance (σ^2) of observations in a population is the arithmetic mean of the squared deviations of each observation (x) from the population mean (μ). However, the observer rarely knows the true population mean. More likely, the observer has some estimate of this quantity, the sample mean (x). Thus, just as the population mean is estimated by the sample mean, so the population variance is estimated by the sample variance (σ^2). Although the sample variance measures the extent of variation in values of a set of observations, it is described in units of squared deviation or squares of the original numbers.

To obtain a measure of dispersion in terms of the units of the original data, the positive square root of the variance is taken. The resultant measure is known as the standard deviation. Numerically, the standard error of the mean of a sample is calculated as the estimated standard deviation divided by the square root of the number of observations:

$$\text{Standard error} = \frac{\text{Standard deviation}}{\sqrt{n}}$$

Statistical Analyses

Chi-Square Tests

Chi-square (χ^2) tests provide a basis for judging whether more than two sampled population proportions can be considered equal. The mathematical derivations behind chi-square tests are beyond the scope of this text. However, two fundamental generalities are at its heart: tests of goodness of fit and tests of independence. *Tests of goodness of fit* provide the method for deciding whether a particular theoretical probability distribution (such as a normal curve) is a close enough approximation to a sample frequency distribution for that theoretical distribution to describe the population from which the sample was drawn. *Tests of independence* help the statistician to decide whether a hypothesis of independence between different variables is tenable. The entire chi-square sequence tests the equality of more than two population proportions. Thus, chi-square tests may reveal that a set of observed frequencies differs so greatly from a set of theoretical frequencies that the hypothesis under which the theoretical frequencies were derived should be rejected.

The chi-square test is a useful, simple test, but it has limited power. For example, following cataract extraction, the expected incidence of cystoid macular edema (CME) is 15%. In a series of 100 patients pretreated with aspirin, CME occurred in 10 patients. Does that observation indicate a statistically significant benefit for treatment? (Chi-square = 0.25, $P < .70$.) This result means that 7 out of 10 times, this result would be caused by chance alone, with no real benefit from the aspirin pretreatment. If only five patients developed CME ($\chi^2 = 1.1$, $P < .30$), the same results would occur less than 30% of the time just from chance. In contrast, if only one patient developed CME ($\chi^2 = 13.32$, $P < .001$), it could mean that if the experiment were repeated 1000 times, this result would occur less than once by chance alone.

In general, statistical significance is considered reasonable by chi-square testing at the $P < .05$ level or less. Because the sampling distribution of the chi-square statistic only approximates a theoretical random distribution, the sample size usually must be large enough for an approximation to be good. Therefore, in the case of contingency tables, samples with expected frequencies of less than five in any cell should be measured with a more exact test than the chi-square.

t-Tests

The Student's *t*- and paired *t*-tests are more powerful tests of statistical significance. They attempt to answer the question of whether the *means* of two normally distributed populations are far enough apart to conclude that the distributions are different. From the *t*-statistic, a *P* value is generated. If the *P* value is sufficiently small, the observer concludes that there is sufficient evidence to reject the hypothesis and that there is no difference in the means. What makes this *t*-test useful is the underlying assumption that populations treated differently tend to have different means and that populations treated in an identical manner (ie, a treatment had no effect) have the same means. Again, the *t*-test examines the difference between the *means* obtained from samples from two normal populations. Note that this difference is weighed only statistically. Statistical significance does not imply clinical importance, which must be scrutinized by the clinical investigator.

Researchers must know something about the variability of a normal population in order to completely specify it, so the *t*-test has different forms depending on the assumption made about the variances of the two groups. The two groups themselves may differ in character. For example, two data samples may consist of pairs of observations made on the same individual. Under these circumstances, the values of observations in one sample may not be independent of values in the other. The researcher may take advantage of this interdependence in the construction of the statistical test, thereby serving to increase the power of the test. In the paired *t*-test, increased power is a result of the incorporation of the correlation between the two samples into the statistical test.

For example, consider a researcher who measures the IOP of 10 patients before and after each patient is given a mydriatic eyedrop in the hope of determining if, on the average, the mydriatic changes the IOP. That researcher can analyze the data by computing the average IOP before instillation of the mydriatic and again after instillation and then comparing these two means by using a Student's *t*-test. However, in doing so, the researcher assumes that the two samples are independent (ie, knowledge of a patient's IOP prior to mydriatic instillation does not help predict the postinstillation result). Because this assumption is false, any statistical test based on it can be misleading.

The appropriate procedure in this example would be to compute the difference between the premydriatic and postmydriatic IOP of each patient. The analysis is still based on the mean difference between the pressures before and after instillation, but by computing the variance of the mean difference from the difference obtained from each patient, the researcher reduces the variance of the estimate considerably, depending on the correlation between premydriatic and postmydriatic IOP. By decreasing the variance of the estimate, the researcher has increased the likelihood of detecting a mydriatic effect and has thus enhanced the power of the test.

Analysis of variance

A powerful generalization of the *t*-test, analysis of variance simultaneously examines samples from several normal distributions by asking whether the means of these normal distributions are identical. A researcher starting with samples from each of k populations could address this question by performing *t*-tests on all of the possible sample pairings from the k distributions. However, this process would result in k(k − 1) *t*-tests, each of which would require interpretation, a tedious task that often results in misleading conclusions. The analysis of variance test leads to just one *P* value, examining whether the means of the k normal distributions are identical. Thus, despite its name, the analysis of variance test is really a test of means. Many different types of analysis of variance tests can be used (eg, Latin squares, repeated measures), but they all address essentially the same question: are the means of the groups under observation different?

Correlation Coefficient

The fundamental objective of *correlation analysis* is to obtain a measure of the degree of association between two variables—that is, to find out how well the variables correlate with each other. *Regression analysis*, by contrast, provides the basis for predicting values of a variable from values of one or more other variables. In general, for many medical and biological systems, a simple two-variable correlation model is assumed. One objective of regression analysis is to estimate values of the dependent variable from values of the independent variable. Most commonly, this estimation is accomplished by a *regression line*, a line "best fitted" to the scattered entries of data. This regression line displays mean values of Y for given values of X. Because the line has a simple equation of the form

Y = mX + b, the equation provides estimates of the dependent variable when values of X are inserted.

Correlation analysis attempts to measure the degree of association or correlation between two variables. The coefficient of correlation measures, in part, the strength of the linear relationship between two variables: a coefficient of 1.0 would indicate a perfect correlation, whereas a coefficient of 0 would indicate no correlation. The slope of the best-fitted straight line is the correlation coefficient multiplied by the ratio of the standard deviation of the dependent variable to the standard deviation of the independent variable. It is important to note the difference between correlation and causation. Variables may be uncorrelated but strongly related.

Multivariable Analysis

Many researchers have come to realize that relationships between variables can be complicated. For example, the likelihood of a patient suffering from a myocardial infarction depends not only on that patient's age but also on gender, smoking habits, glucose metabolism, cholesterol and triglyceride levels, blood pressure, and family history of vascular disease and diabetes, among other factors. All of these factors must be examined simultaneously to fully appreciate their total impact on the outcome event. To this end, a number of multivariable procedures have been developed. *Multiple regression analysis*, *logistic regression*, and *Cox hazard functions* represent a subset of a class of powerful statistical procedures. Their definitions and applications are beyond the scope of this summary. However, when combined with the computing capability of the mini- or microcomputer, these procedures provide a readily available set of tools with which the clinical investigator can further elucidate the complicated interdependencies of many pertinent risk factors on the outcome of the variable of interest.

Data From Follow-Up Studies

In describing the results from long-term follow-up studies, more complex statistical methods besides simple frequency distributions and estimates of the mean may be necessary. Patients are enrolled at various points in time and observed for months or years for the occurrence of the outcome measurement (eg, vision loss). Unfortunately, investigators often summarize the results of such a study with a statement like this: "125 patients with retinal disease were observed from 6 months to 7 years (mean follow-up, 26.5 months). 25 of the 125 patients (20%) experienced severe visual loss during the follow-up period." Such statements are not informative and may be misleading.

Survival, or life-table, analyses are more appropriate because they have the advantage of using the full information on patients followed for varying lengths of time. In these analyses, all patients are followed until the *event*, or outcome measurement of interest, occurs or until the date of the analysis. The length of follow-up is then computed for each patient from enrollment to the event or date of analysis. Life tables are usually presented in graph form, displaying either the cumulative proportion with an event or the proportion surviving without an event.

Use of One or Two Eyes in Data Analyses

A common statistical problem encountered by the clinical researcher in the field of ophthalmology is the issue of using one eye versus two eyes in the same individual. Because eyes are highly correlated in the same individual, each eye is not counted twice in the sample size calculation because they are not independent entities. How does the researcher deal with such data? The following options are available:

- Use the right eye
- Use the left eye
- Select one eye randomly
- Use the mean of two eyes
- Use both eyes, accounting for correlation between the eyes

The final option has the advantage of accommodating all the available data. Methods such as *generalizing estimating equations* (also known as *GEE*) are beginning to be used in the ophthalmic literature. The explanation of the theories behind the use of such methods is beyond the scope of this chapter. The interested reader is referred below to other literature. The use of generalizing estimating equations is also helpful in situations in which the data collected are not "independent" but are correlated, such as longitudinal studies in which a patient is examined at several time points, familial studies, and multiple measurements at a single time. A study of familial aggregation of lens opacities in the Framingham Eye Study used such a method to show the strong associations between siblings for nuclear and posterior subcapsular opacities.

Finally, if one eye is randomly assigned to receive the treatment while the fellow eye is designated to be the control eye, the sample size may be reduced because the basic systemic parameters are identical in the same individual. Such paired analyses may be useful in studies in which the treatment is local and does not have a cross-over or systemic effect.

The Framingham Offspring Eye Study Group. Familial aggregation of lens opacities: the Framingham Eye Study and the Framingham Offspring Eye Study. *Am J Epidemiol.* 1994; 140:550–564.

Glynn RJ, Rosner B. Accounting for the correlation between fellow eyes in regression analysis. *Arch Ophthalmol.* 1992;110:381–387.

Statistical Association

Using descriptive studies, researchers can generate hypotheses based on data that demonstrate significant etiologic or therapeutic factors. Such hypotheses can be tested by an analytic study, which ultimately leads to the determination of the presence or absence of a *statistical association.* This association may be correct, but alternative explanations such as chance, bias, and confounding must be ruled out.

Chance

In epidemiologic studies, it is not feasible to study every member of the population of interest. Instead, a subgroup of the entire population is studied. Inferences about the characteristics of the population are based on information collected on the subgroup. Such inferences may not be correct because of random sampling variability or chance (luck of the draw). The deviation of the sample values from the true population values decreases as the sample size and the representativeness of the subgroup increases.

Tests of statistical significance and quantification of the sampling variability are involved in evaluating the role of chance. Hypothesis testing begins with the *null hypothesis,* which states that there is no association between the factor and the disease. The *alternative hypothesis* states that there is indeed a relationship between the factor and the disease. For example, the investigators in the Diabetic Retinopathy Study hoped to be able to demonstrate the efficacy of treatment and thus reject the null hypothesis that there is no difference between the rates of severe visual loss in the treated and untreated groups.

Tests of significance generally lead to a probability statement, or *P* value. This *P* value is the probability of obtaining by chance alone a result at least as extreme as that observed. A *P* value of 0.05 means that there is a 5% probability of mistakenly rejecting the null hypothesis. That is, in "truth" there is no association between the disease and the risk factor studied, but a difference as large as that found in the study could be found by chance alone, 1 time out of 20. Chance can never be completely excluded as an explanation for a study's findings, and thus the null hypothesis can never be unequivocally rejected. However, as the *P* values become smaller, such as 0.01 or 0.001, it becomes less likely that the difference found in the experiment is a result of chance. The smaller the *P* value, the less likely the null hypothesis is true and the less likely random chance explains the findings.

The calculated *P* value is related to the size of the difference found in the study and the standard error of that difference. Small *P* values are the result of large study differences, small standard errors, or both. The *standard error* is related both to the variability of observation and the total number of persons in the study (the study *sample size*). In general, a study involving a small number of subjects can reach a *P* value small enough to reject the null hypothesis only if a large study difference (difference between the study groups) is present. However, a small study difference may result in a statistically significant *P* value in a study with a large sample size because the standard error decreases with increasing sample size. Thus, a study could attain statistical significance, and the null hypothesis could be rejected, but the difference between the groups could be so small as to be essentially meaningless clinically. For example, a researcher might undertake a large study to evaluate the side effects of intracapsular versus extracapsular cataract surgery. The study might show that 94% of one group compared with 93% of the other group had good visual acuity outcomes. If the sample size was large enough, this difference would be statistically significant, but such a difference is unlikely to be clinically meaningful.

Another way of evaluating a statistical association is via the *confidence interval.* The study difference is bracketed by a range of values known as the confidence interval. A 95% confidence interval indicates that if the experiment were repeated 20 times, 19 out of the 20 tries would result in a value within this interval. If the null value (no difference) is included in the confidence interval, it is inappropriate to reject the null hypothesis at the $P \leq .05$ level. The confidence interval decreases with a larger sample size, which leads to less variability and more precision. Both the P value and its close relative, the confidence interval, provide an estimate of the role of chance in the results of a study.

Bias

Bias is any systematic error in a study that results in an incorrect measurement of the association between the disease and the risk factor. Bias may be introduced by the investigator or by participants in the study. Generally, it can be divided into selection or information bias.

Selection bias

Selection bias occurs when the subjects in the study are not representative of the proposed study population. Measurements made on this study group are not representative of treatment effects or associations that would be true for the targeted study population. Some study designs are more likely to suffer from selection bias than others. In a cohort study, the population free of the disease under study is defined at the outset. These subjects are followed over time for the development of this disease, and the prevalence of various risk factors in those who develop the disease is then compared with the prevalence in those who did not develop the disease. These associations are not affected by selection bias because the population was selected prior to the development of disease.

Studies of cases and controls, in contrast, are particularly vulnerable to selection bias. Generally, all available cases are selected, most of them having been referred because of the presence of the disease. Matching these referred cases with comparable persons is difficult. Ideally, controls should be randomly drawn from the same population that the cases came from, but this is generally not possible. When evaluating the associations found in case-control studies, the researcher must always keep in mind that the association may result from the fact that a variable is a risk factor for the disease or that the control group was selected from a special subgroup of the population. Consider a case-control study of open-angle glaucoma in which the controls were selected from a retina clinic. The finding of an increased prevalence of myopia in the control group compared with the subjects with glaucoma could indicate that hyperopia is associated with the development of glaucoma or could indicate that myopia is especially prevalent among patients with retinal disease. In this example, the increased prevalence of myopia in the control group is probably a result of the special subgroup that served as the source of controls.

Information bias

Information bias is introduced into a study when the data collection method lacks completeness or comparability in each of the study groups. Both the subjects and the examiners are potential sources of this bias. One type of subject bias is called *recall bias*, typically a problem in studies of cases and controls when historical information is being collected. Persons with a disease are often more likely to remember possible factors associated with the development of the disease than are persons in the control group.

For example, a subject with an ocular malignancy may tend to report completely or even overestimate exposure to x-rays compared with someone who does not have a malignancy. Similarly, a subject with AMD may be more likely to be aware of a family member with the disease than would the normal control. Affected subjects are more likely to have asked family members about signs and symptoms of the disease, and they are more likely to have discussed this disease with their eye doctors, than are family members of persons without AMD.

Exposure identification is often determined through an interview. If the interviewer knows the identity of the cases and controls, his or her prejudices concerning potential risk factors and aggressiveness in ascertaining the histories in the cases and controls may distort the collection of data.

Because information bias can also occur in clinical trials, *masking* is an important aspect of the randomized clinical trial. Sometimes it is possible to maintain the *double-blind*, or *double-masked*, situation. In surgical trials, patients undergoing surgical treatment know that they are in the treated group. Having undergone surgery, they may be particularly likely to try harder during testing and to minimize losses on historical data collection. Persons collecting data in a trial can also be affected by the knowledge of whether an ocular or a systemic treatment has been given. They may urge the treated patients to try harder in the measurement of the outcome variable in an attempt to find beneficial results of treatment. This effort may be on a subconscious level with no intent to purposely distort the data, but their honest desire to find a successful treatment prejudices their attempts to collect the data. If the double blind is not possible, attempts should be made to ensure that the person assessing the outcome variable is masked as to treatment status.

Sommer A. *Epidemiology and Statistics for the Ophthalmologist.* New York: Oxford University Press; 1980.

Confounding

Confounding can occur when multiple factors are associated with the development of the disease or the outcome under study. To affect the study results, the confounder must be associated with both the exposure under study and the disease. In a case-control study of smoking and AMD, age may be a confounding factor. The researcher might find a definite association between smoking and AMD. However, a strong relationship between age and AMD may also be found. If age and smoking were related (eg, if older patients were more likely to smoke than young patients), the association of smoking and AMD could be the result of the confounding factor *age* rather than a direct relationship between smoking itself and macular degeneration. That is, smoking itself has an apparent association with AMD but actually has nothing to do with the development of AMD; rather, both smoking and AMD are more common in older people than in younger people. This confounding effect can be tested by stratifying the study group by age and looking in groups matched for age for an increased prevalence of smoking in the cases compared with the controls. If confounding had been responsible for the original association, no new association within age strata would then be observed.

Confounding has also been termed the *mixing of effects.* The mixing of factors both positively and negatively associated with the disease can mask true associations. Thus, confounders can be responsible for positive or negative associations and can be responsible for apparent lack of association.

In the design of studies, confounding is controlled by three methods: randomization, restriction, and matching. *Randomization* in a clinical trial of sufficient sample size makes it likely that all potential confounding factors, both recognized and unrecognized, are equally distributed in the study groups. When the confounding factors are balanced, differences between the groups cannot be related to the confounding factor. *Restriction* is a term that describes the enforcement of strict eligibility criteria in the creation of homogeneous study groups. The price paid for restriction is the reduction of eligible subjects, making recruitment difficult. Also, when the study group is restricted (eg, to a group of a specific age), age cannot be evaluated as a potential factor. Generalizability of study results may also be limited in the restricted study. *Matching,* the pairing of an affected case to one or more controls, is a technique used frequently in case-control studies and occasionally in clinical trials. With this technique, subjects (either cases and controls in a case-control study or treated and untreated patients in a clinical trial) are paired on the basis of their similarity with respect to specific selective variables such as age, sex, and race. This is a laborious, expensive technique to control for confounding, and it can seriously limit recruitment. Furthermore, in a case-control study, matching prevents the researcher from evaluating the effect of a factor that has been matched on.

Confounding may be controlled retrospectively in the analysis phase of the study by *stratification,* the evaluation of the association within groups or within the strata of the confounding variable. Age-, sex-, and race-adjusted strata-specific estimates would be calculated. The disadvantage with this method is that only a small number of potential known confounders can be controlled simultaneously. Multivariable analysis, however, allows for the determination of association while controlling for a larger number of known factors simultaneously.

Validity, Generalizability, Consistency

To assess the validity of the study, the factors of chance, bias, and confounding must be evaluated as possible alternative explanations for the results of the study. Once validity is established, the results are then considered for their generalizability to populations other than the targeted study population. For example, the Framingham Heart Study involved a mostly white population. Generalizability of the Framingham results to the black population would be a matter of speculation. The consistency of associations between risk factors and a particular disease from one study to another provides further evidence that a relationship is true and not a chance association. For example, the association of hyperopia with AMD found in the case-control study of Hyman and co-workers was also found in two other case-control studies. This consistent finding supports the credibility of a probably true association between hyperopia and AMD.

Sample Size and Power

As previously mentioned, the sample size of a study greatly influences the magnitude of the study's P value. An important initial aspect of a study design includes the sample size and power calculations to determine the number of persons required to detect a statistically significant effect of a given magnitude. The *type I error*, or α *error*, is associated with the null hypothesis. The probability of making a type I error is equal to the P value. For example, at the 5% level, there is a 5% (or 1 in 20) risk of erroneously rejecting the null hypothesis when the null hypothesis is indeed true. The *type II error*, or β *error*, is the chance of erroneously failing to reject the null hypothesis when it is false. In other words, this error describes the chance of failing to show a difference that in fact exists.

The *power* of a study is the probability of rejecting the null hypothesis when indeed there is a difference of specified size between the study groups. The power is the complement of the β error, or

$$1 - \beta = \text{power of the study}$$

If $\beta = 0.20$, the power of the study is $1.00 - 0.20 = 0.80$, indicating an 80% chance of detecting a difference if the "true" difference between groups is equal to or greater than the magnitude of the difference specified during the study design phase.

The *sample size calculation* begins with the alternative hypothesis—that is, the expected magnitude of the effect of the treatment or of the association with the risk factor being studied. These values are often estimated from previously published reports or, if such reports are unavailable, the investigators may choose a minimum effect that might be considered clinically meaningful. This is an important step, requiring the clinician's careful judgment. The total sample size is related to the significance level, or α; the power $(1 - \beta)$; and the magnitude of the effect. The necessary sample size increases if the power of the study increases or the significance level α decreases.

The medical literature, including ophthalmic literature, unfortunately has a sizable number of studies with negative results, frequently the consequence of inadequate sample size. Studies that fail to find a clinical and statistical difference should include the intended sample size and power calculation. Numerous formulas are found in statistical textbooks and computer programs that can generate sample size calculations. It is beyond the scope of this section to provide such material. More important, it must be stressed that clinical research is a collaborative effort among clinicians, statisticians, and epidemiologists. Expertise from each of these disciplines should be used in the development phase of any study.

Colton T. *Statistics in Medicine*. Boston: Little Brown; 1974.

Snedecor GW, Cochran WG. *Statistical Methods*. 6th ed. Ames, IA: Iowa State University Press; 1968.

Basic Texts

General Medicine

Adams RD, Victor M, Ropper AH, eds. *Principles of Neurology.* 7th ed. New York: McGraw-Hill, 2001.

Beers MH, Berkow R, eds. *The Merck Manual of Diagnosis and Therapy.* 17th ed. Rahway, NJ: Merck Research Laboratories; 1999.

Braunwald E, Zipes DP, Libby P, eds. *Heart Disease: A Textbook of Cardiovascular Medicine.* 6th ed. Philadelphia: Saunders; 2001.

Cecil RL, Goldman L, Bennett JC. *Cecil Textbook of Medicine.* 21st ed. Philadelphia: Saunders; 1996.

Cancer: Rates and Risks. 4th ed. Bethesda, MD: National Institutes of Health; 1996.

Diabetes in America. 2nd ed. Bethesda, MD: National Institutes of Health; 1995.

DeVita VT Jr, Hellman S, Rosenberg SA, eds. *Cancer: Principles and Practice of Oncology.* 6th ed. Philadelphia: Lippincott Williams & Wilkins; 2001.

Harrison TR, Braunwald E, eds. *Harrison's Principles of Internal Medicine.* 15th ed. New York: McGraw-Hill; 2001.

Kelley WN, Harris ED Jr, Ruddy S, et al, eds. *Textbook of Rheumatology.* 5th ed. Philadelphia: Saunders; 1997.

Mandell GL, Douglass RG, Bennett JE, Dolin R, eds. *Mandell, Douglas and Bennett's Principles and Practice of Infectious Diseases.* 5th ed. New York: Churchill Livingstone; 2000.

Wilson J, Foster DW, Kronenberg H, et al, eds. *Williams Textbook of Endocrinology.* 9th ed. Philadelphia: Saunders; 1998.

Credit Reporting Form

Basic and Clinical Science Course, 2005–2006
Section 1

The American Academy of Ophthalmology is accredited by the Accreditation Council for Continuing Medical Education to provide continuing medical education for physicians.

The American Academy of Ophthalmology designates this educational activity for a maximum of 30 category 1 credits toward the AMA Physician's Recognition Award. Each physician should claim only those hours of credit that he/she actually spent in the activity.

The American Medical Association has determined that non-US licensed physicians who participate in this CME activity are eligible for AMA PRA category 1 credit.

If you wish to claim continuing medical education credit for your study of this section, you may claim your credit online or fill in the required forms and mail or fax them to the Academy.

To use the forms:

1. Complete the study questions and mark your answers on the Section Completion Form.
2. Complete the Section Evaluation.
3. Fill in and sign the statement below.
4. Return this page and the required forms by mail or fax to the CME Registrar (see below).

To claim credit online:

1. Log on to the Academy website (www.aao.org).
2. Go to Education Resource Center; click on CME Central.
3. Follow the instructions.

Important: These completed forms or the online claim must be received at the Academy within 3 years of purchase.

I hereby certify that I have spent ______ (up to 30) hours of study on the curriculum of this section and that I have completed the Study Questions.

Signature: ____
                                                                              Date

Name: ____

Address: ____

City and State: _____________________________________ Zip: _______________

Telephone: (________) _________________ Academy Member ID# _______________
                     area code

Please return completed forms to: **Or you may fax them to:** 415-561-8575
American Academy of Ophthalmology
P.O. Box 7424
San Francisco, CA 94120-7424
Attn: CME Registrar, Customer Service

2005–2006
Section Completion Form

Basic and Clinical Science Course

Answer Sheet for Section 1

Question	Answer	Question	Answer	Question	Answer
1	a b c d	18	a b c d	35	a b c d
2	a b c d	19	a b c d	36	a b c d
3	a b c d	20	a b c d	37	a b c d
4	a b c d	21	a b c d	38	a b c d
5	a b c d	22	a b c d	39	a b c d
6	a b c d	23	a b c d	40	a b c d
7	a b c d	24	a b c d	41	a b c d
8	a b c d	25	a b c d	42	a b c d
9	a b c d	26	a b c d	43	a b c d
10	a b c d	27	a b c d	44	a b c d
11	a b c d	28	a b c d	45	a b c d
12	a b c d	29	a b c d	46	a b c d
13	a b c d	30	a b c d	47	a b c d
14	a b c d	31	a b c d	48	a b c d
15	a b c d	32	a b c d	49	a b c d
16	a b c d	33	a b c d	50	a b c d
17	a b c d	34	a b c d		

Section Evaluation

Please complete this CME questionnaire.

1. To what degree will you use knowledge from BCSC Section 1 in your practice?
   ☐ Regularly
   ☐ Sometimes
   ☐ Rarely

2. Please review the stated objectives for BCSC Section 1. How effective was the material at meeting those objectives?
   ☐ All objectives were met.
   ☐ Most objectives were met.
   ☐ Some objectives were met.
   ☐ Few or no objectives were met.

3. To what degree is BCSC Section 1 likely to have a positive impact on health outcomes of your patients?
   ☐ Extremely likely
   ☐ Highly likely
   ☐ Somewhat likely
   ☐ Not at all likely

4. After you review the stated objectives for BCSC Section 1, please let us know of any additional knowledge, skills, or information useful to your practice that were acquired but were not included in the objectives. [Optional]

5. Was BCSC Section 1 free of commercial bias?
   ☐ Yes
   ☐ No

6. If you selected "No" in the previous question, please comment. [Optional]

7. Please tell us what might improve the applicability of BCSC to your practice. [Optional]

Study Questions

Although a concerted effort has been made to avoid ambiguity and redundancy in these questions, the authors recognize that differences of opinion may occur regarding the "best" answer. The discussions are provided to demonstrate the rationale used to derive the answer. They may also be helpful in confirming that your approach to the problem was correct or, if necessary, in fixing the principle in your memory. Where relevant, additional references are given. The following study questions and discussions were submitted by Edward J. Rockwell, MD, on behalf of the Self-Assessment Committee.

1. Which one of the following bacteria evades phagocytosis in the absence of antibody and complement because of polysaccharide encapsulation?

   a. *Staphylococcus aureus*

   b. *Staphylococcus epidermidis*

   c. *Streptococcus pneumoniae*

   d. *Pseudomonas aeruginosa*

2. Which one of the following antibiotics is the treatment of choice for life-threatening *Staphylococcus aureus* systemic infection?

   a. Penicillin

   b. Vancomycin

   c. Gentamicin

   d. A cephalosporin

3. Which one of the following antibiotics is the treatment of choice for *Streptococcus pyogenes* infections (eg, strep throat, impetigo)?

   a. Penicillin

   b. Vancomycin

   c. Gentamicin

   d. A cephalosporin

4. All except which one of the following is true about Lyme disease?

   a. It is tick-borne.

   b. Late manifestations are seen in the skin, joints, and nervous system.

   c. It is usually diagnosed by bacterial culturing.

   d. The organism is sensitive to tetracycline.

5. Which one of the following statements is not correct about herpes zoster?

   a. Primary infection usually occurs in childhood in the form of chickenpox (varicella).

   b. No systemic antiviral treatment exists at this time.

   c. Postherpetic neuralgia may occur.

   d. Herpes zoster occurs after a reactivation of a latent nerve infection.

6. Health care workers exposed to HIV may be given immediate treatment with which one of the following medications?

   a. Zidovudine (Retrovir)

   b. Saquinavir (Invirase)

   c. Ganciclovir (Cytovene)

   d. HIV vaccine

7. β-Adrenergic receptor site stimulation causes all except which one of the following?

   a. Vasoconstriction

   b. Tachycardia

   c. Increased myocardial contractility

   d. Bronchoconstriction

8. The annual mortality rate of patients with asymptomatic carotid bruit has been estimated at 4%. The most likely cause of death is which one of the following?

   a. Nonhemorrhagic stroke

   b. Hemorrhagic stroke

   c. Subarachnoid hemorrhage

   d. Complications of heart disease

9. Which one of the following is most sensitive in distinguishing a myocardial infarction from unstable angina or noncardiac chest pain?

   a. Elevation of the ST segment on the electrocardiogram

   b. Echocardiogram

   c. Elevated serum cardiac enzymes

   d. Depression of the ST segment on exercise stress testing

10. All but which one of the following may be indicated for the management of congestive heart failure?

    a. α-Adrenergic antagonists

    b. Digitalis

    c. The calcium channel blocker diltiazem (Cardizem)

    d. β-Adrenergic antagonists

11. Which one of the following does not increase serum high-density lipoprotein cholesterol (HDL-C)?

    a. Aerobic exercise

    b. Moderate alcohol consumption

    c. Gemfibrozil (Lopid)

    d. Lovastatin (Mevacor)

12. Hypercholesterolemia is a risk factor for all but which one of the following?

    a. Arteritic ischemic optic neuropathy

    b. Ischemic heart disease

    c. Cerebrovascular disease

    d. Peripheral vascular disease

13. Which one of the following is most indicative of restrictive pulmonary disease?

    a. Abnormal-appearing chest radiograph

    b. FEV_1 less than 80% predicted

    c. Low PO_2 in arterial blood gas

    d. Total lung capacity less than 70% predicted

14. Which one of the following is the best test to monitor heparin therapy?

    a. Prothrombin time (PT)

    b. Partial thromboplastin time (PTT)

    c. Bleeding time

    d. Platelet count

15. Which one of the following is not used to dissolve existing clots?

    a. Streptokinase

    b. Urokinase

    c. Heparin

    d. Tissue plasminogen activator

16. Which one of the following statements is not correct about rheumatoid arthritis?

    a. It tends to affect the large joints.

    b. Approximately 80% of patients are positive for rheumatoid factor.

    c. Stiffness at rest often improves with use.

    d. Extra-articular disease may be found.

17. A 50-year-old white male presents with acute nongranulomatous anterior uveitis. He has had chronic back pain for years. Which one of the following does not fit with his clinical syndrome?

    a. Sacroiliitis on radiography

    b. Spinal ankylosis on radiography

    c. Positive HLA-DR4

    d. Restrictive lung disease

18. Which one of the following is the most common ophthalmologic manifestation of systemic lupus erythematosus?

    a. Cranial nerve palsies

    b. Retinal vascular disease

    c. Cortical blindness

    d. Sjögren syndrome

19. Renal disease is associated with all but which one of the following diseases?

    a. Rheumatoid arthritis

    b. Scleroderma

    c. Polyarteritis nodosa

    d. Wegener granulomatosis

20. Which one of the following is most effective for treating Wegener granulomatosis?

    a. Aspirin

    b. Nonsteroidal anti-inflammatory agents

    c. Cyclophosphamide

    d. Methotrexate

21. The definitive test for giant cell arteritis is which one of the following?

    a. Wintrobe sedimentation rate

    b. Westergren sedimentation rate

    c. C-reactive protein

    d. Temporal artery biopsy

22. In addition to uveitis, with or without hypopyon, which one of the following is the most common ophthalmic manifestation of Behçet syndrome?

    a. Glaucoma

    b. Retinal vasculitis

    c. Corneal disease

    d. Eyelid ulcers

23. Nonsteroidal anti-inflammatory agents include all but which one of the following?

    a. Aspirin

    b. Ibuprofen (Advil, Motrin)

    c. Cyclosporine

    d. Rofecoxib (Vioxx)

24. Type 2 diabetes is characterized by all but which one of the following?

    a. Genetic predisposition

    b. Low basal insulin secretion early in the disease

    c. Later age of onset than with type 1 diabetes

    d. Increased visceral fat

25. The Diabetes Control and Complications Trial showed a decreased risk of all but which one of the following?

    a. Hypoglycemia

    b. Development and progression of retinopathy

    c. Development and progression of nephropathy

    d. Development and progression of neuropathy

26. Which one of the following is not used to diagnose diabetes mellitus?

    a. Random blood glucose exceeding 200 mg/dL

    b. Glucose level exceeding 200 mg/dL during glucose tolerance test

    c. Glycosylated hemoglobin (HbA_{1c})

    d. Fasting serum glucose exceeding 126 mg/dL

27. Which one of the following is the leading cause of death in the United States of America?

    a. Coronary artery disease

    b. Stroke

    c. Cancer

    d. Accidents

28. Which one of the following choices is preferred for a diabetic patient about to undergo major surgery?

    a. Light breakfast with full regular insulin dose in early AM

    b. Fasting with reduced insulin dose in AM

    c. Fasting, withhold insulin, and in preoperative area start a dextrose IV and give half of an insulin dose

    d. Switch from insulin to oral hypoglycemic agent preoperatively

29. The most sensitive and specific test(s) for screening for thyroid disease is which one of the following choices?

    a. T_3 level

    b. Free T_4 and sensitive TSH levels

    c. Radioactive iodine uptake

    d. Thyroid-binding globulin level

30. Which one of the following ocular structures is the most radiosensitive?

    a. Lens

    b. Cornea

    c. Retina

    d. Optic nerve

31. Cancer is predominantly a genetic disease. Which one of the following cancers may have a viral cause?

    a. Breast

    b. Colon

    c. Lung

    d. Cervical

32. Which one of the following statements is not correct about bipolar disorder, formerly known as *manic depression?*

    a. It is the most common form of depression.

    b. There may be alternating periods of depression and elevated mood.

    c. It is treated with psychotherapy.

    d. It is treated with lithium.

33. Which one of the following best describes the patient who claims to be unable to work but has no organic basis for visual loss?

    a. Conversion disorder

    b. Hypochondriasis

    c. Factitious disorder

    d. Malingering

34. Fetal alcohol syndrome includes all but which one of the following?

    a. Blepharophimosis

    b. Cataract

    c. Telecanthus

    d. Optic nerve hypoplasia

35. The barbiturates have all but which one of the following effects?

    a. Sedative

    b. Hypnotic

    c. Antidepressive

    d. Anticonvulsive

36. Antidepressants include all but which one of the following?

    a. Lithium

    b. Monoamine oxidase inhibitors

    c. Fluoxetine (Prozac)

    d. Haloperidol (Haldol)

37. Parkinson disease is characterized by all but which one of the following?

    a. Increased rigidity

    b. Excess dopamine production

    c. Potential worsening of symptoms with neuroleptic drugs

    d. Loss of neurons in the substantia nigra

38. Alzheimer disease is characterized by all but which one of the following?

    a. Neurofibrillary tangles

    b. Progressive dementia in later life

    c. A toxic cause in most cases

    d. Extraneuronal amyloid plaques

39. Vaccines are currently available for all but which one of the following?

    a. Rabies

    b. Influenza types A and B

    c. *Meningococcus*

    d. *Haemophilus influenzae*

40. Which one of the following would argue against widespread screening for a disease?

    a. It is treatable or preventable.

    b. It has a low prevalence.

    c. It is generally asymptomatic.

    d. The cost of the disease and its complications is high.

41. Which one of the following is not a risk factor for breast cancer?

    a. Fibrocystic disease

    b. First-degree relative with breast cancer

    c. Early menarche

    d. Nulliparity

42. Which one of the following is the most preventable cancer in the United States?

    a. Prostate

    b. Colon

    c. Lung

    d. Breast

43. Routine childhood vaccinations include all but which one of the following?

    a. HiB

    b. Varivax

    c. HepB

    d. Influenza

44. Which one of the following should be immediately available during an edrophonium (Tensilon) test?

    a. Atropine sulfate

    b. Epinephrine

    c. Pyridostigmine (Mestinon)

    d. Propranolol

45. An anesthesiologist would avoid which one of the following in a patient with history of malignant hyperthermia?

    a. Thiopental sodium

    b. Nitrous oxide

    c. Midazolam (Versed)

    d. Succinylcholine

46. Which one of the following medications would be the most important for a preoperative patient to take the morning of surgery?

    a. Antihypertensive agent

    b. Digoxin

    c. Thyroid medication

    d. Estrogen supplements

47. Which one of the following studies would best demonstrate the incidence of a disease?

    a. Case series

    b. Case-control study

    c. Cohort study

    d. Randomized, prospective, controlled clinical trial

48. Advantages of interventional studies include all but which one of the following?

    a. Low cost

    b. Low risk of bias

    c. Best way to establish efficacy of treatment

    d. Effective for establishing rates of complications of treatment

49. For populations with a normal distribution, the range of observations with a mean ± 3 standard deviations would include what percentage of observations?

    a. 68.3%

    b. 95.5%

    c. 99.7%

    d. 100%

50. Which one of the following statistical tests would be best for studying the effects of gender, smoking, cholesterol levels, blood pressure, diabetes, and family history of heart disease on the incidence of heart attack?

    a. Student's t-test

    b. Chi-square test

    c. Analysis of variance

    d. Multivariable analysis

Answers

1. Answer—c. Of the four choices, only *Streptococcus pneumoniae* has a polysaccharide coating that prevents phagocytosis in the absence of antibody and complement.

2. Answer—b. The high percentage of methicillin-resistant strains of *Staphylococcus aureus* has reduced the usefulness of penicillin for these infections. Gentamicin has good gram-negative but less gram-positive antibacterial activity. A cephalosporin may be successful, although *S aureus* resistance to this group is increasing. Vancomycin is the antibiotic of choice for life-threatening staphylococcal infections, pending antibiotic sensitivity studies. Emerging resistance to vancomycin may change this.

3. Answer—a. Most isolates of *Streptococcus pyogenes* remain highly susceptible to penicillin. Unless there is an allergy to one or more of the penicillins, it remains the treatment of choice for *S pyogenes* infections.

4. Answer—c. Lyme disease is a bacterial disease transmitted to humans from deer by a tick vector. Late manifestations of the disease include skin, joint, and nervous system manifestations. The organism *Borrelia burgdorferi* is a spirochete that is difficult to culture. Serologic tests such as ELISA are usually used to confirm the diagnosis of Lyme disease.

5. Answer—b. Primary infection with herpes zoster occurs as chickenpox (varicella) in childhood. The virus remains dormant in dorsal root nerve ganglia. A severe postherpetic neuralgia may last for months or years after herpes zoster manifestation ("shingles"). The systemic antiviral agents famciclovir, valacyclovir, and acyclovir are used to treat systemic herpes zoster infection.

6. Answer—a. At this time, there is no proven effective HIV vaccine. Ganciclovir has been used as a first-line treatment for cytomegalovirus infections. The protease inhibitor saquinavir is used in multidrug therapy for HIV infection. Zidovudine is used for prophylaxis in health care workers who are exposed occupationally to HIV. Combination therapy with zidovudine, lamivudine, and ritonavir may be used.

7. Answer—d. β-Adrenergic receptor stimulation causes vasoconstriction, increased heart rate, and increased myocardial contractility. Stimulation of β_2-adrenergic receptor sites causes bronchodilation, not bronchoconstriction.

8. Answer—d. The annual stroke rate in patients with asymptomatic bruit is about 1.5%. Most patients do not die. Intracranial hemorrhage after stroke occurs in about 15% of acute cerebrovascular disorders. Such a hemorrhage may be subarachnoid, intracerebral, or intraventricular. Interestingly, in patients with an asymptomatic bruit, the risk of death from complications of heart disease is greater than from stroke or its complications.

9. Answer—c. Electrocardiographic changes, whether on static examination or in exercise stress testing, may be seen with noninfarctive cardiac ischemia. Echocardiography may show cardiac changes after myocardial infarction (MI), including ventricular or valvular dysfunction, ventricular septal defect, and ventricular aneurysm, but is not diagnostic for acute MI. Acute elevation of cardiac enzymes is a better indicator of acute MI.

10. Answer—c. Digitalis, α-adrenergic antagonists (prazosin, clonidine), and β-adrenergic antagonists (carvedilol, metoprolol) can be used to successfully manage congestive heart failure (CHF). Diltiazem, a calcium channel blocker, is associated with increased mortality when used in patients with CHF. Amlodipine is the only calcium channel blocker that has been shown to be safe in patients with CHF.

11. Answer—d. Aerobic exercise, moderate alcohol consumption, and gemfibrozil have all been demonstrated to increase serum high-density lipoprotein cholesterol (HDL-C), which may have a beneficial effect against atherogenesis. High levels of LDL-C and low levels of HDL-C have been shown to increase the risk of coronary artery disease. Lovastatin reduces serum LDL-C but does not increase HDL-C.

12. Answer—a. Hypercholesterolemia is a risk factor for ischemic heart disease, cerebrovascular disease, peripheral vascular disease, and nonarteritic ischemic optic neuropathy. Arteritic ischemic optic neuropathy is seen in giant cell arteritis, a vascular inflammatory condition, associated with polymyalgia rheumatica.

13. Answer—d. Low arterial PO_2 can have a number of causes and is not specific for the type of pulmonary disease. An abnormal-appearing chest radiograph may show severe kyphosis, one cause of restrictive lung disease, but is not usually diagnostic of restrictive lung disease. An FEV_1 less than 80% of predicted suggests obstructive pulmonary disease. A total lung capacity less than 70% predicted suggests restrictive pulmonary disease, such as pulmonary fibrosis.

14. Answer—b. Heparin therapy is monitored by the partial thromboplastin time (PTT). Prothrombin time or the International Normalized Ratio (INR) is used to monitor oral warfarin therapy. Bleeding time is a function of platelet count and function. Platelet abnormalities do not affect the PTT.

15. Answer—c. Urokinase, streptokinase, and tissue plasminogen activator can be used to dissolve clots. Heparin and warfarin are used to prevent the formation of new clots or the propagation of existing clots.

16. Answer—a. Patients with rheumatoid arthritis (RA) often have stiffness at rest that improves with activity (morning stiffness), and extra-articular disease (lungs, skin, cardiac, ocular) may be seen. RA tends to involve the small joints of the fingers and feet, but all joints may be affected.

17. Answer—c. Patients with ankylosing spondylitis may have anterior nongranulomatous uveitis and axial skeletal disease manifested as sacroiliitis as well as bony fusion (ankylosis), which may cause restrictive lung disease. Men are more often affected than women. HLA-B27 is associated with ankylosing spondylitis, and HLA-DR4 with rheumatoid arthritis.

18. Answer—b. Sjögren syndrome, cranial nerve palsies, and cortical blindness may be seen in systemic lupus erythematosus. However, retinal vascular disease is the most common ophthalmologic manifestation of systemic lupus erythematosus.

19. Answer—a. Renal disease is generally not seen in rheumatoid arthritis but is seen in scleroderma, polyarteritis nodosa, and Wegener granulomatosis.

20. Answer—c. Aspirin and nonsteroidal anti-inflammatory agents may be helpful in the management of many forms of arthritis and other inflammatory disorders. Methotrexate is beneficial for some patients with severe rheumatoid arthritis. Wegener granulomatosis is a potentially fatal systemic disease. Cyclophosphamide and prednisone are usually used in the management of Wegener granulomatosis.

21. Answer—d. C-reactive protein, the Westergren sedimentation rate, and the Wintrobe sedimentation rate may each be elevated in giant cell arteritis. However, temporal artery biopsy is the definitive test for giant cell arteritis.

22. Answer—b. In addition to uveitis, with or without hypopyon, retinal vasculitis is the most common ophthalmic manifestation of Behçet syndrome. Corneal disease and glaucoma may result from chronic intraocular inflammation. Oral and genital ulcers, not eyelid ulcers, are common in Behçet syndrome.

23. Answer—c. Aspirin, ibuprofen, and rofecoxib, a cyclooxygenase-2 inhibitor, are all nonsteroidal anti-inflammatory agents. Cyclosporine is an immunosuppressive alkylating agent.

24. Answer—b. Type 2 diabetes is characterized by later age of onset than type 1 (formerly *juvenile*) diabetes and increased visceral fat. Both type 1 and type 2 diabetes have a genetic predisposition. Type 1 diabetes is characterized by reduced insulin production, usually with destruction of insulin-producing β-cells in the pancreas. Early in the course of type 2 diabetes, basal insulin secretion is usually normal or increased.

25. Answer—a. The Diabetes Control and Complications Trial showed decreased risk of development and progression of retinopathy, nephropathy, and neuropathy but a threefold increase in the risk of hypoglycemia.

26. Answer—c. Fasting blood glucose, random glucose, and a glucose tolerance test can be used to diagnose diabetes mellitus. Glycosylated hemoglobin (HbA_{1c}) is used to monitor glucose control in the treated diabetic patient rather than to diagnose diabetes mellitus.

27. Answer—a. Coronary artery disease is the leading cause of death in the United States. Cancer is the second and cerebrovascular disease the third most frequent cause of death in the United States.

28. Answer—c. Of the choices given, the preferred preoperative routine for a diabetic about to undergo major surgery is to have the patient fast, withhold insulin, and start IV dextrose and give half an insulin dose in the preoperative area. Patients should never be told to fast and use insulin during the morning of surgery. A reduced insulin dose in the fasting diabetic patient can safely be administrated once IV dextrose (usually 5%) has been started. A switch from insulin to oral hypoglycemic agents is not indicated.

29. Answer—b. Radioactive iodine uptake measures the thyroid gland's ability to concentrate a dose of radioactive iodine. It is not a good measure of thyroid metabolic status. Thyroid binding globulin and T_3 levels vary in many other disease states, but the free T_4 level may be normal. Free T_4 and sensitive TSH have a sensitivity of 99.5% and a specificity of 98% in screening for thyroid disease and are better measures for thyroid disease.

30. Answer—a. The lens is the most radiosensitive structure in the eye, followed in order by the cornea, the retina, and the optic nerve.

31. Answer—d. Breast and colon cancer have a genetic basis in many patients. The incidence of colon cancer may also be affected by diet. Lung cancer, especially squamous cell carcinoma, is associated with cigarette smoking. Carcinoma of the cervix may be associated with herpes infection.

32. Answer—a. In bipolar disorder, formerly known as *manic depression*, periods of depression often alternate with elevated mood, although this pattern varies. Lithium is the cornerstone of therapy, and psychotherapy is used as an adjunct. Major depression is far more common than bipolar disorder.

33. Answer—d. The patient who claims to be unable to work but has no organic basis for the visual loss is most likely malingering. This is the intentional production of symptoms or loss of function for secondary gain. In a conversion disorder, which is usually due to psychosocial stress, the patient is unaware of the loss of function *(hysterical blindness)*. *Hypochondriasis* is a preoccupation with the fear of having or developing an illness. In a *factitious disorder*, symptoms are willfully produced, usually because of a psychological need to assume a sick role.

34. Answer—b. Fetal alcohol syndrome may include blepharophimosis, telecanthus, ptosis, optic nerve hypoplasia or atrophy, and tortuosity of the retinal arteries and veins. Cataract is not a part of fetal alcohol syndrome.

35. Answer—c. The barbiturates have anticonvulsive, sedative, and hypnotic effects. They are not used as antidepressive agents.

36. Answer—d. Monoamine oxidase inhibitors, fluoxetine, and lithium are used to treat depression. Haloperidol is a major tranquilizer.

37. Answer—b. Parkinson disease is characterized by tremor, bradykinesia, akinesia, rigidity, and a shuffling and stooped gait. Neuroleptic drugs may cause Parkinson disease. Parkinson disease leads to a loss of neurons in the substantia nigra with decreased, not increased, production of dopamine. Levodopa (L-dopa) is commonly used to treat Parkinson disease.

38. Answer—c. Alzheimer disease is characterized by progressive dementia, usually in patients over age 65 years. Extraneuronal amyloid plaques and neurofibrillary tangles are seen histopathologically. Alzheimer disease has genetic factors that follow either a familial autosomal dominant or sporadic autosomal dominant inheritance pattern. Toxins and free radicals may also play a role in the pathogenesis of Alzheimer disease.

39. Answer—a. Vaccines are currently available for influenza, meningococcus, and *Haemophilus influenzae*. There currently is no vaccine for rabies.

40. Answer—b. Ideal diseases to screen for are the ones that are reliably detectable, treatable or preventable, progressive (especially if untreated), and generally asymptomatic. A high, rather than low, prevalence argues in favor of screening. For a rare disease, screening may not prove cost-effective.

41. Answer—a. Nulliparity, early menarche, and history of a first-degree relative with breast cancer are all risk factors for breast cancer. Fibrocystic disease is not a risk factor for breast cancer.

42. Answer—c. Lung cancer is the most preventable of the four cancers listed because it is largely caused by cigarette smoking. Screening and early testing for breast, colon, and prostate cancers can lead to their early detection and more favorable outcomes. Colonoscopy and sigmoidoscopy can be used to remove adenomas and prevent some colon cancers.

43. Answer—d. HepB, DTaP, HiB, IPV (or OPV), and Varivax are important childhood vaccines. Influenza vaccine is not routinely recommended in children but may be indicated in selected cases such as children with chronic or debilitating diseases.

44. Answer—a. Atropine sulfate (0.4–0.5 mg) should be immediately available during an edrophonium (Tensilon) test. The anticholinergic agent atropine can block adverse cholinergic effects of edrophonium. Mestinon, a cholinesterase inhibitor, is used to treat patients with myasthenia gravis. Epinephrine would not be as useful as atropine, and propranolol could worsen bradycardia caused by edrophonium.

45. Answer—d. An anesthesiologist would avoid succinylcholine in a patient with history of malignant hyperthermia. There would be no contraindication to the use of the other agents. The inhaled agents halothane, enflurane, and isoflurane also may trigger malignant hyperthermia.

46. Answer—a. Of the listed medications, antihypertensive agents are the most important to take the morning of surgery. Rebound hypertensive crises can be precipitated by abrupt withdrawal of β-blockers, clonidine, or angiotensin-converting enzyme inhibitors. However, diuretics can usually be withheld the morning of surgery. Digoxin and thyroid or estrogen supplements have a long half-life and can be resumed after surgery.

47. Answer—c. A cohort study would be the best study to demonstrate the incidence of a disease. In a cohort study, persons who are initially free of the disease are followed over time, during which time some subjects develop the disease. A case series or case-control study would not be capable of determining the incidence of a disease. A randomized, prospective, controlled clinical trial is the best way to compare different treatments or treatment versus no treatment, but such a trial is not good for establishing the incidence of a disease.

48. Answer—a. Interventional studies are excellent for establishing the efficacy of treatment and for establishing the rates treatment complications. The design of these studies greatly reduces the risk of bias. Unfortunately, they are expensive and time-consuming.

49. Answer—c. The mean ± 1 standard deviation would include 68.3% of observations, the mean ± 2 standard deviations would include 95.5% of observations, and the mean ± 3 standard deviations would include 99.7% of observations.

50. Answer—d. A multivariable analysis is the best statistical test for studying the effects of gender, smoking, cholesterol levels, blood pressure, diabetes, and family history of heart disease on the incidence of heart attack. The t-test is used to determine whether the means of two normally distributed populations are significantly different. The chi-square test is used to determine whether two sampled population proportions are different. Analysis of variance is used to establish the significance of the difference of means of multiple normal distributions.

Index

(i = image; *t =* table)

Abacavir, 29
Abciximab, 100
Absence epilepsy, 240
Absorptiometry, dual-photon x-ray, 204
Abstinence syndrome, 228
Abuse, elder, 197–198
Acarbose, 183
Accolate. *See* Zafirlukast
Accupril. *See* Quinapril
ACE inhibitors. *See* Angiotensin-converting enzyme
   (ACE) inhibitors
Acebutolol, 70*t*
Acetohexamide, 181*t*
ACLS. *See* Advanced cardiac life support
Acquired immunodeficiency syndrome (AIDS), 24–37
   CDC definition of, 26–27, 27*t*
   classification of, 27, 27*t*
   clinical syndrome of, 26–27, 27*t*
   etiology of, 25
   incidence of, 24–25
   occupational exposure to, 28
      prophylaxis for, 32, 33*t*
      precautions in health care setting and, 41
   ophthalmologic considerations and, 36
   opportunistic infections associated with, 32–36
   pathogenesis of, 25–26
   prognosis of, 28–32
   seroepidemiology of, 27–28
   syphilis in, 14
   transmission of, 28
   treatment of, 28–32
   tuberculosis and, 19, 20
ACS. *See* Acute coronary syndromes
Actinomycin-D, 222
Activase. *See* Tissue plasminogen activator
Activated protein C resistance, 149
Active immunization, 256
Actos. *See* Pioglitazone
Acular. *See* Ketorolac tromethamine
Acute coronary syndromes, 90, 91–93. *See also*
   Myocardial infarction
   hypercholesterolemia and, 119
   management of, 99–103
Acyclovir, 49*t*, 60
   for herpes simplex virus infections, 20–21, 60
   for herpes zoster, 21, 60
Acylureidopenicillins, 51–52
AD. *See* Alzheimer disease
Adalat. *See* Nifedipine
Adalimumab, 169
Adefovir, 29, 60
Adenoma, thyroid hormone-producing, 192
Adenosine, in atrial flutter diagnosis, 115
Adnexa (ocular)
   radiation affecting, 216–217
   in systemic malignancies, 224
Adrenergic inhibitors. *See* Alpha blockers; Beta
   blockers
Adriamycin. *See* Doxorubicin

Adult Treatment Panel (ATP) III report, 119, 120
Advance directives, surgery in elderly patients and, 199
Advanced cardiac life support (ACLS), 268–269
Advil. *See* Ibuprofen
Affective disorders (mood disorders), 226–227
Afterload, 106
   reduction of for heart failure, 107
Age-Related Eye Disease Study, 300
Agenerase. *See* Amprenavir
Aggrestat. *See* Tirofiban
Aging, 195–210
   anemia and, 141
   elder abuse and, 197–198
   falls and, 208, 209*t*
   medication use and, 197
   osteoporosis and, 202–208, 203*t*, 205*t*, 207*t*
   outpatient visits and, 197
   physiologic/pathologic eye changes and, 196
   psychology/psychopathology of, 199–202
      normal changes and, 200
   surgical considerations and, 198–199
   systemic disease incidence and, 208–210
Agnosia, visual, in Alzheimer disease, 245
AIDS. *See* Acquired immunodeficiency syndrome
AIDS-dementia complex (HIV encephalopathy), 26.
   See also Acquired immunodeficiency syndrome
AIDS-related virus (ARV), 25
Akinetopsia, cerebral, in Alzheimer disease, 245
Albumin, thyroxine bound to, 188–189
Albuterol, 132–133, 133*t*, 134, 137*i*
Alcohol (ethanol)
   cholesterol levels affected by, 119, 125
   drug interactions and, 53
   hypertension affected by, 67
   use/abuse of, 229*t*, 230
Aldactazide. *See* Spironolactone
Aldactone. *See* Spironolactone
Aldochlor. *See* Methyldopa
Aldomet. *See* Methyldopa
Aldoril. *See* Methyldopa
Alendronate, 206, 207*t*
Aleve. *See* Naproxen
Alfenta. *See* Alfentanil
Alfentanil, perioperative, 284*t*, 287
Alkeran. *See* Melphalan
Alkylating agents, for cancer chemotherapy, 217, 218*t*
Allergic granulomatosis (Churg-Strauss angiitis), 161*t*,
   162
Allergic reactions
   anaphylaxis as, 270–272
   to insulin, 180
   to latex, ocular surgery and, 282
   to local anesthetics, 273
   to penicillin, 52
Allergic (hypersensitivity/leukocytoclastic) vasculitis,
   161, 161*t*
Allylamines, 48*t*, 59
Alpha agonists, drug interactions and, 79*t*
Alpha-antagonists central, for hypertension, 70*t*

Alpha blockers
cholesterol levels affected by, 125
for heart failure, 107
for hypertension, 70*t*, 71*t*, 75
interactions of, 79*t*
Alpha (α) error (type I error), 315
Alpha-glucosidase inhibitors, 183
Alpha (α)-hemolytic bacteria, endocarditis prophylaxis and, 4, 5–8*t*
Alpha (α)-interferon
in cancer therapy, 223
for hepatitis C, 23
Alpha (α)-synuclein, mutation in gene for, in Parkinson disease, 237
Alpha-Tocopherol, Beta Carotene Cancer Prevention Study, 304
Alprazolam, ocular effects of, 276*t*
Altace. *See* Ramipril
Alternative hypothesis, 311
sample size calculation and, 315
Alzheimer disease, 242–245
Amantadine, 49*t*, 60
for Parkinson disease, 238
Amaryl. *See* Glimepiride
Amaurosis fugax, carotid artery disease and, 86
AmBisome. *See* Amphotericin B
AMD-3100, 30
American Society of Anesthesiologists, patient physical status classification of, 280*t*
Amikacin, 46*t*, 54
Amikin. *See* Amikacin
Amiloride, 69*t*, 73*t*
Aminocyclitols. *See* Aminoglycosides
Aminoglycosides, 45–46*t*, 54. *See also specific agent*
resistance to, 11
Aminopenicillins, 51
Aminophylline, for medical emergencies, 268*t*
Amiodarone
for heart failure, 108–109
ocular effects of, 277*t*
for ventricular tachycardia, 116
Amlodipine
for angina, 98
for heart failure, 107
for hypertension, 71*t*, 73*t*
Amoxicillin, 40*t*, 51
with clavulanic acid, 40*t*, 53
for endocarditis prophylaxis, 7*t*, 8*t*
ocular surgery and, 284–285
Amoxil. *See* Amoxicillin
Amphetamines, abuse of, 229*t*, 230
Amphotec. *See* Amphotericin B
Amphotericin B, 18, 48*t*, 59
Ampicillin, 40*t*, 51
for endocarditis prophylaxis, 7*t*, 8*t*
ocular surgery and, 284–285
Haemophilus influenzae resistance and, 8
with sulbactam, 40*t*, 53–54
Amprenavir, 30
β-Amyloid, in Alzheimer disease, 242–243
Amyloid plaques, in Alzheimer disease, 242–243
Amyloid precursor protein (APP), 242, 243
Amyloidosis/amyloid deposits, 145
ANA. *See* Antinuclear (antineutrophil) antibodies

Ana-Kit, 271–272
Analgesics, ocular effects of, 276*t*
Analysis of variance, 308
Analytic epidemiology/studies, 291, 292, 296–304. *See also specific type*
Anaphylactoid reactions, 271
Anaphylaxis, 270–272
local anesthetics causing, 273
Anaplastic carcinoma, of thyroid gland, 194
Anaprox. *See* Naproxen
Ancef. *See* Cefazolin
Ancobon. *See* 5-Fluorocytosine
Ancotil. *See* 5-Fluorocytosine
Ancrod, for stroke, 84
Anemia, 140–142
of chronic disease, 141
iron deficiency differentiated from, 139, 141
in elderly patients, 141
ocular manifestations of, 142
physiologic, 141
sickle cell, 141–142
treatment of, 142
Anesthesia (anesthetics)
local (topical/regional)
adverse reactions to, 273–275, 286
allergic, 273, 282–283
toxic, 273–275, 288
maximum safe dose of, 273*t*
malignant hyperthermia caused by, 281–282, 288–289, 289*t*
retrobulbar, adverse reactions to, 274, 287–288
sickling crisis and, 142
Aneurysms
berry (saccular), 84–85
cerebral, ruptured, intracranial hemorrhage caused by, 84–85
Angiitis, Churg-Strauss (allergic granulomatosis), 161*t*, 162
Angina pectoris, 90–91. *See also* Ischemic heart disease
ECG changes in, 93
stable, 91, 97–99, 98*t*
management of, 97–99, 98*t*
risk stratification for, 98*t*
unstable, 91
management of, 100–101
variant (Prinzmetal), 91
Angiogenesis inhibitors, in cancer therapy, 211, 223
Angiography
coronary, 97
magnetic resonance, in cerebrovascular ischemia/infarction, 83
in subarachnoid hemorrhage, 85
Angioid streaks, in pseudoxanthoma elasticum, 145
Angiomas, venous, 85
Angiopathies, strokes caused by, 82
Angioplasty, percutaneous transluminal coronary (PTCA/balloon angioplasty)
for angina, 98
for ST segment elevation acute coronary syndromes, 101, 102
troponin levels in determining need for, 94
Angiotensin-converting enzyme (ACE) inhibitors
guidelines for use on day of surgery and, 284
for heart failure, 107

C (parafollicular) cells, 188
C-reactive protein, in giant cell arteritis, 163
CABG. *See* Coronary artery bypass graft
Calan. *See* Verapamil
Calanolide, 30
Calcitonin, for osteoporosis, 206–208, 207*t*
Calcium, for osteoporosis, 205–206
Calcium channel blockers
  for angina, 98
  for heart failure, 107
  for hypertension, 71–72*t*, 73*t*, 75
  interactions of, 79*t*
  for non–ST segment elevation acute coronary
    syndromes, 100
  ocular effects of, 277*t*
Calcium chloride, for medical emergencies, 268*t*
Cancer, 211–224. *See also specific type or organ or
  structure affected*
  chemicals causing, 212–213
  chemotherapy for, 217–222, 218–220*t*
  etiology of, 212–215
  genetic and familial factors in, 211, 212, 214–215,
    224
  in HIV infection/AIDS, 36
  hypercoagulability and, 149
  incidence of, 211
  ophthalmic considerations and, 224
  radiation causing, 213
  radiation therapy for, 215–217
  recent developments in, 211
  screening for, 250*t*, 250–254
  therapy, 215–224, 218–220*t*
    recent developments in, 211
  vaccines against, 224
  viruses causing, 214
Cancer checkup, 250*t*
Cancer chemotherapy. *See* Chemotherapy
Cancer-cluster families, 215
Candida albicans, 17–18
Cannabis use/abuse, 229*t*
Capillary telangiectasias, 85
Capoten. *See* Captopril
Capozide. *See* Captopril
Capravirine, 30
Captopril
  for heart failure, 107
  for hypertension, 72*t*, 73*t*
  for non–ST segment elevation acute coronary
    syndromes, 100
  ocular effects of, 277*t*
Carbacephems, 43*t*, 53
Carbapenems, 53–54. *See also specific agent*
Carbenicillin, 51
Carbepenems, 43–44*t*
Carbocaine. *See* Mepivacaine
Carboxypenicillins, 51
Carcinogenesis, 212–215
  chemical, 212–213
  genetic and familial factors in, 214–215
  radiation in, 213
  viral, 214
Cardene. *See* Nicardipine
Cardiac arrest. *See* Cardiopulmonary arrest
Cardiac disease. *See* Heart disease

Cardiac enzymes, in myocardial infarction, 94
Cardiac failure. *See* Congestive heart failure
Cardiac glycosides. *See* Digitalis/digitoxin/digoxin
Cardiac output, in atrial fibrillation, 115
Cardiac rhythm, disorders of, 109–117. *See also*
  Arrhythmias
Cardiac-specific troponins (troponins T and I), in
  myocardial infarction, 94, 95*i*
Cardiac transplantation, for heart failure, 109
Cardiac valves, replacement of, for heart failure, 109
Cardiogenic shock, 269. *See also* Shock
  after myocardial infarction, 92
Cardiolite scintigraphy. *See* Technetium-99m Sesta-
  MIBI scintigraphy
Cardiopulmonary arrest, 265–269
Cardiopulmonary resuscitation, 265–269
  medications used in, 268*t*
Cardioselective beta blockers, for hypertension, 75
Cardiovascular disorders. *See also specific type*
  hypertension and risk of, 64*t*
  screening for, 248–250
Cardioversion
  for atrial fibrillation, 115
  for atrial flutter, 114–115
  for ventricular tachycardia, 116
Cardizem. *See* Diltiazem
Cardura. *See* Doxazosin
Carmustine, 220*t*
Carotene and Retinol Efficacy Trial, 304
Carotid arteries, disorders of, 82, 86–88
  occlusive. *See* Carotid occlusive disease
Carotid bruits, 86. *See also* Carotid occlusive disease
Carotid endarterectomy, for carotid stenosis, 81, 86–88
Carotid occlusive disease, 86–88
  site of obstruction and, 82
  strokes caused by, 86–88
Carotid stenosis, 86–88. *See also* Carotid occlusive
  disease
Carteolol, 70*t*
Cartrol. *See* Carteolol
Carvedilol
  for heart failure, 108
  for hypertension, 71*t*
Case-control studies, 293*t*, 298–300
  selection bias and, 312
  strengths and weaknesses of, 294*t*, 299–300
Case reports/series, 292–294, 293*t*
  strengths and weaknesses of, 294*t*
Catapres. *See* Clonidine
Cataract
  diabetic, 187
  radiation-induced, 216
Catheter-based reperfusion. *See* Percutaneous
  transluminal coronary angioplasty
CCR-5 receptor, HIV infection/AIDS and, 32
CD4+ T cells, in HIV infection/AIDS, 25, 27*t*, 28, 29
CEA. *See* Carotid endarterectomy
Ceclor. *See* Cefaclor
Cedax. *See* Ceftibuten
CeeNU. *See* Lomustine
Cefaclor, 41*t*
  ocular effects of, 276*t*
Cefadroxil, 41*t*
  for endocarditis prophylaxis, 7*t*

Clofibrate, for hypercholesterolemia, 123
Clomid. *See* Clomiphene
Clomiphene, ocular effects of, 277*t*
Clonidine
  guidelines for use on day of surgery and, 284
  for heart failure, 107
  for hypertension, 70*t*, 73*t*
Clopidogrel
  for carotid disease, 86, 88
  for stroke prevention, 83
Clostridium difficile, 5–7
Clotrimazole, 48*t*
Clotting. *See* Coagulation
Cloxacillin, 39*t*, 51
CMV. *See* Cytomegalovirus
Coactinon. *See* Emivirine
Coagulation. *See also* Hemostasis
  disorders of, 147–150
    acquired, 147–148
    hereditary, 147
  laboratory evaluation of, 144
  pathways of, 142, 143*i*
Coagulation factors, 142–143, 143*i*
  abnormalities/deficiencies of, 147
Cocaine, abuse of, 229*t*, 230–231
Cogan syndrome, 162
Cognex. *See* Tacrine
Cohort studies (follow-up studies), 293*t*, 296–298
  analysis of data from, 309–310
  strengths and weaknesses of, 294*t*
Colestipol, for hypercholesterolemia, 122–123
Colitic (enteropathic) arthritis, 154–155
Colitis
  granulomatous (Crohn disease), 154
  ulcerative, 154
    arthritis associated with, 154–155
Colon cancer. *See* Colorectal cancer
Colonoscopy, in cancer screening, 247, 253
  virtual, 247, 253
Colony-forming unit–culture, 139
Colony-forming unit–erythroid, 139
Colony-forming unit–spleen, 139
Colony-stimulating factors, in cancer therapy, 223
Color flow Doppler imaging, in ischemic heart disease, 95
Colorectal cancer
  incidence of, 252
  screening for, 252
Coma
  myxedema, 193
  nonketotic hyperglycemic-hyperosmolar, 184
Combipres. *See* Clonidine
Combivir. *See* Lamivudine (3TC), with zidovudine
Complete (third-degree) atrioventricular block, 111
Completed stroke, 82
Compliance with therapy, 231, 236
Computed tomography (CT scan)
  dual-energy quantitative, in osteoporosis, 204
  in ischemic heart disease, 96
  in pulmonary diseases, 131
Conduction disturbances, cardiac, 110–112
Confidence interval, 311–312
Confounding, 291, 313–314
Confusion, postoperative, in elderly, 199

Congenital syphilis, 11
Congestive heart failure, 103–109
  atrial fibrillation and, 115
  classification of, 103*t*, 105
  clinical course of, 106
  clinical signs of, 104
  compensated, 103
  decompensated, 103
  diagnosis of, 104
  epidemiology of, 104–105
  etiology of, 105
  high-output, 105
  ischemic heart disease causing, 104, 105
  management of
    invasive or surgical, 109
    medical and nonsurgical, 107–109
  after myocardial infarction, 92, 93
  pathophysiology of, 106
  refractory, 103
  symptoms of, 103–104
Conjunctivitis, in reactive arthritis, 154
Connective tissue disorders, mixed, 158
Consistency, of experimental study, 314
Contact lenses, for trial fitting, disinfection of, 36
Continuous positive airway pressure (CPAP), 132
Contraceptives, oral,
  hypercoagulable states and, 150
  ocular effects of, 277*t*
Contractility, myocardial, 106
  reduction of in angina management, 97–98
Conversion disorders, 227
COPD. *See* Chronic obstructive pulmonary disease
Cor pulmonale, 130
Cordarone. *See* Amiodarone
Coreg. *See* Carvedilol
Corgard. *See* Nadolol
Cornea, donor, screening for HIV antibodies and, 36
Corneal pigmentation, antipsychotic drugs causing, 229
Coronary angiography, 97
Coronary angioplasty, percutaneous transluminal (PTCA/balloon angioplasty)
  for angina, 98
  for ST segment elevation acute coronary syndromes, 101, 102
  troponin levels in determining need for, 94
Coronary artery bypass graft (CABG), 99
  troponin levels in determining need for, 94
Coronary artery stenosis, hemodynamically significant, 97
Coronary heart disease (coronary artery atherosclerosis), 90. *See also* Ischemic heart disease
  in diabetes, 181
  hypercholesterolemia and, 119, 120, 121*t*
  risk factors for, 90
  screening for, 249–250
Coronary syndromes, acute. *See* Acute coronary syndromes
Correlation analysis, 308
Correlation coefficient, 308–309
Cortical bone, 202
Corticosteroids (steroids), 165–167
  for anaphylaxis, 271
  for Behçet syndrome, 164, 165
  in cancer chemotherapy, 221